The National Collaborating Centre

for Chronic Conditions

Funded to produce guidelines for the NHS by NICE

TYPE 2 DIABETES

National clinical guideline for management in primary and secondary care (update)

This is an update of the following
NICE (inherited) clinical guidelines on
Type 2 diabetes which were published in 2002:
E – retinopathy; F – renal disease; G – blood glucose;
H – management of blood pressure and blood lipids

Published by

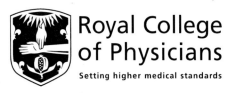

Royal College
of Physicians
Setting higher medical standards

Royal College of Physicians

The Royal College of Physicians plays a leading role in the delivery of high-quality patient care by setting standards of medical practice and promoting clinical excellence. We provide physicians in the United Kingdom and overseas with education, training and support throughout their careers. As an independent body representing over 20,000 Fellows and Members worldwide, we advise and work with government, the public, patients and other professions to improve health and healthcare.

National Collaborating Centre for Chronic Conditions

The National Collaborating Centre for Chronic Conditions (NCC-CC) is a collaborative, multiprofessional centre undertaking commissions to develop clinical guidance for the National Health Service (NHS) in England and Wales. The NCC-CC was established in 2001. It is an independent body, housed within the Clinical Standards Department at the Royal College of Physicians of London. The NCC-CC is funded by the National Institute for Health and Clinical Excellence (NICE) to undertake commissions for national clinical guidelines on an annual rolling programme.

Citation for this document

National Collaborating Centre for Chronic Conditions. *Type 2 diabetes: national clinical guideline for management in primary and secondary care (update)*. London: Royal College of Physicians, reprint 2009.

ISBN 978-1-86016-333-3

ROYAL COLLEGE OF PHYSICIANS
11 St Andrews Place, London NW1 4LE
www.rcplondon.ac.uk

Registered charity No 210508

Typeset by Dan-Set Graphics, Telford, Shropshire

Printed in Great Britain by The Lavenham Press Ltd, Sudbury, Suffolk

Contents

DEVELOPMENT OF THE GUIDELINE

THE GUIDELINE

Members of the Guideline Development Group

Professor Jonathan Mant *(Chair)*
Professor of Primary Care Stroke Research, University of Birmingham

Mrs Lina Bakhshi
Information Scientist, NCC-CC

Mrs Margaret Bannister
Nurse Consultant in Diabetes Care, Bradford and Airedale Primary Care Trust

Mrs Katherine Cullen
Health Economist, NCC-CC

Professor Melanie Davies
Professor of Diabetes Medicine, University of Leicester

Dr Jose Diaz
Health Services Research Fellow in Guideline Development, NCC-CC

Mrs Barbara Elster
Patient and Carer Representative, Essex

Dr Roger Gadsby
General Practitioner and Senior Lecturer in Primary Care, Warwickshire

Dr Anupam Garrib
Health Services Research Fellow, NCC-CC

Ms Irene Gummerson
Primary Care Pharmacist, Yorkshire

Dr Martin Hadley-Brown
General Practitioner Trainer, University of Cambridge

Professor Philip Home
Clinical Advisor to the GDG; Professor of Diabetes Medicine, Newcastle University

Mrs Kathryn Leivesley
Practice Nurse, North Manchester Primary Care Trust

Mrs Emma Marcus
Clinical Specialist Diabetes Dietitian, Hinckley and Bosworth Primary Care Trust

Mr Leo Nherera
Health Economist, National Collaborating Centre for Women's and Children's Health

Ms Roberta Richey
Health Services Research Fellow in Guideline Development, NCC-CC

Mr John Roberts
Patient and Carer Representative, Merseyside

Dr Mark Savage
Consultant Physician, North Manchester General Hospital

Lorraine Shaw
Paediatric Diabetes Clinical Nurse Specialist, Birmingham Children's Hospital

Dr Stuart Smelie
Consultant Chemical Pathologist, Bishop Auckland General Hospital

Ms Nicole Stack
Guideline Development Project Manager, NCC-CC

Ms Claire Turner
Guideline Development Senior Project Manager, NCC-CC

Ms Susan Varney
Health Services Research Fellow in Guideline Development, NCC-CC

Dr Jiten Vora
Consultant Physician Endocrinologist, Royal Liverpool and Broadgreen University Hospital

The following experts were invited to attend specific meetings and to advise the Guideline Development Group:

Dr Julian Barth
Consultant Chemical Pathologist, Leeds NHS Trust attended one meeting as a deputy for Dr Stuart Smellie

Dr Indranil Dasgupta
Consultant Physician and Nephrologist, Birmingham Heartlands Hospital

Dr Michael Feher
Consultant Physician, Chelsea Westminster Hospital attended one meeting as a deputy for Dr Mark Savage

Dr Charles Fox
Consultant Physician, Northampton General Trust attended one meeting as a deputy for Professor Melanie Davies

Natasha Jacques
Principal Pharmacist Medicine, Solihull Hospital attended one meeting as a deputy for Ms Irene Gummerson

Dr Eric Kilpatrick
Consultant Chemical Pathologist, University of Hull attended one meeting as a deputy for Dr Stuart Smellie

Dr Ian Lawrence
Consultant Diabetologist, University of Leicester attended one meeting as a deputy for Professor Melanie Davies and Dr Jiten Vora

Professor Sally Marshall
Professor of Diabetes, Newcastle University

Professor David Wood
Professor of Cardiovascular Medicine, Imperial College London

Acknowledgements

The Guideline Development Group (GDG) is grateful to Bernard Higgins, Jane Ingham, Rob Grant, Jill Parnham and Susan Tann of the NCC-CC for their support throughout the development of the guideline.

The GDG would like to thank the following individuals for giving their time to advise us regarding the design and interpretation of the economic model of analysis of third-line therapy with insulins, glitazones or exenatide in Type 2 diabetes:

- Professor Alastair Gray, University of Oxford
- Dr Philip Clarke, University of Sydney
- Dr Joanne Lord, National Institute for Health and Clinical Excellence.

The GDG would like to thank the following individuals for peer reviewing the guideline:

- Professor Simon Heller, University of Sheffield
- Professor David Owens, Llandough Hospital, Penarth
- Professor Bryan Williams, University of Leicester
- Dr Miles Fisher, Glasgow Royal Infirmary
- Professor Soloman Tesfaye, University of Sheffield
- Mr Irvine Turner, Patient Representative.

Preface

In 2007, the Centers for Disease Control and Prevention in the USA took the step, unusual for a non-infectious disease, of classifying the increase in the incidence of diabetes as an epidemic, their projections suggesting that the prevalence of this already common disease will have doubled by 2050. In the UK, diabetes already affects approximately 1.9 million adults overall, and some estimates suggest that there are an additional 0.5 million with undiagnosed diabetes.* This makes diabetes one of the commonest of all chronic medical conditions, and represents a huge potential problem for our health services.

Over 90% of people with diabetes have Type 2 diabetes. This is still perceived as the milder form, and while this may be true in some respects, such as the risk of ketoacidosis, the causation of Type 2 diabetes is more complex and the management is not necessarily easier. Type 2 diabetes can cause severe complications, affecting the eye, the nervous system and the kidney. The overall risk of cardiovascular disease is more than doubled, and life expectancy is reduced by an average 7 years. In 2002, NICE published a suite of five guidelines dealing with different aspects of the care of Type 2 diabetes. The rising prevalence of the disease, and the range of complications which can arise, reinforce the importance of up-to-date guidance and accordingly NICE have asked the National Collaborating Centre for Chronic Conditions (NCC-CC) to produce this guideline, amalgamating and updating the previously published work.

The guideline is informed by extensive literature and covers many aspects of diabetes management, although it is not intended to be a comprehensive textbook. It covers those topics of particular relevance to life expectancy such as control of cholesterol and lipid levels, and management of hypertension. It deals with major complications such as renal disease. There are also key recommendations in areas of great importance to patients such as structured education and the monitoring of glucose levels. Naturally, there are also sections dealing with control of blood glucose levels and the use of the various drugs available for this purpose.

The guideline development group (GDG) have had a particularly difficult task during development. The remit they were given was unusually large, and I have already mentioned the vast amount of evidence which they were required to consider. They were required to incorporate several existing NICE technology appraisals (TAs) within the guideline. In addition, they had to contend with a major safety scare over one of the glucose lowering agents which evolved over the course of guideline development. It is a measure of their commitment and appetite for hard work that, despite the size of the existing task, they were frustrated rather than relieved at not being able to include information about newer agents such as the DPP-4 inhibitors, the first of which was licensed towards the end of the development process (these agents will be covered at a later date in a separate, short guideline). All at the NCC-CC are extremely grateful to the GDG for the tremendous effort they have put into producing this guideline on schedule. The challenge now is to implement its recommendations and to make a genuine difference to the well-being and health of those with Type 2 diabetes.

Dr Bernard Higgins MD FRCP
Director, National Collaborating Centre for Chronic Conditions

---

* Department of Health. *Health survey for England 2003.* London: Stationary Office, 2004.

DEVELOPMENT OF THE GUIDELINE

1 | Introduction

1.1 Background

Diabetes is a group of disorders with a number of common features, of which raised blood glucose is by definition the most evident. In England and Wales the four commonest types of diabetes are:

- Type 1 diabetes
- Type 2 diabetes
- secondary diabetes (from pancreatic damage, hepatic cirrhosis, endocrinological disease/therapy, or anti-viral/anti-psychotic therapy)
- gestational diabetes (diabetes of pregnancy).

This guideline is concerned only with Type 2 diabetes. The underlying disorder is usually that of a background of insulin insensitivity plus a failure of pancreatic insulin secretion to compensate for this.

The insulin insensitivity is usually evidenced by excess body weight or obesity, and exacerbated by overeating and inactivity. It is commonly associated with raised blood pressure, a disturbance of blood lipid levels, and a tendency to thrombosis. This combination is often recognised as the 'metabolic syndrome', and is associated with fatty liver and abdominal adiposity (increased waist circumference).

The insulin deficiency is progressive over time, such that the high glucose levels usually worsen relentlessly over a timescale of years, requiring continued escalation of blood glucose lowering therapy. The worsening insulin deficiency with age also means that diabetes can appear in elderly people who are quite thin. In some people in middle age the condition can be difficult to distinguish from slow onset Type 1 diabetes.

In people whose hyperglycaemia has yet to be treated, glucose metabolism may be sufficiently disturbed to cause symptoms, typically of polyuria, thirst, weight loss and fatigue. Diabetic coma (ketoacidosis) is uncommon in Type 2 diabetes unless exacerbating factors (infection, drugs) are present, but insulin deficiency and high sugar intake can lead to a related state (hyperosmolar coma).

Type 2 diabetes is notable for the increased cardiovascular risk that it carries. This can be manifest as coronary artery disease (heart attacks, angina), peripheral artery disease (leg claudication, gangrene), and carotid artery disease (strokes, dementia). Many people with Type 2 diabetes have the same risk of a cardiovascular event as someone without diabetes who has already had their first heart attack; people with diabetes and a previous cardiovascular event are at very high risk – around 10 times the background population. Accordingly management of cardiovascular risk factors plays a large part in care of people with Type 2 diabetes, and is particularly cost effective.

Because of the problems of maintaining good blood glucose control associated with the increasing insulin deficiency, the degree of hyperglycaemia occurring in some individuals is sufficient to give rise to a risk of the specific ('microvascular') complications of diabetes. Due to early death caused by cardiovascular disease these are less common than in people with Type 1 diabetes, but include eye damage (sometimes blindness), kidney damage (sometimes requiring dialysis or transplantation), and nerve damage (resulting in amputation, painful symptoms, erectile dysfunction, and other problems).

This situation of multiple vascular risk factors and multiple complications leads to multiple targets for reduction of risk and improvement of health in people with Type 2 diabetes. Such targets for management include obesity, activity levels, plasma glucose control, blood pressure control, blood lipid control, reduction of thrombogenicity, laser therapy for eye damage, drug therapy to delay kidney damage, local foot care, and symptomatic treatments for various types of nerve damage. As a result diabetes care is typically complex and time consuming.

The necessary lifestyle changes, the complexities of management, and the side effects of therapy, together make self-monitoring and education for people with diabetes central parts of management.

1.2   Definition

The GDG worked to the World Health Organization (WHO) definition of diabetes, which requires a degree of high plasma glucose levels sufficient to put the individual at risk of the specific (microvascular) complications of diabetes. Diagnosis is not addressed in this guideline. This definition was reconfirmed by the WHO in 2006, but, like earlier versions, does not contain a specific definition for Type 2 diabetes.[2]

People are normally thought to have Type 2 diabetes if they do not have Type 1 diabetes (rapid onset, often in childhood, insulin-dependent, ketoacidosis if neglected) or other medical conditions or treatment suggestive of secondary diabetes. However, there can be uncertainty in the diagnosis particularly in overweight people of younger age. A further area of confusion is the group of disorders classified as monogenetic diabetes – formally Maturity Onset Diabetes of the Young (MODY) – which are usually not insulin requiring but which present in the first decades of life.

It is noted that Type 1 diabetes with onset after childhood can be confused with Type 2 diabetes. However, lower body weight, more rapid progression to insulin therapy, and absence of features of the metabolic syndrome often give useful distinguishing clues.

1.3   Prevalence

The prevalence of diabetes in the UK is increasing as is the prevalence of obesity, decreased physical activity, but also increased longevity after diagnosis thanks to better cardiovascular risk protection. The current prevalence of Type 2 diabetes is unknown, and will vary with factors such as mix of ethnic groups and degree of social deprivation.

Table 1.1 The prevalence of doctor-diagnosed diabetes (2003)[3]

	Men (≥55 years)	Women (≥55 years)
General population (%)	4.3	3.4
Black Caribbean	10.0	8.4
Black African	5.0	2.1
Indian	10.1	5.9
Pakistani	7.3	8.6
Bangladeshi	8.2	5.2
Chinese	3.8	3.3
Irish	3.6	2.3

Prevalence estimates vary from around 3.5 to 5.0%, the third edition of the International Diabetes Federation (IDF) Atlas suggesting 4.0%, being 1.71 million in the 20- to 79-year-old age group, of whom it is conventional to assume 85% have Type 2 diabetes.[4] Current prevalence estimates are a poor pointer to future burden of diabetes due to their continuing increase. The healthcare burden is also affected by the improved longevity of people with diabetes with better management, which means that overall they carry a larger burden of complications and insulin deficiency needing more complex care.

1.4   Health and resource burden

Type 2 diabetes can result in a wide range of complications (see above), with repercussions for both the individual patient and the NHS. The economic impact of this disease includes at least three factors:

- direct cost to the NHS and associated healthcare support services
- indirect cost to the economy, including the effects of early mortality and lost productivity
- personal impact of diabetes and subsequent complications on patients and their families.

Mortality attributed to people with diabetes is suggested as 4.2% of deaths in men and 7.7% of deaths in women in the UK. These are likely to be underestimates as deaths from vascular events such as stroke and myocardial infarction (MI) are notorious for under-recording of the underlying causative disease. In a population-based study in Cardiff, at a time when population prevalence was only 2.5%, deaths in people with diabetes accounted for over 10% of the total, with around 60% attributable to diabetes.[5] Life years lost vary considerably with factors such as blood glucose, blood pressure and blood lipid control, and smoking, as well as age, and can be estimated by comparing United Kingdom Prospective Diabetes Study (UKPDS) risk engine estimates to UK government statistical tables. Typically a 60-year-old man, newly diagnosed and without existing arterial disease can expect to lose 8–10 years of life without proper management.

The direct cost of Type 2 diabetes to the NHS is unknown, as much is classified as cardiovascular or renal disease. However, with prevalence estimates of 3.5–5.0%, and healthcare costs double those of the background population or more, estimates of 7–12% of total NHS expenditure seem not unreasonable. The IDF Atlas notes that in industrialised countries healthcare costs in people with diabetes tend to be double those of the background population. This suggests a £2.8 billion attributable cost for the UK for 2007.[4]

2 Methodology

2.1 Aim

The aim of the National Collaborating Centre for Chronic Conditions (NCC-CC) is to provide a user-friendly, clinical, evidence-based guideline for the NHS in England and Wales that:

- offers best clinical advice for the management of Type 2 diabetes
- is based on best published clinical and economic evidence, alongside expert consensus
- takes into account patient choice and informed decision making
- defines the major components of NHS care provision for Type 2 diabetes
- details areas of uncertainty or controversy requiring further research
- provides a choice of guideline versions for differing audiences.

2.2 Scope

The guideline was developed in accordance with a scope, which detailed the remit of the guideline originating from the Department of Health (DH) and specified those aspects of Type 2 diabetes care to be included and excluded. The application of the guideline to children has not been excluded but we were not able to specifically search for paediatric literature due to volume of work. When health carers are applying these guidelines to children they need to use their clinical judgement in doing so. For further assistance with applying this guideline to children please refer to the British National Formulary (BNF) for children.[6]

Prior to the commencement of the guideline development, the scope was subjected to stakeholder consultation in accordance with processes established by the National Institute for Health and Clinical Excellence (NICE).[1] The full scope is shown in appendix B. Available at www.rcplondon.ac.uk/pubs/brochure.aspx?e=247

2.3 Audience

The guideline is intended for use by the following people or organisations:

- all healthcare professionals
- people with Type 2 diabetes and their parents and carers
- patient support groups
- commissioning organisations
- service providers.

2.4 Involvement of people with Type 2 diabetes

The NCC-CC was keen to ensure the views and preferences of people with Type 2 diabetes and their carers informed all stages of the guideline. This was achieved by:

- having two people with Type 2 diabetes as patient representatives on the GDG
- consulting the Patient and Public Involvement Programme (PPIP) housed within NICE during the pre-development (scoping) and final validation stages of the guideline project
- the inclusion of patient groups as registered stakeholders for the guideline.

2.5 Guideline limitations

The guideline has the following limitations.

- NICE clinical guidelines usually do not cover issues of service delivery, organisation or provision (unless specified in the remit from the DH).
- NICE is primarily concerned with health services and so recommendations are not provided for social services and the voluntary sector. However, the guideline may address important issues in how NHS clinicians interface with these other sectors.
- Generally, the guideline does not cover rare, complex, complicated or unusual conditions.
- Where a meta-analysis was available, generally the individual papers contained within were not appraised.
- It is not possible in the development of a clinical guideline to complete an extensive systematic literature review of all pharmacological toxicity, although NICE expect their guidelines to be read alongside the summaries of product characteristics (SPCs).

2.6 Other work relevant to the guideline

The guideline will update the following NICE technology appraisals (TAs) but only in relation to Type 2 diabetes:

- 'Guidance on the use of glitazones for the treatment of Type 2 diabetes', *NICE technology appraisal guidance* no. 63 (2003)
- 'Guidance on the use of patient-education models for diabetes', *NICE technology appraisal guidance* no. 60 (2003)
- 'Guidance on the use of long-acting insulin analogues for the treatment of diabetes – insulin glargine', *NICE technology appraisal guidance* no. 53 (2002).

Related NICE public health guidance:

- 'Smoking cessation services, including the use of pharmacotherapies, in primary care, pharmacies, local authorities and workplaces, with particular reference to manual working groups, pregnant smokers and hard to reach communities', *Public health programme guidance* no. PH010 (February 2008)
- 'Physical activity guidance for the Highways Agency, local authorities, primary care, pharmacists, health visitors and community nurses, schools, workplaces, the leisure and fitness industry and sports clubs', *Public health programme guidance* no. PH008 (January 2007).

Related NICE clinical guidelines:

- 'Cardiovascular risk assessment: the modification of blood lipids for the primary and secondary prevention of cardiovascular disease' (expected date of publication May 2008)
- 'Diabetes in pregnancy: management of diabetes and its complications from pre-conception to the postnatal period', *NICE clinical guideline* no. 63 (2008)
- 'Hypertension: management of hypertension in adults in primary care' (partial update of NICE CG18), *NICE clinical guideline* no. 34 (2006)
- 'Obesity: the prevention, identification, assessment and management of overweight and obesity in adults and children', *NICE clinical guideline* no. 43 (2006)
- 'Type 1 diabetes: diagnosis and management of type 1 diabetes in children, young people and adults', *NICE clinical guideline* no. 15 (2004, to be reviewed 2008)
- 'Type 2 diabetes: prevention and management of foot problems', *NICE clinical guideline* no. 10 (2004).

Related TA guidance:

- 'Guidance on the use of ezetimibe for the treatment of primary (heterozygous-familial and non-familial) hypercholesterolaemia', *NICE technology appraisal guidance* no. 132 (2007)
- 'Guidance on the use of statins for the prevention of cardiovascular events in patients at increased risk of developing cardiovascular disease or those with established cardiovascular disease', *NICE technology appraisal guidance* no. 94 (2006)
- 'Guidance on the use of inhaled insulin for the treatment of Type 1 and Type 2 diabetes', *NICE technology appraisal guidance* no. 113 (2006)
- 'Guidance on the use of clopidogrel and dipyridamole for the prevention of artherosclerotic events', *NICE technology appraisal guidance* no. 90 (2005)
- 'Guidance on the use of the clinical effectiveness and cost effectiveness of insulin pump therapy', *NICE technology appraisal guidance* no. 57 (2003).

2.7 Background

The development of this evidence-based clinical guideline draws upon the methods described by the NICE's 'Guideline development methods manual'[1] and the methodology pack[7] specifically developed by the NCC-CC for each chronic condition guideline (see www.rcplondon.ac.uk/clinical-standards/ncc-cc/Pages/NCC-CC.aspx). The developers' role and remit is summarised in table 2.1.

Table 2.1 Role and remit of the developers	
NCC-CC	The NCC-CC was set up in 2001 and is housed within the Royal College of Physicians (RCP). The NCC-CC undertakes commissions received from NICE. A multiprofessional partners' board inclusive of patient groups and NHS management governs the NCC-CC.
NCC-CC Technical Team	The technical team met approximately two weeks before each GDG meeting and comprised the following members: 　GDG Chair 　GDG Clinical Adviser 　Information Scientist 　Two Research Fellows 　Health Economist 　Project Manager.
GDG	The GDG met monthly (June 2006 to July 2007) and comprised a multidisciplinary team of professionals and people with Type 2 diabetes who were supported by the technical team. The GDG membership details including patient representation and professional groups are detailed in the GDG membership table at the front of this guideline.
Guideline Project Executive	The Project Executive was involved in overseeing all phases of the guideline. It also reviewed the quality of the guideline and compliance with the DH remit and NICE scope. The Project Executive comprises: 　NCC-CC Director 　NCC-CC Assistant Director 　NCC-CC Manager 　NICE Commissioning Manager 　Technical Team.
Formal consensus	At the end of the guideline development process the GDG met to review and agree the guideline recommendations.

Members of the GDG declared any interests in accordance with the NICE technical manual.[1] A register is given in appendix D, available online at www.rcplondon.ac.uk/pubs/brochure.aspx?e=247

2.8　The process of guideline development

The basic steps in the process of producing a guideline are:

- developing clinical evidence-based questions
- systematically searching for the evidence
- critically appraising the evidence
- incorporating health economic evidence
- distilling and synthesising the evidence and writing recommendations
- grading the evidence statements
- agreeing the recommendations

- structuring and writing the guideline
- updating the guideline.

▷ Developing evidence-based questions

The technical team drafted a series of clinical questions that covered the guideline scope. The GDG and Project Executive refine and approve these questions, which are shown in appendix A. Available at www.rcplondon.ac.uk/pubs/brochure.aspx?e=247

▷ Searching for the evidence

The information scientist developed a search strategy for each question. Key words for the search were identified by the GDG. In addition, the health economist searched for additional papers providing economic evidence or to inform detailed health economic work (for example, modelling). Papers that were published or accepted for publication in peer-reviewed journals were considered as evidence by the GDG. Conference paper abstracts and non-English language papers were excluded from the searches.

Each clinical question dictated the appropriate study design that was prioritised in the search strategy but the strategy was not limited solely to these study types. The research fellow or health economist identified titles and abstracts from the search results that appeared to be relevant to the question. Exclusion lists were generated for each question together with the rationale for the exclusion. The exclusion lists were presented to the GDG. Full papers were obtained where relevant. See appendix A for literature search details. Available at www.rcplondon.ac.uk/pubs/brochure.aspx?e=247

▷ Appraising the evidence

The research fellow or health economist, as appropriate, critically appraised the full papers. In general, no formal contact was made with authors; however, there were ad hoc occasions when this was required in order to clarify specific details. Critical appraisal checklists were compiled for each full paper. One research fellow undertook the critical appraisal and data extraction. The evidence was considered carefully by the GDG for accuracy and completeness.

All procedures are fully compliant with the:
- NICE methodology as detailed in the 'Guideline Development Methods – Information for National Collaborating Centres and Guideline Developers' Manual[1]
- NCC-CC quality assurance document and systematic review chart available at www.rcplondon.ac.uk/clinical-standards/ncc-cc/Pages/NCC-CC.aspx.

▷ Health economic evidence

Areas for health economic modelling were agreed by the GDG after the formation of the clinical questions. The health economist reviewed the clinical questions to consider the potential application of health economic modelling, and these priorities were agreed with the GDG.

The health economist performed supplemental literature searches to obtain additional data for modelling. Assumptions and designs of the models were explained to and agreed by the GDG members during meetings, and they commented on subsequent revisions.

▷ Distilling and synthesising the evidence and developing recommendations

The evidence from each full paper was distilled into an evidence table and synthesised into evidence statements before being presented to the GDG. This evidence was then reviewed by the GDG and used as a basis upon which to formulate recommendations. The criteria for grading evidence are shown in table 2.2.

Evidence tables are available online at www.rcplondon.ac.uk/pubs/brochure.aspx?e=247

▷ Grading the evidence statements

Table 2.2 Grading the evidence statements[1]	
Level of evidence	**Type of evidence**
1++	High-quality meta-analyses, systematic reviews of RCTs, or RCTs with a very low risk of bias.
1+	Well-conducted meta-analyses, systematic reviews of RCTs, or RCTs with a low risk of bias.
1–	Meta-analyses, systematic reviews of RCTs, or RCTs with a high risk of bias.*
2++	High-quality systematic reviews of case-control or cohort studies. High-quality case-control or cohort studies with a very low risk of confounding, bias or chance and a high probability that the relationship is causal.
2+	Well-conducted case-control or cohort studies with a low risk of confounding, bias or chance and a moderate probability that the relationship is causal.
2–	Case-control or cohort studies with a high risk of confounding, bias or chance and a significant risk that the relationship is not causal.*
3	Non-analytic studies (for example case reports, case series).
4	Expert opinion, formal consensus.

*Studies with a level of evidence '–' are not used as a basis for making a recommendation.
RCT, randomised controlled trial

▷ Agreeing the recommendations

The GDG employed formal consensus techniques to:
- ensure that the recommendations reflected the evidence base
- approve recommendations based on lesser evidence or extrapolations from other situations
- reach consensus recommendations where the evidence was inadequate
- debate areas of disagreement and finalise recommendations.

The GDG also reached agreement on the following:
- five recommendations as key priorities for implementation
- five key research recommendations
- algorithms.

In prioritising key recommendations for implementation, the GDG took into account the following criteria:

- high clinical impact
- high impact on reducing variation
- more efficient use of NHS resources
- allowing the patient to reach critical points in the care pathway more quickly.

Audit criteria for this guideline will be produced for NICE by Clinical Accountability Service Planning and Evaluation (CASPE) Research following publication in order to provide suggestions of areas for audit in line with the key recommendations for implementation.

▷ Structuring and writing the guideline

The guideline is divided into sections for ease of reading. For each section the layout is similar and contains the following parts.
- *Clinical introduction* sets a succinct background and describes the current clinical context.
- *Methodological introduction* describes any issues or limitations that were apparent when reading the evidence base.
- *Evidence statements* provide a synthesis of the evidence base and usually describes what the evidence showed in relation to the outcomes of interest.
- *Health economics* presents, where appropriate, an overview of the cost effectiveness evidence base, or any economic modelling.
- *From evidence to recommendations* sets out the GDG decision-making rationale providing a clear and explicit audit trail from the evidence to the evolution of the recommendations.
- *Recommendations* provide stand alone, action-orientated recommendations.
- *Evidence tables* are not published as part of the full guideline but are available online at www.rcplondon.ac.uk/pubs/brochure.aspx?e=247. These describe comprehensive details of the primary evidence that was considered during the writing of each section.

▷ Writing the guideline

The first draft version of the guideline was drawn up by the technical team in accord with the decisions of the GDG, incorporating contributions from individual GDG members in their expert areas and edited for consistency of style and terminology. The guideline was then submitted for a formal public and stakeholder consultation prior to publication. The registered stakeholders for this guideline are detailed on the NICE website, www.nice.org.uk. Editorial responsibility for the full guideline rests with the GDG.

Table 2.3 Versions of this guideline	
Full version	Details the recommendations, the supporting evidence base and the expert considerations of the GDG. Published by the NCC-CC. Available at www.rcplondon.ac.uk/pubs/brochure.aspx?e=247
NICE version	Documents the recommendations without any supporting evidence. Available at www.nice.org.uk
'Quick reference guide'	An abridged version. Available at www.nice.org.uk
'Understanding NICE guidance'	A lay version of the guideline recommendations. Available at www.nice.org.uk

▷ Updating the guideline

Literature searches were repeated for all of the evidence-based questions at the end of the GDG development process allowing any relevant papers published up until 16 April 2007 to be considered. Future guideline updates will consider evidence published after this cut-off date.

Two years after publication of the guideline, NICE will ask a National Collaborating Centre to determine whether the evidence base has progressed significantly to alter the guideline recommendations and warrant an early update. If not, the guideline will be considered for update approximately 4 years after publication.

2.9 Disclaimer

Healthcare providers need to use clinical judgement, knowledge and expertise when deciding whether it is appropriate to apply guidelines. The recommendations cited here are a guide and may not be appropriate for use in all situations. The decision to adopt any of the recommendations cited here must be made by the practitioner in light of individual patient circumstances, the wishes of the patient, clinical expertise and resources.

The NCC-CC disclaims any responsibility for damages arising out of the use or non-use of these guidelines and the literature used in support of these guidelines.

2.10 Funding

The NCC-CC was commissioned by NICE to undertake the work on this guideline.

3 Key messages of the guideline

3.1 Key priorities for implementation

Offer structured education to every person and/or their carer at and around the time of diagnosis, with annual reinforcement and review. Inform people and their carers that structured education is an integral part of diabetes care.

Provide individualised and ongoing nutritional advice from a healthcare professional with specific expertise and competencies in nutrition.

When setting a target glycated haemoglobin (GHb):
- involve the person in decisions about their individual HbA_{1c} target level, which may be above that of 6.5 % set for people with Type 2 diabetes in general
- encourage the person to maintain their individual target unless the resulting side effects (including hypoglycaemia) or their efforts to achieve this impair their quality of life
- offer therapy (lifestyle and medication) to help achieve and maintain the HbA_{1c} target level
- inform a person with a higher HbA_{1c} that any reduction in HbA_{1c} towards the agreed target is advantageous to future health
- avoid pursuing highly intensive management to levels of less than 6.5 %.

Offer self-monitoring of plasma glucose to a person newly diagnosed with Type 2 diabetes only as an integral part of his or her self-management education. Discuss its purpose and agree how it should be interpreted and acted upon.

When starting insulin therapy, use a structured programme employing active insulin dose titration that encompasses:
- structured education
- continuing telephone support
- frequent self-monitoring
- dose titration to target
- dietary understanding
- management of hypoglycaemia
- management of acute changes in plasma glucose control
- support from an appropriately trained and experienced healthcare professional.

3.2 Algorithms

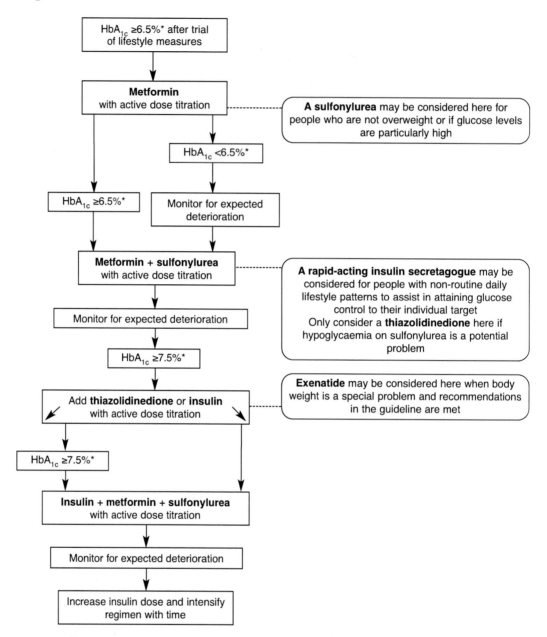

Figure 3.1 Scheme for the pharmacotherapy of glucose lowering in people with Type 2 diabetes
For details see recommendations on glucose lowering targets, clinical monitoring, use of oral agents, and use of insulin
* or as individually agreed

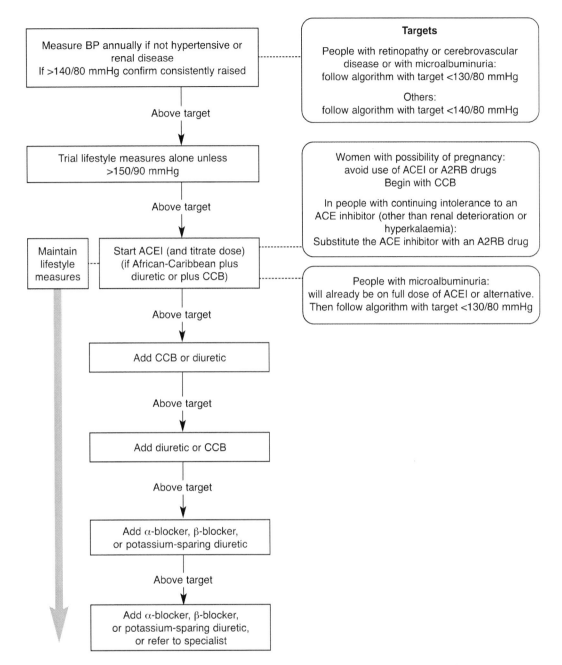

Figure 3.2 Scheme for the management of blood pressure (BP) for people with Type 2 diabetes
ACEI, angiotensin-converting enzyme inhibitor; A2RB, angiotensin 2 receptor blocker (sartan); CCB, calcium channel blocker

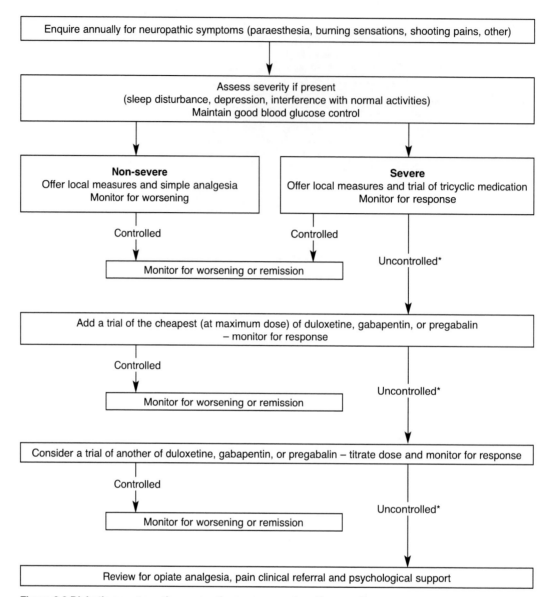

Figure 3.3 Diabetic symptomatic neuropathy management – a therapeutic summary
*Where neuropathic symptoms cannot be adequately controlled it is useful, to help individuals cope, to explain the reasons for the problem, the likelihood of remission in the medium term, the role of improved blood glucose control

4 Glossary and definitions

ACEI	Angiotensin-converting enzyme inhibitor
ACR	Albumin creatinine ratio
ADA	American Diabetes Association
AER	Albumin excretion rate – a measure of kidney damage due to diabetes (and other conditions) and a risk factor for arterial disease.
Albuminuria	The presence of albumin and other proteins in urine.
Alpha-glucosidase inhibitors	Group of drugs which inhibit the digestion of complex carbohydrates in the gut, and thus flatten the post-meal blood glucose excursion.
BMI	Body mass index – a index of body weight corrected for height.
Cohort study	A retrospective or prospective follow-up study. Groups of individuals to be followed up are defined on the basis of presence or absence of exposure to a suspected risk factor or intervention. A cohort study can be comparative, in which case two or more groups are selected on the basis of differences in their exposure to the agent of interest.
CKD	Chronic kidney disease
Confidence interval (CI)	A range of values which contains the true value for the population with a stated 'confidence' (conventionally 95%). The interval is calculated from sample data, and generally straddles the sample estimate. The 95% confidence value means that if the study, and the method used to calculate the interval, is repeated many times, then 95% of the calculated intervals will actually contain the true value for the whole population.
Cochrane review	The Cochrane Library consists of a regularly updated collection of evidence-based medicine databases including the Cochrane Database of Systematic Reviews (reviews of randomised controlled trials prepared by the Cochrane Collaboration).
Concordance	Concordance is a concept reflecting the extent to which a course of action agreed between clinicians and a person with diabetes is actually carried out; often but not solely used in the sense of therapeutic interventions or behavioural changes.
Cost-effectiveness analysis	An economic study design in which consequences of different interventions are measured using a single outcome, usually in natural units (for example, life-years gained, deaths avoided, heart attacks avoided, cases detected). Alternative interventions are then compared in terms of cost per unit of effectiveness.
Cost-utility analysis	A form of cost-effectiveness analysis in which the units of effectiveness are quality adjusted life years.
DCCT	Diabetes Control and Complications Trial – a landmark study of the effects of intensification of diabetes care on development of microvascular complications.

Diabetes centre	A generic term for a source of a unified multidisciplinary diabetes service.
Diabetes mellitus	Chronic condition characterised by elevated blood glucose levels. Diabetes is of diverse aetiology and pathogenesis, and should not be regarded as a single disease. Predominant types are Type 1 diabetes and Type 2 diabetes, diabetes secondary to other pancreatic disease or other endocrine disease, and diabetes of onset in pregnancy.
Diabetes UK	Self-help charity for people with diabetes in the UK, and a professional organisation for diabetes care.
Education	In the context of this guideline, patient education in self-management of everyday diabetes issues like insulin therapy, dietary changes, self-monitoring of glucose level, physical exercise, coping with concurrent illness, how to avoid hypoglycaemia, complications, arterial risk control, jobs, travel, etc.
FBG	Fasting blood glucose level or concentration
FPG	Fasting plasma glucose level or concentration
Framingham equation	A widely known and used calculation of arterial risk, derived from a long-term study in Framingham, Massachusetts. Not valid in people with Type 1 or Type 2 diabetes.
GDG	Guideline Development Group
Glucose excursions	Change in blood glucose levels especially after meals.
GFR	Glomerular filtration rate – a measure of kidney function.
GHb	Glycated haemoglobin – see HbA_{1c}.
GI	Gastrointestinal
HbA_{1c}	The predominant form of glycated haemoglobin, present in red blood cells, and formed when the normal haemoglobin A reacts non-enzymatically with glucose. As the reaction is slow and only concentration dependent, the amount of HbA_{1c} formed is proportional only to the concentration of HbA and glucose. As HbA remains in the circulation for around 3 months, the amount of HbA_{1c} present, expressed as a percentage of HbA, is proportional to the glucose concentration over that time.
HTA	Health Technology Assessment, funded by the NHS Research and Development Directorate.
IDF	International Diabetes Federation – a global federation of diabetes associations.
Incremental cost	The cost of one alternative less the cost of another.
Incremental cost effectiveness ratio (ICER)	The ratio of the difference in costs between two alternatives to the difference in effectiveness between the same two alternatives.
Insulin analogues	A derivative of human insulin in which change of the amino-acid sequence alters duration of action after injection.

20

Insulin regimen	A therapeutic combination of different insulin preparations, including time of injection and frequency during a day.
IHD	Ischaemic heart disease
Meta-analysis	A statistical technique for combining (pooling) the results of a number of studies that address the same question and report on the same outcomes to produce a summary result.
Metabolic syndrome	Overweight (abdominal adiposity), insulin insensitivity, higher blood pressure, abnormal blood fat profile.
Methodological limitations	Features of the design or reporting of a clinical study which are known to be associated with risk of bias or lack of validity. Where a study is reported in this guideline as having significant methodological limitations, a recommendation has not been directly derived from it.
MI	Myocardial infarction
Microalbuminuria	A low but clinically significant level of albumin and other proteins in the urine.
NCC-CC	The National Collaborating Centre for Chronic Conditions, set up in 2000 to undertake commissions from the NICE to develop clinical guidelines for the NHS.
NHS	National Health Service – this guideline is written for the NHS in England and Wales.
NICE	National Institute for Health and Clinical Excellence – a special health authority set up within the NHS to develop appropriate and consistent advice on healthcare technologies, and to commission evidence-based guidelines.
NPH insulin	Neutral protamine Hagedorn insulin – a basal insulin, named after the Danish researcher Hans Christian Hagedorn, and developed in the 1940s. Synonymous with isophane insulin.
NS	Not significant (at the 5% level unless stated otherwise).
NSC	National Screening Committee (UK)
NSF	National Service Framework – a nationwide initiative designed to improve delivery of care for a related group of conditions.
Observational study	Retrospective or prospective study in which the investigator observes the natural course of events with or without control groups, for example cohort studies and case-control studies.
Odds ratio	A measure of relative treatment effectiveness. An odds ratio of 1 means equality between the comparisons in the study, and higher numbers mean greater differences. The odds of an event happening in the intervention group, divided by the odds of it happening in the control group.
PDE5 inhibitors	Phosphodiesterase type 5 inhibitors, a class of drugs developed in recent years to treat erectile dysfunction.

PROCAM	Prospective Cardiovascular Münster Heart Study – an epidemiological study performed in Germany.
Proteinuria	The presence of protein in the urine.
p-values	The probability that an observed difference could have occurred by chance. A p-value of less than 0.05 is conventionally considered to be 'statistically significant'.
Quality of life	A term used to describe an individual's level of satisfaction with their life and general sense of well-being. It is often measured as physical, psychological and social well-being.
Quality of life-adjusted year (QALY)	A measure of health outcome which assigns to each period of time a weight, ranging from 0 to 1, corresponding to the health-related quality of life during that period, where a weight of 1 corresponds to optimal health, and a weight of 0 corresponds to a health state judged equivalent to death; these are then aggregated across time periods.
RCT	Randomised controlled trial. A trial in which people are randomly assigned to two (or more) groups – one (the experimental group) receiving the treatment that is being tested, and the other (the comparison or control group) receiving an alternative treatment, a placebo (dummy treatment) or no treatment. The two groups are followed up to compare differences in outcomes to see how effective the experimental treatment was. Such trial designs help minimise experimental bias.
RR	Relative risk
Sensitivity analysis	A measure of the extent to which small changes in parameters and variables affect a result calculated from them. In this guideline, sensitivity analysis is used in health economic modelling.
Short-form 36 (SF-36)	The SF-36 assesses functioning and well-being in chronic disease. Thirty-six items in eight domains are included, which cover functional status, well-being, and overall evaluation of health.
Specialist	A clinician whose practice is limited to a particular branch of medicine or surgery, especially one who is certified by a higher medical educational organisation.
Stakeholder	Any national organisation, including patient and carers' groups, healthcare professionals and commercial companies with an interest in the guideline under development.
Statistical significance	A result is deemed statistically significant if the probability of the result occurring by chance is less than 1 in 20 ($p<0.05$).
Systematic review	Research that summarises the evidence on a clearly formulated question according to a pre-defined protocol using systematic and explicit methods to identify, select and appraise relevant studies, and to extract, collate and report their findings. It may or may not use statistical meta-analysis.

Technology appraisal	Formal ascertainment and review of the evidence surrounding a health technology, restricted in the current document to appraisals undertaken by NICE.
Thiazolidinediones	A group of drugs which improve insulin sensitivity in people with reduced sensitivity to their own or injected insulin; presently the licensed drugs are both of the chemical group known as trivially 'glitazones' or PPAR-γ agonists.
Type 1 diabetes	Insulin-deficiency disease, developing predominantly in childhood, characterised by hyperglycaemia if untreated, and with a consequent high risk of vascular damage usually developing over a period of decades.
Type 2 diabetes	Diabetes generally of slow onset mainly found in adults and in association with features of the metabolic syndrome. Carries a very high risk of vascular disease. While not insulin dependent many people with the condition eventually require insulin therapy for optimal blood glucose control.
UAER	Urinary albumin excretion rate
UKPDS	United Kingdom Prospective Diabetes Study – a landmark study of the effect of different diabetes therapies on vascular complications in people with Type 2 diabetes.
WHO	World Health Organization

THE GUIDELINE

5 Education

5.1 Structured education

5.1.1 Clinical introduction

Type 2 diabetes mellitus is a progressive long-term medical condition that is predominantly managed by the person with the diabetes and/or their carer as part of their daily life. Accordingly, understanding of diabetes, informed choice of management opportunities, and the acquisition of relevant skills for successful self-management play an important role in achieving optimal outcomes. Delivery of these needs is not always assured by conventional clinical consultations. Structured programmes have been designed not only to improve people's knowledge and skills, but also to help motivate and sustain people with diabetes in taking control of their condition and in delivering effective self-management.

Recent information from the Health Commission survey in 2007 suggests that only 11% of people with Type 2 diabetes report being offered structured education.[8] This suggests that the majority of healthcare providers have found it difficult to implement and resource quality education programmes that meet these standards. There appears to be an urgent need to ensure that all people with Type 2 diabetes are offered high-quality structured education. The aims of structured education and self-management programmes are to improve outcomes through addressing the individual's health beliefs, optimising metabolic control, addressing cardiovascular risk factors (helping to reduce the risk of complications), facilitating behaviour change (such as increased physical activity), improving quality of life and reducing depression. An effective programme will also enhance the relationship between the person with diabetes and their healthcare professionals, thereby providing the basis of true partnership in diabetes management.

The clinical question that has been addressed is how to deliver such education, including what approaches deliver the intended benefits, and what components of the education process best deliver the surrogate, self-care, and quality of life outcomes.

5.1.2 Methodological introduction and evidence statements

Please refer to the Technology Assessment Report 'The clinical effectiveness of diabetes education models for Type 2 diabetes: a systematic review' commissioned by the NHS R&D Health Technology Assessment (HTA) programme on behalf of the NCC-CC. Available at www.ncchta.org/project/1550.asp

5.1.3 Health economic methodological introduction

Two papers were identified in the search for health economics. Neither study was conducted in the UK and the results were not generalisable to the UK setting so both were excluded.[9,10]

5.1.4 From evidence to recommendations

The GDG noted that the last review of this area by a HTA on behalf of NICE in 2003 looked at the evidence for structured education. Little robust evidence of the effectiveness of any particular educational approach for people with Type 2 diabetes was found. One conclusion was that further research was required, but meanwhile that educational programmes with a theoretical basis demonstrated improved outcomes, and that group education was a more effective use of resources and may have additional benefits.

Educational interventions are not only complex in themselves, but they also exist in a complex environment with other aspects of managing a chronic disease. Such interventions will interact with, and support medical management directed at vascular risk factors and that of diabetes complications which have already developed. Their success is likely to depend on the individual's personal and cultural beliefs, the overall healthcare setting, their lifestyles, and perhaps their educational background.

It was noted that to address some of the difficulties in describing and implementing effective structured education and self-management programmes, a Patient Education Working Group (PEWG) had been convened by the Department of Health and Diabetes UK, and had laid out in detail the necessary requirements for developing high-quality patient education programmes. The key criteria had been endorsed by the recent HTA review. The five standards were as follows.

1   Any programme should have an underpinning philosophy, should be evidence-based, and suit the needs of the individual. The programme should have specific aims and learning objectives, and should support development of self-management attitudes, beliefs, knowledge and skills for the learner, their family and carers.
2   The programme should have a structured curriculum which is theory-driven, evidence-based, resource-effective, have supporting materials, and be written down.
3   It should be delivered by trained educators who should have an understanding of the educational theory appropriate to the age and needs of the programme learners, and be trained and competent in delivery of the principles and content of the specific programme they are offering.
4   The programme itself should be quality assured, be reviewed by trained, competent, independent assessors and be assessed against key criteria to ensure sustained consistency.
5   The outcomes from the programme should be regularly audited.

The GDG found no reason to diverge from these principles. The GDG noted and endorsed the importance of quality assurance and audit in this complex area.

As the intervention is complex, the measured outcomes of any particular programme are by nature multifaceted and will vary with such factors as the timing in relation to diagnosis, critical changes of therapy, or other critical clinical findings. Even then, appropriate study outcomes are for the most part interim surrogate measures; no studies included late complications. However, psychological outcomes as well as biomedical outcomes can be appropriately assessed, to include quality of life and change in healthcare behaviours, and aspects of depressed mood. More directly cognitive measures, knowledge, acquisition of skills, and changing health beliefs were found to be useful indicators of a programme's effectiveness.

The HTA commissioned for the current review included 14 studies, of which eight appeared to have been conducted since 2003, and most were for people with established (rather than newly diagnosed) Type 2 diabetes. The GDG noted that, as expected, some studies showed effects on HbA_{1c}, others improved body weight and other lifestyle changes, some improved quality of life or knowledge, and yet others changed health beliefs or reduced depression. This diversity was often simply a reflection of study aims and design. The HTA review acknowledged that health psychology approaches and some methods of health promotion have a good evidence base, but little is incorporated into studies of structured education, even though addressing health beliefs and motivating individuals to change behaviour is a cornerstone of any educational programme. Reported training for diabetes educators was poorly detailed in most studies.

The GDG was concerned that only three studies were UK-based. As cultural issues, patient health beliefs and attitudes are likely to differ from one country to another, applicability of the others may be limited. The GDG noted that the UK Diabetes Education and Self Management for Ongoing and Newly Diagnosed (DESMOND study) found changes in health beliefs, reduction in depression, and increases in self-reported physical activity, reduction in weight and improvement in smoking status. In people with established diabetes there was useful evidence from the X-PERT programme with improvements in HbA_{1c}, reduced diabetes medication, body weight, waist circumference, total serum cholesterol, diabetes knowledge and increase in self-reported physical activity and treatment satisfaction.

Overall the GDG then felt that well-designed and well-implemented programmes were likely to be effective and cost-effective interventions for people with Type 2 diabetes, in line with the NICE TA. For those people in whom education delivered in a group setting is appropriate, it is evidently likely to be more cost effective.

RECOMMENDATIONS

R1   Offer structured education to every person and/or their carer at and around the time of diagnosis, with annual reinforcement and review. Inform people and their carers that structured education is an integral part of diabetes care.

R2   Select a patient-education programme that meets the criteria laid down by the Department of Health and Diabetes UK Patient Education Working Group.

- Any programme should be evidence-based, and suit the needs of the individual. The programme should have specific aims and learning objectives, and should support development of self-management attitudes, beliefs, knowledge and skills for the learner, their family and carers.
- The programme should have a structured curriculum that is theory-driven and evidence-based, resource-effective, has supporting materials, and is written down.
- The programme should be delivered by trained educators who have an understanding of education theory appropriate to the age and needs of the programme learners, and are trained and competent in delivery of the principles and content of the programme they are offering.
- The programme itself should be quality assured, and be reviewed by trained, competent, independent assessors who assess it against key criteria to ensure sustained consistency.
- The outcomes from the programme should be regularly audited.

R3   Ensure the patient education programme provides the necessary resources to support the educators, and that educators are properly trained and given time to develop and maintain their skills.

R4   Offer group education programmes as the preferred option. Provide an alternative of equal standard for a person unable or unwilling to participate in group education.

R5 Ensure the patient-education programmes available meet the cultural, linguistic, cognitive, and literacy needs within the locality.

R6 Ensure all members of the diabetes healthcare team are familiar with the programmes of patient education available locally, that these programmes are integrated with the rest of the care pathway, and that people with diabetes and their carers have the opportunity to contribute to the design and provision of local programmes.

6 Lifestyle management/ non-pharmacological management

6.1 Dietary advice

6.1.1 Clinical introduction

All people with Type 2 diabetes should be supported to:

- try to achieve and maintain blood glucose levels and blood pressure in the normal range or as close to normal as is safely possible
- maintain a lipid and lipoprotein profile that reduces the risk of vascular disease.

Optimal dietary behaviours can contribute to all of these.

Dietary intervention should address the individual's nutritional needs, taking into account personal choices, cultural preferences and willingness to change, and to ensure that quality of life is optimised. It is usual that a registered dietician plays a key role in providing nutritional care advice within the multidisciplinary diabetes team. It is also recognised that all team members need to be knowledgeable about nutritional therapy, and give emphasis to consistent dietary and lifestyle advice.[11]

The management of obesity is not specifically addressed in the current guideline. Readers are referred to the NICE obesity management guideline which addresses the area in some detail.[12]

Smoking cessation is not addressed in the current guideline. Readers are referred to the NICE public health programme guidance on smoking cessation services, including the use of pharmacotherapies, in primary care, pharmacies, local authorities and workplaces, with particular reference to manual working groups, pregnant smokers and hard to reach communities. Guidance was published in February 2008.

Clinical questions arise around the optimal strategies to reduce calorie intake (and thus improve sensitivity to endogenous insulin), to control exogenous delivery of free sugars into the circulation, to control blood pressure, and to optimise the blood lipid profile. Issues specifically related to people with kidney disease or of medical use of fish oils are not considered in this section. Issues specifically related to delivery of patient education are considered in the chapter on Patient Education (see chapter 5).

6.1.2 Methodological introduction

The search attempted to identify RCTs and observational studies conducted in adults with Type 2 diabetes which were assessing different forms of dietary advice targeting weight loss. A sample size threshold of N=50 and a follow-up of at least 3 months were established as cut-off points. Studies evaluating purely pharmacological interventions for weight reduction were excluded.

There were only eight studies that addressed this question.[13–20] Two RCTs were excluded due to methodological limitations.* In all the studies, the intent was for participants to lose weight and thereby improve glycaemic, lipid and blood pressure control.** Among the remaining six studies there were four RCTs and two observational studies. No major methodological limitations were identified across these studies.

▷ RCTs

One RCT[17] compared the effects of a combined intervention; low-calorie diet, sibutramine therapy and meal replacements with an individualised reduced calorie diet, and was the only study to include the use of weight-loss medication.

Two RCTs used the American Diabetes Association (ADA) guidelines as a comparison group to either a soy-based meal replacement intervention,[13] N=104 with a 1-year follow-up, or a low-fat vegan diet,[14] N=99 with a 22-week follow-up.

A further RCT compared a low-fat with a low-carbohydrate diet.[16]

▷ Observational studies

A case series with a follow-up of 6.5 years investigated the onset of diabetic complications and adherence to ADA recommendations.[19] A prospective cohort study addressed the relationship between eating habits and long-term weight gain, following a group of patients being managed in primary care for a period of 4 years.[20]

It should be noted that the results of diet interventions aimed at patients with Type 2 diabetes are difficult to interpret due to differences in the interventions, the populations, the study designs and the outcomes reported.

As is obvious, isolated diet interventions without adequate educational support and concomitant lifestyle changes are very unlikely to reduce risk factors and to improve clinical outcomes and quality of life for patients with Type 2 diabetes.

6.1.3 Health economic methodological introduction

No health economic papers were identified.

6.1.4 Evidence statements

▷ Weight reduction and glycaemic control outcomes

RCTs

Studies that compared a meal replacement intervention with a reduced calorie diet

An RCT comparing a soy-based meal replacement with an individualised diet based on ADA recommendations in obese Type 2 diabetics[13] found that average weight reduction in the meal replacement group was greater than that in the individualised diet group. At 6 months, the meal

---

* One RCT comparing the effects of a high-protein with a low-protein diet[15] and another RCT comparing low-carbohydrate versus conventional weight loss diets in severely obese adults.[18]
** Four studies focused on the effects of diet in obese Type 2 diabetics.

replacement group had lost on average 5.24±0.60 kg, and the individualised diet group had lost an average of 2.85±0.67 kg (p=0.0031). At 1 year this difference was not significant with the meal replacement group losing on average 4.35±0.81 kg and the individualised diet group losing an average of 2.36±0.76 kg (p=0.0670). **Level 1+**

The same RCT reported that similar changes were observed in the body mass index (BMI) at 12 months with a reduction of 1.47±0.27 kg/m^2 in the meal replacement group and 0.77±0.25 kg/m^2 in the individualised diet group. Although these values were significantly different from their baseline values, none were significantly different from each other (p=0.0687). **Level 1+**

With respect to glycaemic control, the RCT found that mean HbA$_{1c}$ levels were significantly lower in the meal replacement than in the individualised diet group, 0.49±0.22% (p=0.0291), for the entire study period. Plasma glucose concentrations were significantly lower in the meal replacement group than in the individualised diet group at 3 (p=0.04) and 6 (p=0.002) months, but not at 12 months (p=0.595). **Level 1+**

The study by Redmon[17] reported on a combination intervention including sibutramine, an intermittent low-calorie diet with the use of meal replacements for 1 week every 2 months, and the use of meal replacements between the low-calorie diet weeks. The comparison group received an individualised diet plan with a 500–1,000 kcal energy deficit per day.

The study reported that at 1 year of follow-up, the combination therapy group had a significantly greater weight loss of 7.3±1.3 kg than the standard therapy group 0.8±0.9 kg (p<0.001), with most weight loss occurring during the low-calorie weeks and some weight gain occurring in between the low-calorie weeks. **Level 1+**

In relation to glycaemic control, the study showed that at 1 year, HbA$_{1c}$ had declined from a baseline of 8.1±0.2% to 7.5±0.3% in the combination therapy group but had remained unchanged at 8.2±0.2% in the standard therapy group, and this difference was significant (p=0.05). After adjusting for medication changes, this difference remained significant. In an analysis of those participants whose medication had not changed, it was found that there was a significant positive linear association between change in weight at 1 year and change in HbA$_{1c}$ (r=0.53; p=0.006). A 5 kg decrease in weight at 1 year was associated with a 0.4% decrease in HbA$_{1c}$. **Level 1+**

Studies comparing a low-carbohydrate with a low-fat diet

One RCT[16] examined the short-term effects, participants were followed up for 3 months, of a low-carbohydrate diet compared with a reduced portion low-fat diet in obese Type 2 diabetics. There was a significantly larger mean weight reduction in the low-carbohydrate arm (N=51) of their RCT, 3.55±0.63 kg, than in the low-fat arm (N=51) which showed a mean reduction of 0.92±0.40 kg (p=0.001). **Level 1+**

The same RCT reported that glycaemic control improved in both arms of the trial. Improvements were greater in the low-carbohydrate arm, HbA$_{1c}$ decreased from a baseline of 9.00±0.20%, by 0.55±0.17%, but this did not reach statistical significance. In the low-fat arm HbA$_{1c}$ decreased from a baseline of 9.11±0.17% by 0.23±0.13% (p=0.132). **Level 1+**

Studies comparing low- or modified-fat diets with reduced calorie diets

Barnard et al.[14] investigated the effects of a low-fat vegan diet compared with a diet based on ADA guidelines, on body weight and glycaemic control in an RCT with 99 Type 2 diabetics, followed up for 22 weeks. During the study period, 43% (21/49) of vegan participants and 26% (13/50) of ADA participants reduced their diabetic medications, mainly as a result of hypoglycaemia. Eight per cent in each group, 4/49 of the vegan group and 4/50 of the ADA group, increased their medications.

The study concluded that for the whole sample, body weight was reduced in both groups by 5.8 kg in the vegan group and 4.3 kg in the ADA group, but this difference was not statistically significant (p=0.082). In those whose medication was stable this difference was significant with a 6.5 kg reduction in the vegan group, and 3.1 kg in the ADA group, p<0.001. BMI declined by 2.1 ± 1.5 kg/m^2 in the vegan group and by 1.5 ± 1.5 kg/m^2 in the ADA group (p=0.08). The waist-to-hip ratio declined in the vegan group 0.02 ± 0.01 but not in the ADA group (p=0.003). **Level 1+**

With respect to glycaemic control, the RCT stated that while the HbA$_{1c}$ decline in both groups was statistically significant from their baseline values with a decline of 0.96% (p<0.0001) in the vegan group and 0.56% (p=0.0009) in the ADA group, there was no significant difference between the groups (p=0.089). Again the results were different in those participants whose medication was unchanged. The HbA$_{1c}$ decline was greater in the vegan group, 1.23 ± 1.38%, than in the ADA group, 0.38 ± 1.11%, (p=0.01). **Level 1+**

Table 6.1 Summarised results for body weight reduction and glycaemic control across RCTs					
RCTs	**T=**	**Comparison**	**Comparison**	**Weight/BMI**	**Glycaemic control**
Li (2005)[13]	1 year	Soy-based meal replacement	Individualised diet	Weight and BMI=NS	HbA$_{1c}$ significantly lower in meal replacement arm
Redmon (2003)[17]	1 year	Sibutramine + low-calorie diet + meal replacement	Individualised diet	Weight reduction significantly higher in combination arm	HbA$_{1c}$ significantly lower in combination arm*
Daly (2006)[16]	3 months	Low-carbohydrate diet	Reduced portion low-fat diet	Weight reduction significantly higher in carbohydrate arm	HbA$_{1c}$=NS
Barnard (2006)[14]	22 weeks	Low-fat vegan diet	Diet based on ADA guidelines	Weight=NS	HbA$_{1c}$=NS

* A 5 kg decrease in weight at 1 year was associated with a 0.4% decrease in HbA$_{1c}$.

Observational studies

In an observational study with 4 years of follow-up,[20] the authors investigated the association between eating behaviour and long-term weight gain. Ninety-seven Type 2 diabetics were recruited at diagnosis and after initial nutrition advice were followed up for a period of 4 years.

The study found that at the end of follow-up, mean body weight change in men was a gain of 1.3 ± 5.4 kg, whereas in women, there was a mean body weight reduction of -1.1 ± 5.0 kg. These changes were not statistically significant, (p values not given). Similarly, BMI increased in men by 0.42 ± 1.76 kg/m^2 and decreased in women by 0.40 ± 1.89 kg/m^2, (p values not given). Glycaemic outcomes were not reported. **Level 2+**

In the second observational study,[19] weight loss over the 6.5-year follow-up is not reported. However, metabolic control did improve in patients over the period, with the proportion of patients with HbA_{1c} <7% increasing from 52.4% to 64.3% in men and from 43.9 to 50.9% in women. It was not reported whether or not this was significant. **Level 3**

▷ Blood pressure and blood lipid control outcomes

RCTs

Studies that compared a meal replacement intervention with a reduced calorie diet

The RCT by Li et al.,[13] reporting on the comparison of a soy-based meal replacement plan with an individualised diet plan, did not report on changes in blood pressure during the study.

For the blood lipid control outcomes, while there were no significant differences between groups during the study for lipid parameters, there were differences within the groups when compared to baseline values. In the meal replacement group, there were decreases in total cholesterol, triglycerol, low-density lipoprotein (LDL) and high-density lipoprotein (HDL) at the end of the study, however these changes were only significant in the triglycerol group with an overall decrease from baseline of 28.00 mg/dl (p=0.038). Decreases in total cholesterol were significant at 3 (p<0.0001) and 6 (p=0.0037) months, but at 12 months with a reduction of 10.76 mg/dl from baseline, this was not significant (p=0.084). LDL decreased by 11.04 mg/dl at 3 months (p=0.024), but at 12 months the change from baseline had reduced to 6.10 mg/dl (p=0.255). HDL had decreased by 0.97 mg/dl at 12 months (p=0.345). In the individualised diet plan group, after initial decreases at 3 or 6 months, at 12 months there were increases in total cholesterol by 5.26 mg/dl (p=0.396), LDL by 8.76 mg/dl (p=0.129) and HDL by 2.26 mg/dl (p=0.012). Only in triglycerol levels was there a sustained decreased at 12 months with a reduction from baseline of 28.89 mg/dl (p=0.119). **Level 1+**

In the study by Redmon[17] which compared a combined intervention (described above) with an individualised diet plan, at 1 year there were reductions in systolic and diastolic blood pressure in both groups, although this did not differ between the groups. Systolic blood pressure reduced in the combination group by 6±3 mmHg and by 6±2 mmHg in the comparison group. Diastolic blood pressure reduced in the combination group by 3±1 mmHg and by 6±2 mmHg in the comparison group. **Level 1+**

At 1 year, changes in fasting cholesterol, HDL, LDL and fasting triglycerides did not differ between groups. There were reductions from baseline values in fasting cholesterol and LDL cholesterol in both groups, with a decrease in fasting cholesterol of 6±8 mg/dl in the combination therapy group and 17±9 mg/dl in the comparison group (p=0.90). LDL decreased by 12±5 mg/dl in the combination therapy group and 13±6 mg/dl in the comparison group (p=0.89). Fasting triglycerides decreased by 46±24 mg/dl in the combination group compared to an increase of 8±18 mg/dl in the comparison group, however this was not significant (p=0.07). **Level 1+**

Studies comparing a low-carbohydrate with a low-fat diet

At 12 weeks of follow-up, in the low-carbohydrate arm of this RCT[16] there was a reduction in systolic blood pressure of 6.24±2.96 mmHg and a reduction of 0.39±2.64 mmHg in the low-fat arm, with no significant difference between the arms (p=0.147). **Level 1+**

With respect to lipid parameters, there was a greater reduction in the total cholesterol: HDL ratio in the low-carbohydrate arm, mean reduction of 0.48, than in the low-fat arm, mean reduction 0.10 (p=0.011). There were also reductions in triglycerides in both arms, 0.67 mmol/l in the low-carbohydrate arm and 0.25 in the low-fat arm, which did not approach statistical significance (p=0.223). **Level 1+**

Studies comparing low- or modified-fat diets with reduced calorie diets

In the RCT comparing the low-fat vegan diet with the ADA diet,[14,20] there were non-significant reductions in systolic and diastolic blood pressure in both groups. In the vegan group systolic blood pressure decreased by 3.8±12.6 mmHg (p<0.05) compared with baseline and in the ADA group by 3.6±13.7 mmHg from baseline, with no significant difference between the groups (p=0.93). Similarly the reduction in diastolic blood pressure was greater in the vegan group, 5.1±8.3 mmHg (p<0.0001) than in the ADA group 3.3±8.8 mmHg (p<0.05) although this was not different between groups (p=0.30). **Level 1+**

For the entire sample, although lipid parameters decreased significantly from baseline values, there were no significant differences between groups. Among those whose lipid controlling medications remained constant (vegan N=39/49; ADA N=41/50), total cholesterol reduced in the vegan groups by 33.5±21.5 mg/dl (p<0.0001), in the ADA group by 19.0±28.5 mg/dl (p<0.0001) and this was a significantly different between groups (p=0.01). Reductions in HDL cholesterol were not significantly different between the groups.

Reductions in non-HDL cholesterol were significantly lower than baseline in the vegan groups 27.6±21.1 mg/dl (p<0.0001) and in the ADA group 16.3±30.1 mg/dl (p<0.05), but not significantly different between the groups (p=0.05).

LDL cholesterol reduced in the vegan group by 22.6±22.0 mg/dl (p<0.0001) and in the ADA group by 10.7±23.3 mg/dl (p<0.05), and was significantly different between the groups (p=0.02). The total-to-HDL cholesterol ratio and triglyceride concentrations fell for both groups, but there was no difference between the groups. **Level 1+**

Table 6.2 Summarised results for blood pressure and lipid levels across RCTs

RCTs	T=	Comparison	Comparison	Blood pressure	Lipid levels
Li (2005)[13]	1 year	Soy-based meal replacement	Individualised diet	No changes	NS differences
Redmon (2003)[17]	1 year	Sibutramine + low calorie diet + meal replacement	Individualised diet	NS differences	NS differences
Daly (2006)[16]	3 months	Low-carbohydrate diet	Reduced portion low-fat diet	NS differences	TC:HDL ratio significantly lower in carbohydrate arm
Barnard (2006)[14]	22 weeks	Low-fat vegan diet	Diet based on ADA guidelines	NS differences	NS differences

Observational studies

In the observational study investigating the effect of eating behaviours on weight,[20] changes in blood pressure or lipid profiles were not reported.

In the diabetes nutrition and complications trial[19] changes in blood pressure were reported as the proportion of patients who had a systolic blood pressure <130 mmHg, which decreased from 28.6% at baseline to 11.9% at the end of the study. Similarly in women there was a decrease from 15.8% at baseline to 8.8% after 6.5 years. The proportion of patients with a diastolic blood pressure of <80 mmHg decreased from 26.2% to 21.4% and from 31.6% to 28.1% in men and women respectively.

In this study they reported the number of patients who were adherent to the ADA diet recommendations and were able to achieve the recommended intakes of various types of fats. They found that levels of adherence to the recommendations was low with only 26.6% of patients consuming the recommended amount of saturated fatty acids (SFAs), 13.0% consuming the recommended ≥10% of dietary energy from polyunsaturated fats, and 38.5% consuming the recommended ≥60% of dietary energy from carbohydrates and monounsaturated fats. They also estimated that 46.4% of patients consumed a ratio of polyunsaturated fatty acids (PUFAs)/SFAs >0.4 and 69% consumed a ratio of monounsaturated fats (MUFAs)/SFAs >1.5. Patients who consumed MUFAs/SFAs <1.5 had a 3.6–4.7 times greater risk of developing diabetic complications (confidence intervals (CIs) not presented). Patients who consumed PUFAs/SFAs <0.4 were 3.4–8.2 times more at risk of developing diabetic complications. **Level 3**

6.1.5 From evidence to recommendations

The GDG noted that there was little new evidence to warrant any change to previous views in this field. The major consensus-based recommendations from the UK and USA emphasise sensible practical implementation of nutritional advice for people with Type 2 diabetes. Other relevant NICE guidance should be considered where relevant, including clinical guideline no. 43 on the assessment and management of overweight and obesity in adults and children and clinical guideline no. 48 which gives dietary and lifestyle advice post-MI. Overlap with the NICE/RCP Type 1 diabetes guideline was noted. Management otherwise will concentrate on principles of healthy eating (essentially those for optimal cardiovascular risk protection), and reduction of high levels of free carbohydrate in food that are hyperglycaemic in the presence of defective insulin secretory reserve.

If people are currently gaining weight, weight maintenance is advantageous.

The GDG noted that in some people with Type 2 diabetes and weight problems it might be appropriate to consider pharmacotherapy, however this was not within the clinical questions addressed.

As with Patient Education (see chapter 5) delivery of dietary advice was noted to depend not only on specific skills, but also required all members of the diabetes care team to be familiar with local policy and thus delivering consistent advice.

Concerns continue to be noted over the promotion of 'diabetic foods' which may be low in classical sugars but high in calories and thus unsuitable as well as unnecessary for the overweight. While reduction in weight was clearly understood to be beneficial through improvements in insulin insensitivity (whether relying on endogenous or exogenous insulin), low-carbohydrate diets were noted to be of unproven safety in the long term and thus could not be endorsed. Similarly high-protein diets are acknowledged as promoting short-term weight loss, but cannot be recommend as safe in the long term.

A dietary plan for people with diabetes would follow the principles of healthy eating in the population, and thus include carbohydrate from fruits, vegetables, wholegrains, and pulses (and thus high fibre and low glycaemic index), reduction in salt intake, the inclusion of low-fat milk and oily fish, and control of saturated and trans fatty acid intake.

The importance of advice on alcohol to the overweight and to those prone to hypoglycaemia through use of insulin secretagogues or insulin was judged important.

RECOMMENDATIONS

R7   Provide individualised and ongoing nutritional advice from a healthcare professional with specific expertise and competencies in nutrition.

R8   Provide dietary advice in a form sensitive to the individual's needs, culture and beliefs being sensitive to their willingness to change, and the effects on their quality of life.

R9   Emphasise advice on healthy balanced eating that is applicable to the general population when providing advice to people with Type 2 diabetes. Encourage high-fibre, low glycaemic index sources of carbohydrate in the diet, such as fruit, vegetables, wholegrains and pulses; include low-fat dairy products and oily fish; and control the intake of foods containing saturated and trans fatty acids.

R10   Integrate dietary advice with a personalised diabetes management plan, including other aspects of lifestyle modification, such as increasing physical activity and losing weight.

R11   Target, for people who are overweight, an initial body weight loss of 5–10%, while remembering that lesser degrees of weight loss may still be of benefit and that larger degrees of weight loss in the longer term will have advantageous metabolic impact.

R12   Individualise recommendations for carbohydrate and alcohol intake, and meal patterns. Reducing the risk of hypoglycaemia should be a particular aim for a person using insulin or an insulin secretagogue.

R13   Advise individuals that limited substitution of sucrose-containing foods for other carbohydrate in the meal plan is allowable, but that care should be taken to avoid excess energy intake.

R14   Discourage the use of foods marketed specifically for people with diabetes.

R15   When patients are admitted to hospital as inpatients or to any other institutions, implement a meal planning system that provides consistency in the carbohydrate content of meals and snacks.

6.2 Management of depression

6.2.1 Clinical introduction

Psychological well-being is clearly part of being healthy. It is an important part of healthcare management of any condition where psychological health is impaired or where it has particular impact on clinical management.

There is evidence of a high prevalence of psychological ill-health in people with diabetes, notably for depression,[21] which is often under-recognised.[22] Additionally because of the importance of self-care to the management of the condition, there is evidence that psychological ill-health is associated with adverse effects on other aspects of the long-term health of people with Type 2 diabetes.[23–25]

Formal assessment of psychological well-being is not a standard part of practice in diabetes care in the UK. Other guidelines, including the NICE guideline for people with Type 1 diabetes, have emphasised the importance of recognising and managing depression. Only general recommendations have been made regarding being alert to problems, availability of skills to manage routine psychological disorders, and of appropriate referral to those with special expertise where the condition is more severe.[26] NICE has recently published a guideline on the management of depression.[27]

No evidence search has been performed for the purpose of the current guideline due to the availability of the NICE depression guideline. People with Type 2 diabetes with psychological and/or depressive disorders should be identified by continuing professional awareness, and managed in accordance with current national guidelines.

7 Glucose control levels

7.1 Clinical monitoring of blood glucose control

7.1.1 Clinical introduction

The risk of arterial disease and microvascular complications in people with diabetes are known to be related to the extent of hyperglycaemia with time. While the lifestyle, oral agent, and injectable therapies discussed in this guideline can improve blood glucose control, their efficacy is limited, as the underlying pathogenesis of diabetes worsens with time. As symptoms are not a reliable guide to blood glucose control in people on therapy, it is important to have an accurate means of measuring blood glucose control over time, to enable decision-making.

This section addresses the clinical questions as to the tests of blood glucose control best predictive of future vascular damage from diabetes, the nature of the relationship between test results and such vascular risk, how tests should be deployed in clinical practice, and how they might be interpreted.

7.1.2 Methodological introduction

The UKPDS is a large (N=3,867) landmark study with a 10-year follow-up period. It evaluated whether in people newly diagnosed with Type 2 diabetes more intense therapy to achieve tighter glycaemic control would result in a greater reduction in the incidence of microvascular and macrovascular complications than would conservative therapy. Due to the size and duration of this study, other studies published from 2001 onwards in this area were only considered if they had a sample size of at least N=2,000 people with Type 2 diabetes, or mixed Type 1 and 2 diabetes populations. Studies were not reviewed if they simply found significant associations between HbA_{1c} and diabetes complications without giving further information about that association.

Published results from the UKPDS were included in this review if they specifically reported results on the relationship between HbA_{1c} and microvascular and/or macrovascular complications. One prospective observational study[28] was identified which analysed the UKPDS glucose control results in terms of both macrovascular and microvascular complications.

A meta-analysis[29] was also identified which assessed the association between glycosylated haemoglobin and cardiovascular (CV) disease in people with diabetes. This included an analysis of 10 studies specifically of people with Type 2 diabetes. As some of the cohorts included in this analysis were participants in the UKPDS study, it is necessary to be alert to double-counting.

Other observational studies identified, which were not published results of the UKPDS study or included in the meta-analysis, considered the relationship between glycaemic control and CV and renal risk,[30] and between glycaemic control and heart failure.[31]

7.1.3 Health economic methodological introduction

One paper was identified which was excluded from further consideration as it was not possible to compare the costs between patients with good or poor control because the well-controlled patients were probably earlier in the course of the disease.[32] Two evaluations based on the UKPDS were identified that were considered to be of good quality.[33]

7.1.4 Evidence statements

- The risk of each of the microvascular and macrovascular complications of Type 2 diabetes and cataract extraction was strongly associated with hyperglycaemia as measured by updated mean HbA_{1c}.

- There was no indication of a threshold for any complication below which risk no longer decreased, nor a level above which risk no longer increased.

Table 7.1 UKPDS study[28]
N=3,642 included in the analysis of relative risk
Level of evidence 2++

Microvascular/macrovascular complications or mortality	1% reduction in updated mean HbA_{1c} was associated with reductions in risk of*
Any endpoint related to diabetes (MI, sudden death, angina, stroke, renal failure, lower extremity amputation or death from peripheral vascular disease, death from hyperglycaemia or hypoglycaemia, heart failure, vitreous haemorrhage, retinal photocoagulation, and cataract extraction)	21%, 95% CI 17% to 24% (p<0.0001)
For deaths related to diabetes (MI, sudden death, stroke, lower extremity amputation or fatal peripheral vascular disease, renal disease, hyperglycaemia or hypoglycaemia)	21%, 95% CI 15% to 27% (p<0.0001)
All cause mortality	14%, 95% CI 9% to 19% (p<0.0001)
MI (fatal MI, non-fatal MI, and sudden death)	14%, 95% CI 8% to 21% (p<0.0001)
Stroke (fatal and non-fatal stroke)	12%, 95% CI 1% to 21% (p=0.035)
Peripheral vascular disease (lower extremity amputation or death from peripheral vascular disease)	43%, 95% CI 31% to 53% (p<0.0001)
Microvascular complications (retinopathy requiring photocoagulation, vitreous haemorrhage, and fatal or non-fatal renal failure)	37%, 95% CI 33% to 41% (p<0.0001)
Heart failure (non-fatal, without a precipitating MI)	16%, 95% CI 3% to 26% (p=0.016)
Cataract extraction	19%, 95% CI 11% to 26% (p<0.0001)

The adjusted incidence rates for any endpoint related to diabetes increased with each higher category of updated mean HbA_{1c}, with no evidence of a threshold and with a three-fold increase over the range of updated mean HbA_{1c} of less than 6%, to equal to, or more than, 10%.

* Data adjusted for age at diagnosis of diabetes, sex, ethnic group, smoking, presence of albuminuria, systolic blood pressure, high and low density lipoprotein cholesterol and triglycerides

- There was an increase in CV risk with increasing levels of glycosylated haemoglobin in persons with Type 2 diabetes.

Table 7.2 Meta-analysis of prospective cohort studies[29]
N=10 studies in people with Type 2 diabetes
Level of evidence 2+

Cardiovascular complications or mortality	Pooled RR for each 1 percentage point increase in glycosylated haemoglobin*
Total CV (combining 10 studies of coronary heart disease alone, stroke alone, and stroke and coronary heart disease combined)	1.18 (95% CI 1.10 to 1.26)
Coronary heart disease (combining five studies of MI, angina and IHD)	1.13 (95% CI 1.06 to 1.20)
Fatal coronary heart disease (combining five studies of fatal MI, angina and IHD)	1.16 (95% CI 1.07 to 1.26)
Cerebrovascular disease (combining three studies of fatal and non-fatal stroke)	1.17 (95% CI 1.09 to 1.25)
Peripheral arterial disease (combining three studies of lower extremity peripheral arterial disease, amputation and claudication)	1.28 (95% CI 1.18 to 1.39)

* All RR estimates in the pooled analyses were from the most fully adjusted multivariate model
IHD, ischaemic heart disease; RR, relative risk

- There was an independent progressive relationship between GHb and incident cardiovascular events, renal disease and death.

Table 7.3 Prospective observational study of participants in the Heart Outcomes Prevention Evaluation (HOPE) study[30]
N=3,529
Level of evidence 2+

Cardiovascular and renal complications	A 1% absolute rise in updated glycated haemoglobin was associated with relative risks of*
Future CV events (the first occurrence of one or more of the following: non-fatal MI, stroke or CV death)	1.07, 95% CI 1.01 to 1.13 (p=0.014)
Death	1.12, 95% CI 1.05 to 1.19 (p=0.0004)
Hospitalisation for heart failure	1.20, 95% CI 1.08 to 1.33 (p=0.0008)
Overt nephropathy	1.26, 95% CI 1.17 to 1.36 (p=0.0001)

There was a consistent and progressive relationship between the GHb level (both baseline and updated) and the age and sex adjusted relative hazard of the above outcomes. All showed significant trends with the strongest relationships being seen with the updated GHb level

* After adjusting for age, sex, diabetes duration, blood pressure, BMI, hyperlipidaemia and ramipril

- There was an independent graded association between glycaemic control and incidence of hospitalisation and/or death due to heart failure.

Table 7.4 Observational study of participants on the Kaiser Permanente Medical Care Program of Northern California diabetes registry[31]
N=48,858
Level of evidence 2+

Cardiovascular complications	The relative risk associated with a 1% increase in HbA_{1c}*
Composite of hospitalisation for heart failure or death with heart failure as the underlying cause	1.08, 95% CI 1.05 to 1.12

A concentration of HbA_{1c} more than or equal to 10% relative to HbA_{1c} less than 7%, was associated with a 1.6 fold increased heart failure risk (for hospitalisation or death)

* This model was adjusted for age, sex, ethnicity, education level, smoking, alcohol consumption, self-reported hypertension, obesity, cardioprotective medicine used at baseline, type of diabetes and treatment, duration of diabetes and incidence of MI during follow-up

7.1.5 Health economic evidence statements

The UKPDS included an analysis of intensive blood glucose control with metformin for overweight patients compared to conventional treatment primarily with diet. The study included 753 overweight (>120% ideal body weight) patients with newly diagnosed Type 2 diabetes from 15 hospital-based clinics in England, Scotland and Northern Ireland. Of these patients 342 were allocated to an intensive blood glucose control policy with metformin and 411 were allocated to conventional treatment, primarily with diet alone. The study was conducted from 1977 to 1991. The median follow-up period was 10.4 years.

In the conventional policy group the glycaemic goal was to obtain the lowest fasting plasma glucose (FPG) attainable with diet alone. In the intensive policy group the aim was a FPG of less than 6.0 mmol/l by increasing the dose of metformin from 500 to 2,550 mg a day as required. Use of metformin for intensive blood glucose control in overweight patients was found to confer a 32% risk reduction for any diabetes related endpoint and a 42% risk reduction for diabetes related deaths compared with a conventional policy.

In the 2001 cost-effectiveness analysis, intensive treatment with metformin cost on average £258 less than conventional treatment, and resulted in a longer life expectancy of 0.4 years.[34]

In the 2005 cost-utility analysis the discounted cost (6% discount rate) of an intensive blood glucose control policy with insulin or sulphonylureas was on average £884 more per patient and the discounted benefits gained were 0.15 quality of life-adjusted year (QALY), a cost per QALY gained of £6,028.[33]

The discounted cost of intensive blood glucose control policy with metformin in overweight patients was on average £1,021 less than the conventional policy and had a longer discounted life expectancy of 0.55 QALYs, making this intensive treatment strategy both cost-saving and more effective.[34]

7.1.6 From evidence to recommendations

There were a number of difficulties agreeing the level at which therapeutic interventions should begin or be enhanced. It was agreed that people with diabetes and the professionals advising them needed a reference level if optimum glucose control is to be obtained. It was noted that treat-to-target studies achieved much better outcomes than studies with less well defined aims.

The evidence base has not significantly moved on since the earlier guideline, except to support the conclusions of the UKPDS epidemiological analysis (that CV risk fell linearly well into the normal range of HbA_{1c}). A single target figure is unhelpful as this may vary in individuals depending on the:

- quality of life that might have to be sacrificed in reaching the target
- extent of side effects
- resources available for management.

An individual requiring insulin for adequate control, who is at risk and prone to hypoglycaemia would have a higher personal target of glucose control than someone newly diagnosed who had adopted significant lifestyle changes.

Microvascular risk data suggests higher glucose control targets. This led to a stronger recommendation in the NICE/RCP Type 1 diabetes guideline for those at no added macrovascular disease risk. Most of those with Type 2 diabetes can be regarded as at high macrovascular risk, by reason of phenotype or age.

Cardiovascular risk can be reduced by 10–15% per 1.0 % reduction of HbA_{1c}, the treatment effect and epidemiological analysis of UKPDS giving the same conclusions. Mean levels of close to 6.5 % were achieved in the first 5 years of the UKPDS in both the main glucose study and the obese ('metformin') study in the active treatment arms. The epidemiological analysis supports a linear fall in macrovascular risk down to 6.0 % or below, and this will largely reflect data from the more actively managed group.

However, expensive therapies or very intensive interventions are required to achieve glucose control in the normal range in most people with diabetes. Consequently a population target should not be any tighter than the HbA_{1c} of 6.5 % previously chosen for those at macrovascular risk. Nearly all people with Type 2 diabetes are of high CV risk, usually in association with insulin insensitivity, but if not with age. Additionally there has been very recent concern (no evidence yet to review) about pursuing very intensive glucose control (target <6.0 %) in people with higher CV risk and longer duration of diabetes, mostly on multiple insulin injection therapy.[35]

The GDG were made aware of the issue of postprandial plasma glucose control, and that it could be specifically targeted in some circumstances and with some interventions. A review of the literature in this regard had not been performed for the present guideline. However, the GDG were informed that an evidence-based guideline had been published by the IDF since completion of the current guideline draft, and that no RCTs addressing the question with true health outcomes as an endpoint had been identified. Accordingly a view to treat this aspect specifically relied on weaker evidence. Accordingly the GDG were content only to make recommendations on the identification of pre-meal and postprandial hyperglycaemia, and levels for intervention.

The GDG expressed concern that intervention levels for enhancement of therapy should not be confused with audit or reimbursement standards. These types of standards are set with much greater attention being paid to attainability.

RECOMMENDATIONS

R16   When setting a target glycated haemoglobin HbA_{1c}:

- involve the person in decisions about their individual HbA_{1c} target level, which may be above that of 6.5 % set for people with Type 2 diabetes in general
- encourage the person to maintain their individual target unless the resulting side effects (including hypoglycaemia) or their efforts to achieve this impair their quality of life
- offer therapy (lifestyle and medication) to help achieve and maintain the HbA_{1c} target level
- inform a person with a higher HbA_{1c} that any reduction in HbA_{1c} towards the agreed target is advantageous to future health
- avoid pursuing highly intensive management to levels of less than 6.5 %.

R17   Measure the individual's HbA_{1c} levels at:

- 2–6-monthly intervals (tailored to individual needs), until the blood glucose level is stable on unchanging therapy; use a measurement made at an interval of less than 3 months as an indicator of direction of change, rather than as a new steady state
- 6-monthly intervals once the blood glucose level and blood glucose lowering therapy are stable.

R18   If HbA_{1c} levels remain above target levels, but pre-meal self-monitoring levels remain well controlled (<7.0 mmol/l), consider self-monitoring to detect postprandial hyperglycaemia (>8.5 mmol/l), and manage to below this level if detected (see chapters 9–11).

R19   Measure HbA_{1c} using high-precision methods and report results in units aligned with those used in DCCT Trial (or as recommended by national agreement after publication of this guideline).[218]

R20   When HbA_{1c} monitoring is invalid (because of disturbed erythrocyte turnover or abnormal haemoglobin type), estimate trends in blood glucose control using one of the following:

- fructosamine estimation
- quality-controlled plasma glucose profiles
- total glycated haemoglobin estimation (if abnormal haemoglobins).

R21   Investigate unexplained discrepancies between HbA_{1c} and other glucose measurements. Seek advice from a team with specialist expertise in diabetes or clinical biochemistry.

8 | Self-monitoring of plasma glucose

8.1.1 Clinical introduction

Self-monitoring is the only direct method by which a person with diabetes can be aware of their level of control of blood glucose. It has utility when used with therapies of erratic effect, those requiring considerable dose adjustment (notably insulin), and in those whose therapies put them at risk of hypoglycaemia. More controversial, except for people using insulin, is the use of self-monitoring to provide feedback on the impact of lifestyle measures on blood glucose control, and as part of the overall educational package designed to enhance self-care. Indirect monitoring using urine glucose tests is cheaper, but also delivers less information than plasma glucose monitoring.

This section addresses the clinical question of the role of self-monitoring of plasma glucose in people at different stages of the condition and on different therapies, and its integration with other key processes of care such as patient education.

8.1.2 Methodological introduction

Three recent systematic reviews[36–38] were identified which compared self-monitoring of blood glucose (SMBG) with usual care and/or with self-monitoring of urine glucose (SMUG) in patients with Type 2 diabetes not using insulin. One was a Cochrane review[38] of six RCTs without a meta-analysis. The same authors also published a second review[37] with the same studies including a meta-analysis. The third review was a meta-analysis of eight RCTs.[36] Although all of these reviews were of high methodological quality, this was not true of the studies included within them. In two reviews,[37,38] four out of six studies were found to be of low quality and in the other review,[36] five of the eight studies were judged to be of moderate risk of bias and three to be of high risk of bias. A further systematic review and meta-analysis included Type 2 diabetic patients that were on insulin treatment and used Bayesian methods to conduct a mixed treatment comparison.[39]

It should be noted that the two Cochrane reviews published by the same authors[37,38] did not perform a meta-analysis because they considered the studies they had identified to have 'clinical heterogeneity', in terms of baseline data of the patients and type of interventions between the studies. With regard to the interventions, the authors concluded that there were also discrepancies in monitoring frequency, training the patient in terms of the technique and educating the patient on how the data should be acted upon.

The meta-analysis by Jansen[39] scored the included studies for internal validity and adjusted for this in sensitivity analysis. This was also the only new study that compared the effects of urine versus blood self-monitoring on glycaemic control, albeit in an indirect comparison.

A protocol for a new 4-year UK trial in this area (the Diabetes Glycaemic Education and Monitoring (DiGEM) trial)[40] was identified and the results of this, once available, should clarify if and how to use SMBG, as part of a self-management programme. In one arm, a self-monitoring group will receive support in interpreting and applying the results of blood testing to enhance motivation and maintain adherence to diet, physical activity and medication regimens.

Two RCTs were identified which compared SMBG with no monitoring.[41,42] One study did not include insulin-treated patients.[42] The other included patients treated with insulin and the use of blood glucose monitoring in one arm of the study.[41]

Four cohort studies were also identified.[43–46] As noted in the previous guideline, it can be argued that limited credence can be given to observational study associations between blood glucose control and self-monitoring as those patients and healthcare professionals who advocate self-monitoring may be the same people who are motivated to achieve better control.

One cross-sectional study[47] and one case-series[48] were also identified.

The GDG requested for a separate qualitative search to be conducted on this topic. This search identified two papers which considered self-monitoring from a patient perspective.[49,50] The papers reported results from the same qualitative Scottish study although the papers had slightly different aims. One explored the respective merits of urine testing and SMBG from the perspective of newly diagnosed patients with Type 2 diabetes[49] whilst the other explored the pros and cons of self-blood glucose monitoring from the patients' perspective.[50]

8.1.3 Health economic methodological introduction

One cost-effectiveness analysis was identified in the search.[51] It did not include enough detail on the costs and utilities to adequately interpret the results.

A cost analysis of implementing intensive control of blood glucose concentration in England identified increased frequency of home glucose tests as a main contributor to the total costs of intensive control.[52] It was estimated that the additional management costs of implementing intensive control policies would be £132 million per year, of which £42.2 million would be on home glucose tests. The sensitivity analysis results found that changes in the unit cost of home blood glucose strips (baseline cost £0.27, range tested £0.16–£0.40) in the proportion of patients already being managed intensively, and the costs of intensifying management, had the largest impact on the cost of implementation.

8.1.4 Evidence statements

(See the methodological introduction for commentary on systematic reviews of RCTs.)

Even though the Cochrane reviews[37,38] were not able to meta-analyse the data (due to clinical and methodological heterogeneity) the authors concluded that SMBG might be effective in improving glycaemic control in patients with Type 2 diabetes who are not using insulin. Authors also stated that a well designed large RCT assessing the benefits (including patient-related outcomes) of SMBG alongside patient education is required. **Level 1+**

The other review[36] concluded that, 'in the short term, and when integrated with educational advice, self-monitoring of blood glucose as an adjunct to standard therapy, may contribute to improving glycaemic control among non-insulin requiring Type 2 diabetes patients'. **Level 1+**

In an indirect analysis, Jansen[39] found a non-significant reduction in HbA_{1c} of 0.3% when interventions with SMBG were compared with those associated with SMUG.

The study by Jansen also reported that interventions with SMBG were found to be more effective in reducing HbA_{1c} than interventions without self-monitoring. The reduction in HbA_{1c} was statistically significant and it was estimated to be around 0.4%. This effect was increased when regular feedback was added to the SMBG and was shown in both an insulin-treated Type 2 diabetes group, and in a group of Type 2 diabetes patients that included those being treated with oral agents. **Level 1+**

An RCT looking at the effects of an education manual[41] on blood glucose monitoring found that the greatest reduction in HbA_{1c} occurred in the education manual group ($-0.13\pm1.28\%$) compared with both the SMBG ($-0.04\pm1.31\%$) and standard care ($0.04\pm1.10\%$) groups. The authors did not report whether there was a significant difference between groups. **Level 1+**

A second multicentre RCT[42] found a significantly greater reduction in HbA_{1c} in the SMBG compared to the non-SMBG group (p=0.0086). **Level 1+**

A retrospective cohort study performed in the USA (N=976) found that duration of SMBG (0–3 years) was not a significant predictor of HbA_{1c} values in those with Type 2 diabetes on oral medication.[45] **Level 2+**

In a German retrospective cohort study of 1,609 patients with Type 2 diabetes, hazard ratios indicated that SMBG was associated with a 32% reduction in morbidity for combined macrovascular (MI and stroke) and microvascular (foot amputation, blindness or end-stage renal failure) non-fatal endpoints (HR=0.68, 95% CI 0.51–0.91, p=0.009). This was despite an increase of microvascular events, and a 51% reduction in mortality over the observation period (HR=0.49, 95% CI 0.31–0.78, p=0.003) where mean follow-up was 6.5 years. In those not receiving insulin, SMBG was associated with a 28% reduction in combined non-fatal endpoints (HR=0.72, 95% CI 0.52–0.99, p=0.0496) and a 42% reduction in mortality over the observation period (HR=0.58, 95% CI 0.35–0.96, p=0.035).[44] **Level 2+**

A retrospective cohort study of people with diabetes in a US medical care programme[43] found greater SMBG practice frequency among new users, which was associated with a graded decrease in HbA_{1c} (relative to non-users) regardless of diabetes therapy (p<0.001). Changes in SMBG frequency among prevalent users were associated with an inverse graded change in HbA_{1c} but only among pharmacologically-treated patients (p<0.0001). **Level 2+**

A study including patients from the Fremantle Diabetes Study (FDS) cohort[46] over 5 years of follow-up did not find any difference in HbA_{1c} or in fasting plasma glucose, either overall or within treatment groups in patients who used SMBG than those who did not (p≥0.05). There were also no differences in HbA_{1c} or FPG between SMBG adherent and non-adherent users by treatment group (p≥0.09). **Level 2+**

In a qualitative study performed in Scotland of newly diagnosed Type 2 diabetics, 'patients reported strongly negative views of urine testing, particularly when they compared it with self-monitoring of blood glucose. Patients perceived urine testing as less convenient, hygienic and accurate than self-monitoring of blood glucose. Most patients assumed that blood glucose meters were given to those with a more advanced or serious form of diabetes. Patients often interpreted negative urine results as indicating that they did not have diabetes.[49]

A Scottish qualitative study sought newly diagnosed Type 2 diabetes patients' perspectives on the pros and cons of SMBG.

Pros of self-monitoring:

- provides a heightened awareness of, and evidence of, the condition
- when readings are within advised guidelines and fluctuations are easily interpretable, patients emphasise the positive role that monitoring has in their diabetes management. Low readings are a high point giving personal gratification
- cultivates independence from health services and enhances self-regulation.

Cons of self-monitoring:

- potentially, self-monitoring can raise anxiety about readings
- blood glucose parameters were found to be problematic by patients when they felt they were receiving contradictory information about upper thresholds or no guidance about ideal parameters
- lack of awareness as to how to manage hyperglycaemia
- increased self-responsibility accompanied by increased self-blame and negative emotional reactions to high glucose readings
- counter-intuitive readings could be sources of distress and anxiety, in some cases adversely effecting adherence to diabetic regimens by promoting nihilistic attitudes
- healthcare professionals were not interested in readings.[50]

8.1.5   From evidence to recommendations

The newer meta-analyses did not add significantly to the views expressed in the previous Type 2 diabetes guideline. The findings of the ROSSO study[44] and the data from the large Kaiser Permanente cohorts[43] added considerable confidence to the view that SMBG was an integral part of effective patient education packages and enabled the effective use of many other therapies and lifestyle interventions. The view in the previous guideline that self-monitoring of plasma glucose is not a stand-alone intervention was endorsed.

Concern was expressed over a number of issues surrounding the successful use of self-monitoring, and recognised that its cost meant that it had to be effectively deployed. It should only be supported in the context of a provision of a package of care, including structured education, from a primary or secondary diabetes care team. The initial education should be provided by a properly trained and skilled professional with understanding of the problems of the technology. Also, the skills of people with diabetes in using the technology should be the subject of regular quality assurance (together with the devices) perhaps as part of the regular annual review process. Devices should be calibrated to plasma glucose levels in line with 2006 WHO recommendations.

The importance of self-monitoring to the effective use of insulin therapy and for those at risk of hypoglycaemia through leisure or work activities (including driving) on oral medications was noted. The frequency of monitoring that is useful to someone with diabetes is highly individual and it is inappropriate to put an artificial restriction on this. The usefulness of self-monitoring, is dependent on the ability of users and health professionals to interpret the data particularly in the early stages of use by a person with diabetes, implying proper education and professional training on these aspects.

Qualitative studies from Scotland suggested that people with diabetes disliked monitoring of urine glucose compared to the self-monitoring of plasma glucose, and did not find it useful.

Hyperglycaemic complications were related to exposure to high glucose levels in plasma, and there were no major studies like the ROSSO and Kaiser studies for urine glucose monitoring. The evidence that plasma glucose monitoring could be replaced by urine glucose monitoring was found to be poor.

Although the DiGEM study was published after the evidence cut-off date, it had been identified as potentially important on the basis of earlier information. However, at review the GDG felt that a study which viewed self-monitoring as a stand-alone intervention, and not as an element of a full educational programme, could not properly inform the appropriate use of self-monitoring. The GDG further noted that people who might already have benefited from self-monitoring were excluded from participation.

Adverse effects of self-glucose monitoring (inconvenience, finger pricking) limited the use and cost-effectiveness of the technology. Obsessional and psychological problems relating to use of self-monitoring were rare in real clinical practice.

RECOMMENDATIONS

R22   Offer self-monitoring of plasma glucose to a person newly diagnosed with Type 2 diabetes only as an integral part of his or her self-management education. Discuss its purpose and agree how it should be interpreted and acted upon.

R23   Self-monitoring of plasma glucose should be available:
- to those on insulin treatment
- to those on oral glucose lowering medications to provide information on hypoglycaemia
- to assess changes in glucose control resulting from medications and lifestyle changes
- to monitor changes during intercurrent illness
- to ensure safety during activities, including driving.

R24   Assess at least annually and in a structured way:
- self-monitoring skills
- the quality and appropriate frequency of testing
- the use made of the results obtained
- the impact on quality of life
- the continued benefit
- the equipment used.

R25   If self-monitoring is appropriate but blood glucose monitoring is unacceptable to the individual, discuss the use of urine glucose monitoring.

9 Oral glucose control therapies (1): metformin, insulin secretagogues, and acarbose

9.1 Clinical introduction

Maintenance of glucose control to target levels is achieved in only very few people with Type 2 diabetes for more than a few months using lifestyle measures alone.[53,54] Oral glucose-lowering drugs are then indicated, and the choice, order and combination in which these are used will reflect evidence of:

- prevention of microvascular and arterial damage
- control of blood glucose levels
- assessment of the inconvenience
- risks of side effects.

Glucose control deteriorates continually with time in most people with Type 2 diabetes – it is not a chronic stable condition.[53,54] This is known to be due to progressive failure of insulin secretion.[55] Accordingly therapy has to be stepped up with time, one drug added to another until such time as only exogenous insulin replacement will suffice.

The evidence of efficacy and side effects differs between drug classes, and to a lesser extent between members of the same class. Since their introduction was over 40 years ago the cost of some generic drugs is low whilst newer drugs have inevitably incurred high development costs and are relatively expensive. Cost-effectiveness is then a relevant issue too. The parent guideline suggested the long established biguanides (metformin) and sulfonylureas as the usual choice of first- and second-line oral glucose-lowering therapy when indicated. These, and other insulin secretagogues working through the same mechanisms as sulfonylureas, are considered in this chapter, and the more expensive newer glucose-lowering drugs in the next chapter.

The clinical questions concern the order with which these oral glucose-lowering medications should be introduced and added to one another in different groups of people with Type 2 diabetes. Because such people vary in attributes (such as body weight) which can affect choice of medication, and because some medication side effects can have consequences for aspects of daily living (such as driving motor vehicles), blanket recommendations cannot be made for everyone with Type 2 diabetes.

9.2 Metformin

9.2.1 Methodological introduction

A large number of RCTs were identified in this area; included trials were limited to participants with Type 2 diabetes, a trial duration of at least 12 weeks and a sample size of 300 or more. Studies with smaller sample sizes were only included if there were no other larger studies for a particular comparison.

Two Cochrane reviews were identified.[56,57] One considered the effectiveness of metformin monotherapy compared with placebo or any active combination.[56] The other review included studies of metformin alone or in combination with other treatments compared with placebo or a range of other treatments, with the aim of reporting deaths due to lactic acidosis and non-fatal cases of lactic acidosis.[57] Similarly, an RCT was identified which compared serious adverse events (AEs) and plasma lactate levels between metformin and non-metformin treated groups.[58]

We identified a further five RCTs which compared metformin monotherapy with pioglitazone,[59] glimepiride,[60] metformin plus rosiglitazone,[61] metformin and rosiglitazone as a fixed-dose combination,[62] and metformin plus nateglinide.[63] Two of these studies had methodological limitations and were not considered further.[60,61]

In one RCT, metformin and biphasic insulin was compared with biphasic insulin alone.[64]

An additional RCT was identified and included which compared metformin immediate-release (MIR) with metformin extended-release (MXR).[65] The GDG subsequently felt that there might be relevant and important information in existence on the AE profile of these two formulations which had not been found during our search. Thus a focused call for evidence to all stakeholders was made. Following this, the GDG considered two RCTs (published in the same paper) which compared MXR against placebo,[66] and to a retrospective chart review comparing immediate-release and extended-release formulations.[67] Consideration was also given to four abstracts; however their usefulness is limited by the small number of patients included and the lack of detail inhibiting any assessment of study quality.[68–71]

It should be noted that differing dosing and titration regimens and the differing populations included in all the studies, may limit direct comparison between studies.

9.2.2 Health economic methodological introduction

Five papers were identified in the literature search, of these three compared metformin monotherapy with metformin in combination and so were thought to be more appropriate evidence for other questions.[72–74] One paper included a subgroup analysis of metformin monotherapy compared to nateglinide monotherapy, although the results of this analysis were not reported.[75] Two evaluations based on the UKPDS were identified that were considered to be of good quality.[33]

9.2.3 Evidence statements

▷ Mortality and morbidity

In terms of mortality and morbidity, a Cochrane review[56] looked at the events listed in the Clinical Endpoint Analyses from the UKPDS* (UKPDS-34 1998). The systematic review found five studies providing data on mortality and/or morbidity outcomes (four RCTs in addition to the UKPDS).

In the UKPDS (median follow-up 10.7 years), among overweight (54% with obesity) participants allocated to intensive blood glucose control, metformin (N=342) showed a greater

---

* According to the Cochrane review, the UKPDS is the unique trial that has been specifically designed to determine whether tight glycaemia control decreases complications related to diabetes and increases life expectancy.

benefit than chlorpropamide, glibenclamide, or insulin (N=951) for any diabetes-related outcomes, and for all-cause mortality. For other outcomes including diabetes-related death, MI, stroke, peripheral vascular disease and microvascular, there were no significant differences between both comparison arms. **Level 1++**

In the same vein, the UKPDS found that overweight participants assigned to intensive blood glucose control with metformin (N=342) showed a greater benefit than overweight patients on conventional treatment (non-intensive blood glucose control, mainly with diet), (N=411), for any diabetes-related outcomes, diabetes-related death, all-cause mortality, and MI. For the rest of the outcomes such as stroke, peripheral vascular disease and microvascular, there were no significant differences between both comparison arms. **Level 1++**

After pooling data from the four non-UKPDS trials, the Cochrane review did not find significant differences among comparisons either for all-cause mortality or for ischemic heart disease (study durations ranged from 24 weeks to 2 years). **Level 1++**

Table 9.1 Metformin mortality and morbidity studies

Study/comparison	Outcome	Effect size (RR)
UKPDS: metformin vs sulfonylureas or insulin	Any diabetes-related outcomes	0.78 (95% CI 0.65 to 0.94) p=0.009
	All-cause mortality	0.73 (95% CI 0.55 to 0.97) p=0.03
	Diabetes-related death	NS
	Myocardial infarction	NS
	Stroke	NS
	Peripheral vascular disease	NS
	Microvascular	NS
UKPDS: metformin vs conventional (non-intensive blood glucose control, mainly with diet)	Any diabetes-related outcomes	0.74 (95% CI 0.60 to 0.90) p=0.004
	Diabetes-related death	0.61 (95% CI 0.40 to 0.94) p=0.03
	All-cause mortality	0.68 (95% CI 0.49 to 0.93) p=0.01
	Myocardial infarction	0.64 (95% CI 0.45 to 0.92) p=0.02
	Stroke	NS
	Peripheral vascular disease	NS
	Microvascular	NS
Non-UKPDS trials: metformin vs comparison	All-cause mortality	NS
	Ischaemic heart disease	NS

▷ Glucose control

Overall, the evidence appraised suggested that monotherapy with metformin produced significantly greater improvements in glycaemic control (i.e. HbA$_{1c}$ and FPG/fasting blood glucose (FBG)) when it was compared with placebo, diet and sulfonylureas. Head-to-head comparisons with other antidiabetic agents (i.e. alpha-glucosidase inhibitors, thiazolidinediones, meglitinides and insulin) and extended-release formulations of metformin, failed to show more benefit for glycaemic control than standard monotherapy with metformin. In addition metformin used in combination with different doses of nateglinide produce significantly lower glycaemic values than metformin monotherapy.

▷ Body weight/body mass index

Overall, the evidence demonstrated a significant difference in terms of body weight/BMI reduction favouring metformin monotherapy when compared with sulfonylureas, glitazones and insulin therapies. Non-significant differences were found in head-to-head comparisons between metformin against placebo, diet, alpha-glucosidase inhibitors, meglitinides and treatment with extend-release formulation of metformin. Combination of metformin and different doses of nateglinide produced a significant reduction in body weight when compared with metformin monotherapy. **Level 1+**

▷ Lipid profile

Non-significant differences in terms of lipid profile were found when metformin was compared with placebo or meglitinides. **Level 1++**

Studies evaluating other comparisons found differences in specific lipid profile parameters.

When compared to diet, metformin significantly reduced total cholesterol (TC), however in a comparison with a α-glucosidase inhibitor, metformin significantly increased TC.[56] **Level 1++**

The meta-analysis of studies comparing metformin to sulfonylureas found significant benefits for metformin in terms of low-density lipoprotein cholesterol (LDL-C) and triglycerides.[56] **Level 1++**

In a comparison of metformin against insulin, significant benefits for metformin were found in terms of total and LDL-C levels but not high-density lipoprotein cholesterol (HDL-C).[56] **Level 1++**

In a study which compared metformin with pioglitazone,[59] pioglitazone was significantly more beneficial in terms of triglycerides and HDL-C, however metformin was more beneficial for LDL-C levels. The TC/HDL-C ratio did not differ significantly between the groups. **Level 1++**

A study which compared metformin monotherapy with metformin and nateglinide[63] found no differences across the lipid profile between these two groups except for triglycerides which were reduced significantly in the metformin and nateglinide group (nateglinide 120 mg tablets thrice daily). **Level 1+**

Where MIR was compared with MXR treatment, lipid profiles were similar between groups (statistical significance not reported) except for triglycerides where the mean change from baseline in the immediate-release group was 1 mg/dL; but was 34 mg/dl in the MXR 1,000 mg arm, and 42 mg/dl in the MXR 1,500 mg arm.[65] **Level 1+**

Table 9.2 Metformin comparison studies

Comparison	Study	Change in HbA$_{1c}$ (%)	FPG	Post load glucose/ PPBG/ PPGE	BMI (kg/m^2)	Body weight (kg)	TC	LDL	TG	HDL
Head-to-head comparisons										
Metformin vs placebo	Cochrane systematic review[56] 12 studies N=1,587	SMD −0.97 (95% CI −1.25 to −0.69)	SMD −0.87 (95% CI −1.13 to −0.61)	NE	NS	–	NS Four studies N=906	NS Four studies N=418	NS Three studies N=374	NS Four studies N=418
Metformin vs diet	Cochrane systematic review[56] Three studies N=914	SMD −1.06 (95% CI −1.89 to −0.22)	NS	NE	NS	–	SMD −0.59 (95% CI −0.90 to −0.27) Two studies N=161	NS One study N=61	NS Two studies N=161	NS One study N=61
Metformin vs alpha-glucosidase inhibitors	Cochrane systematic review[56] Two studies N=223	NS	NS	NE	NS	–	1.32 (95% CI 0.77 to 1.87) One study N=62	SMD One study N=62	NS One study N=62	NS NS One study N=62
Metformin vs sulfonylureas	Cochrane systematic review[56] 12 studies N=2,376	SMD −0.14 (95% CI −0.28 to −0.01)	SMD −0.16 (95% CI −0.27 to −0.05)	NE	SMD −0.45 (95% CI −0.80 to −0.10)	–	NS 10 studies N=1,150	SMD −0.29 (95% CI −0.52 to −0.07) Six studies N=793	SMD −0.22 (95% CI −0.43 to −0.02) 10 studies N=1,150	NS Eight studies N=1,069
Metformin vs meglitinides	Cochrane systematic review[56] Two studies N=413	NS	SMD −0.31 (95% CI −0.51 to −0.12)	NE	NS	–	NS One study N=56	NS One study N=56	NS One study N=56	NS One study N=56

continued

Table 9.2 Metformin comparison studies – continued

Comparison	Study	Change in HbA1c (%)	FPG	Post load glucose/ PPBG/ PPGE	BMI (kg/m²)	Body weight (kg)	TC	LDL	TG	HDL
Head-to-head comparisons – continued										
Metformin vs glitazones	Cochrane systematic review[56] Three studies N=260	SMD –0.28 (95% CI –0.52 to –0.03)	NS	NE	NS	–	NE	NE	NE	NE
	Metformin vs pioglitazone One study[59] N=1,199	NS	–0.3 mmol/l, p=0.016 in favour of pioglitazone	NE	NE	Mean body weight increased by 1.9 kg compared to a decrease of 2.5 kg with metformin*	NS (TC/HDL-C ratio)	+0.27 mmol/l change from baseline for pioglitazone vs –0.12 mmol/l metformin p=0.001	–0.61 mmol/l change from baseline for pioglitazone vs –0.3 mmol/l metformin p=0.001	+0.16 mmol/l change from baseline for pioglitazone vs +0.08 mmol/l metformin p=0.001
Metformin vs insulin	Cochrane systematic review[56] Two studies N=811	NS	NS	NE	SMD –0.91 (95% CI –1.44 to –0.37)	–	SMD –0.77 (95% CI –1.29 to –0.24) One study N=60	SMD –0.83 (95% CI –1.35 to –0.30) One study N=60	SMD NS One study N=60	SMD 0.65 (95% CI 0.13 to 1.17) One study N=60

continued

Table 9.2 Metformin comparison studies – continued

Head-to-head comparisons – continued

Comparison	Study	Change in HbA$_{1c}$ (%)	FPG	Post load glucose/ PPBG/ PPGE	BMI (kg/m^2)	Body weight (kg)	TC	LDL	TG	HDL
MIR vs MXR (MXR – 1,000 mg and 1,500 mg)	One study[65] N=217	NS	Mean FPG concentrations increased in all three treatment groups at week 24. The mean increases were smaller in the MXR groups compared with the MIR group (statistical significance not reported)	NE	NE	NS	Change from baseline MIR –1 mg/dl, MXR 1,000 +2 mg/dl and –3 mg/dl MXR 1,500*	Change from baseline –4 mg/dl with MIR and –6 mg/dl in both MXR groups*	Change from baseline MIR +1 mg/dl, MXR 1,000 +34 mg/dl and +42 mg/dl MXR 1,500*	Change from baseline MIR +2 mg/dl, MXR 1,000 mg/dl and –1 mg/dl MXR 1,500*
Rosiglitazone/ metformin (FDC) vs metformin	One study[62] N=569	Treatment difference –0.22% (95% CI –0.36 to –0.09%, p=0.001)	–18.3 mg/dL 95% CI –23.5 to –13.2; p<0.0001 in favour of rosiglitazone/ metformin	NE	NE	There was a mean size effect increase from baseline in weight in the RSG/MET group (1.3 (0.22) kg) and a mean decrease in the MET group (–0.9 (0.26) kg)*	0.1% change from baseline for MET vs 10.7% RSG/ MET*	3.4% change from baseline for MET vs 14.5% RSG/ MET*	–8.5% change from baseline for MET vs 1.2% RSG/ MET*	–1.3% change from baseline for MET vs 4.1% RSG/ MET*

continued

Table 9.2 Metformin comparison studies – *continued*

Comparison	Study	Change in HbA1c (%)	FPG	Post load glucose/ PPBG/ PPGE	BMI (kg/m²)	Body weight (kg)	TC	LDL	TG	HDL
Head-to-head comparisons – *continued*										
Metformin vs metformin + nateglinide (60 mg and 120 mg)	One study[63] N=467	Nateglinide 60 mg −0.36%, p=0.003 nateglinide 120 mg −0.51%, p<0.001	−0.8 mmol/l, (p=< 0.01) in favour of metformin + nateglinide 120 mg	NE	NE	0.9 kg increase was observed in the nateglinide 120 mg-group (over that in the metformin group) (p<0.001)	NS	NS	Metformin plus nateglinide 120 mg vs metformin (mean difference −0.2 p=0.042)	NS
Combinations										
Metformin + insulin biphasic vs insulin biphasic	One study[64] N=341	0.39%, p=0.007	NE	PPBG NS	NE	NS	NE	NE	NS	NS

MET, metformin; NE, not evaluated; NS, non-significant; PBG, postprandial blood glucose; PPBG, postprandial blood glucose; PPGE, postprandial glucose excursion; RSG, rosiglitazone; SMD, standardised mean difference; TG, triglycerides
*Indicates statistical significance tests not reported/performed

▷ Adverse events

The main differences across all the different treatment groups were:

- the high frequency of gastrointestinal (GI) complaints reported by metformin-treated patients
- the high frequency of hypoglycaemic events reported by sulfonylurea-treated patients
- the high number of episodes of oedema reported by glitazone-treated patients
- the high number of cases of upper respiratory infection in patients treated with meglitinides.

Level 1+

In the only RCT[65] directly comparing MIR and MXR, more diarrhoea, flatulence and abdominal pain were experienced in the extended-release group whilst more or equivalent proportions of patients, experienced nausea/vomiting, headache and dyspepsia/heartburn in immediate-release group (significance tests not performed). In placebo-controlled studies, patients on MXR always experienced more GI AEs than those on placebo.[66] Level 1+

A retrospective chart review[67] found a significantly reduced frequency of GI AE in a cohort of patients when they were switched from MIR to MXR. A cohort of patients taking metformin for the first time also experienced less GI AEs if they were commenced on MXR rather than the immediate-release formulation. Level 2+

Table 9.3 Metformin adverse events

Comparison	Study	Size effect
Head-to-head comparisons		
Metformin vs placebo	Cochrane systematic review[56]	Hypoglycaemia NS GI discomfort NS Diarrhoea Two studies N=639 3.09 (95% CI 1.58 to 6.07)
Metformin vs diet	Cochrane systematic review[56]	Hypoglycaemia One study N=811 4.21 (95% CI 1.40 to 12.66)
Metformin vs alpha-glucosidase inhibitors	Cochrane systematic review[56]	GI discomfort Two studies N=223 0.26 (95% 0.07 to 0.91)
Metformin vs glitazones	Cochrane systematic review[56]	NE
Metformin vs pioglitazone	One study[59] N=1,199	Diarrhoea* Metformin 11.1% Pioglitazone 3.2% Oedema* Metformin 1.7% Pioglitazone 4.5%

continued

Table 9.3 Metformin adverse events – *continued*

Comparison	Study	Size effect
Head-to-head comparisons – *continued*		
MIR vs MXR (MXR – 1,000 mg and 1,500 mg)	One study[65] N=217	Hypoglycaemia* Metformin MIR 1.4% Metformin MXR 1,000 mg 1.3% For other AEs* (Metformin IR 500 mg BD vs Metformin XR 1,000 mg od) Diarrhoea 3% vs 5% Flatulence 1% vs 4% Abdominal pain 1% vs 4% Nausea/vomiting 4% vs 3% Headache 4% vs 4% Dyspepsia/heartburn 6% vs 3%
MXR 1,000 mg (protocol 1) or 500–2,000 mg (protocol 2) vs placebo	Two studies[66]	Protocol 1 All-cause AEs were reported by 59.5% of patients treated with placebo and by 63.5% of patients treated with MXR For GI AEs (placebo vs MXR) Abdominal pain 5.1% vs 7.5% Diarrhoea 5.1% vs 6.9% Nausea/vomiting 3.8% vs 9.4% Protocol 2 All-cause AEs were reported by 59.5% of patients treated with placebo and by 65.85% of patients treated any dosage of MXR For GI AEs (placebo vs MXR) Abdominal pain 2.6% vs 5.1% Diarrhoea 3.4% vs 12.9% Nausea/vomiting 1.7% vs 8.2%
MIR (mean dose 1,282 mg) vs MXR (mean dose 1,258 mg)	One cohort study[67]	Overall in the MXR vs MIR cohorts: frequency of any GI AEs within the first year of treatment NS. Patients switched from MIR to MXR: Frequency of any GI AEs 26.45% on MIR vs 11.71% after switching to MXR; p=0.0006) Frequency of diarrhoea 18.05% vs 8.29%; p=0.0084) Comparison of patients new to metformin treatment with either MIR or MXR % of patients reporting a GI AE during the first year of treatment with MIR 19.83% vs 9.23% MXR (p=0.04) Frequency of diarrhoea (13.5% vs 3.08, p=0.0169)

continued

Table 9.3 Metformin adverse events – *continued*		
Comparison	**Study**	**Size effect**
Head-to-head comparisons – *continued*		
Rosiglitazone/metformin (FDC) vs metformin	One study[62] N=569	Hypoglycaemia* Metformin 0.4% Rosiglitazone/metformin 1% Diarrhoea* Metformin 14% Rosiglitazone/metformin 6% Oedema* Metformin 1% Rosiglitazone/metformin 3%
Metformin vs metformin + nateglinide (60 mg and 120 mg)	One study[63] N=467	Hypoglycaemia* Placebo group 3.9% Nateglinide 60 mg 8.4% Nateglinide 120 mg 15.6% Diarrhoea* Placebo group 7.9% Nateglinide 60 mg 5.8% Nateglinide 120 mg 5.6% Upper respiratory infection* Placebo group 4.6% Nateglinide 60 mg 9.7% Nateglinide 120 mg 8.1%
* Indicates statistical significance tests not reported/performed		

▷ Lactic acidosis

A Cochrane review[57] looked at the risk of lactic acidosis in patients treated with metformin. There were no cases of fatal or non-fatal lactic acidosis reported. **Level 1+**

In addition, one RCT[58] did not find a significant difference in plasma lactate levels between metformin-treated patients and patients treated with other antidiabetic agents. **Level 1+**

9.2.4 Health economics evidence statements

The UKPDS included an analysis of intensive blood glucose control with metformin for overweight patients compared to conventional treatment primarily with diet. The study included 753 overweight (more than 120% ideal body weight) patients with newly diagnosed Type 2 diabetes from 15 hospital-based clinics in England, Scotland and Northern Ireland. Of these patients 342 were allocated to an intensive blood glucose control policy with metformin and 411 were allocated to conventional treatment, primarily with diet alone. The study was conducted from 1977 to 1991. The median follow-up period was 10.4 years.

In the conventional policy group the glycaemic goal was to obtain the lowest FPG attainable with diet alone. In the intensive policy group the aim was a FPG of less than 6.0 mmol/l by increasing the dose of metformin from 500 to 2,550 mg a day as required. Use of metformin for intensive blood glucose control in overweight patients was found to confer a 32% risk reduction for any diabetes-related endpoint and a 42% risk reduction for diabetes-related deaths compared with a conventional policy.

Resource use was routinely collected as part of the study. Non-inpatient resource use data was collected using a questionnaire distributed between January 1996 and September 1997. The incremental costs reported in the analysis have the study protocol driven costs removed. These were replaced with a pattern of clinic visits reflecting general practitioner and specialist clinical opinion on the implementation of intensive policy.

Where a patient was still alive at the end of the follow-up, a simulation model was used to estimate the time from end of follow-up to death. It was assumed that there would be no continuation of benefit of therapy beyond the trial period in both evaluations.

The data was used in a cost-effectiveness analysis[34] and a cost–utility analysis.[33] Both evaluations showed intensive blood glucose control with metformin for overweight patients to be cost-saving compared to conventional treatment.

In the cost-utility analysis, within trial costs and projected costs were included. In the cost-effectiveness analysis only costs incurred during the trial period were included.

Table 9.4 Results: Clarke (2001)[34]

	Mean cost per patient (1997 cost year)		Mean cost difference (95% CI) per patient
	Conventional	Metformin	
Total costs, 3% discount per year	£6,878	£6,607	−£271 (−£1,345, £801)
Total costs, 6% discount per year	£5,893	£5,635	−£258 (−£1,171, £655)

Table 9.5 Results: Clarke (2001)[34]

	Mean (95% CI) life expectancy (years) per patient		Mean difference (95% CI) per patient
	Conventional	Metformin	Difference
Not discounted	21.3	22.3	1.0 (−0.0,2.1)
3% discount per year	15.1	15.7	0.6 (0.0,1.2)
6% discount per year	11.3	11.7	0.4 (0.0, 0.8)

Table 9.6 Results: Clarke (2005)[33]

	Mean cost per patient (2004 cost year)		Mean cost difference (95% CI) per patient
	Conventional	Metformin	
Total cost of treatment (3.5%)	£16,941	£15,290	−£1,021 (−£4,291, £2,249)
Total cost of treatment (6%)	£12,798	£11,792	−£1,006 (−£3,251, £1,239)

Table 9.7 Results: Clarke (2005)[33]			
	Mean (95% CI) QALY per patient		Mean difference (95% CI) per patient
	Conventional	Metformin	
Mean QALYs per patient (not discounted)	16.44	17.32	0.88 (–0.54, 2.29)
3.5% discount rate	–	–	0.55 (–0.10, 1.20)
6% discount rate	–	–	0.40 (–0.01, 0.80)

In the cost-effectiveness model with costs and effects discounted at a 6% rate, there was a 71% probability that metformin would prove to be cost-saving compared with a conventional policy.[34]

If additional costs of intensive policy with metformin were 50% more than assumed in the baseline estimates then the cost per life-year gained would be £948.

In the cost-utility model there was a 77% probability that metformin would prove to be cost-saving compared with a conventional policy.[33] Sensitivity analyses were performed for anti-diabetic therapy cost (±50%); standard practice costs (±50%); cost of complications (±50%); utility of one when free of complications; no treatment benefit and continuing benefit beyond the trial. Metformin was consistently shown to be a cost-reducing intervention.

9.3 Insulin secretagogues

9.3.1 Methodological introduction

A large volume of RCTs were identified in this area as the sulfonylurea and meglitinide drug classes include nine different agents (chlorpropamide, glibenclamide, gliclazide, glimepiride, glipizide, gliquidone, tolbutamide, nateglinide and repaglinide). Head-to-head comparisons with metformin were excluded as this is addressed in a previous question. Comparisons with the thiazolidinediones (the glitazones) were also excluded, as this will be addressed as part of a separate evidence review (see section 10.2).

Twenty-one studies were identified, four of which were excluded due to methodological limitations.[76–79]

Table 9.8 The various comparisons made in the included RCTs

	Reference
Nateglinide vs placebo	80,81
Repaglinide vs placebo	82
Repaglinide vs nateglinide	83
Repaglinide vs glimepiride	84
Repaglinide vs glipizide	85
Repaglinide vs glibenclamide	8
Repaglinide + bedtime NPH vs gliclazide + bedtime NPH	87
Nateglinide + metformin vs repaglinide + metformin	88
Nateglinide + metformin vs glibenclamide + metformin	89
Nateglinide + metformin vs gliclazide + metformin	90
Nateglinide + metformin vs nateglinide vs metformin	91
Nateglinide + insulin glargine vs placebo + insulin glargine	92
Gliclazide modified release vs glimepiride	93
Gliclazide modified release vs gliclazide immediate release	94
Glimepiride vs metformin vs glimepiride + metformin	95
Glibenclamide vs insulin lispro	96

One cohort study on UKPDS data compared patients treated with diet alone vs sulfonylurea vs metformin vs insulin monotherapy.[97]

There is a paucity of studies for some comparisons, for example there are no head-to-head studies of the sulfonylureas (excluding studies of gliclazide-modified release) and only one study which compares a meglitinide with a sulfonylurea.[84]

Differing study populations, dose and titration regimens may limit direct comparison between studies.

9.3.2 Health economic methodological introduction

Thirteen papers were identified in the literature search. Of these, three were considered of good quality and relevant to the guideline. Two UKPDS papers were identified; a cost-utility analysis[33] and a cost-effectiveness[98] analysis of intensive blood glucose control.

Metformin monotherapy was compared with nateglinide plus metformin in the UK.[74]

9.3.3 Evidence statements

▷ Metiglinides (repaglinide and nateglinide) vs placebo

Overall, metiglinides produced a significantly greater glycaemic control and a higher incidence of hypoglycaemic events when compared with placebo. No differences were found in terms of body weight and lipid profile.

Table 9.9 Nateglinide (120 mg) vs placebo
1 study[81] N=47
Level of evidence 1+

HbA1c	Nateglinide –3.6% Placebo +5.6% p=0.02			
FPG	NS			
Post load glucose/PPBG	NE			
Lipid profile	**TC** NS	**LDL** NS	**TG** NS	**HDL** NS
Body weight/BMI	**BMI** NE	**Body weight** NE		
AEs	AE data not reported			

Table 9.10 Nateglinide (30, 60, 120 mg) vs placebo
1 study[80] N=675
Level of evidence 1+

HbA$_{1c}$	Nateglinide relative to placebo (–0.26±0.05, –0.31±0.04, –0.39±0.05 for 30 mg, 60 mg and 120 mg respectively) were significant (p<0.001)			
FPG	Modest but statistically significant and dose-related reduction of FPG relative to placebo (p<0.001 vs placebo for all dose strengths)			
Post load glucose/PPBG	NE			
Lipid profile	**TC** NE	**LDL** NE	**TG** NE	**HDL** NE
BMI/body weight	**BMI** NE	**Body weight** NS		
AEs	Hypoglycaemia There was a dose-related increase in symptomatic hypoglycaemia but the incidence of confirmed hypoglycaemia in nateglinide-treated patients was much lower than symptomatic hypoglycaemia			

	Symptomatic	Confirmed
Placebo	4.9%	(1.2%)
30 mg nateglinide	12%	(2.4%)
60 mg nateglinide	11.4%	(4.0%)
120 mg nateglinide	22.8%	(5.3%)

Table 9.11 Repaglinide vs placebo 1 study[82] N=408 Level of evidence 1+				
HbA$_{1c}$	Final HbA$_{1c}$ levels were significantly greater for repaglinide monotherapy than nateglinide monotherapy (−1.57 vs −1.04%, p=0.002)			
FPG	Significantly greater efficacy for repaglinide than nateglinide (−57 vs −18 mg/dl, p<0.001			
Post load glucose/PPBG	NS			
Lipid profile	**TC** NE	**LDL** NE	**TG** NE	**HDL** NE
BMI/body weight	**BMI** NE	**Body weight** Mean weight gains from baseline to study end were +1.8 kg for repaglinide and +0.7 kg for nateglinide, p=0.04		
AEs	The most common AEs (3–10% of patients in both groups) were upper respiratory tract infection, sinusitis, constipation, arthralgia, headache and vomiting but there was no notable difference in the pattern between the two groups Hypoglycaemia There were 7% of repaglinide patients who had minor hypoglycaemic episodes and 0% for nateglinide (this is 0.016 events per patient per months for repaglinide vs 0 for nateglinide p=0.3, NS)			

▷ Repaglinide vs nateglinide

When repaglinide was compared with nateglinide in people with Type 2 diabetes previously treated with diet and exercise:

- repaglinide and nateglinide had similar postprandial glycaemic effects. However, repaglinide was more effective than nateglinide in reducing HbA$_{1c}$ and FPG values
- a greater weight gain (p=0.04) was seen in repaglinide-treated patients when compared to nateglinide-treated patients
- hypoglycaemic events were more frequently reported by patients receiving repaglinide (non-significant difference between the two groups).

Table 9.12 Repaglinide vs nateglinide
1 study[83] N=150
Level of evidence 1+

HbA$_{1c}$	Final HbA$_{1c}$ levels were 0.99% lower in the repaglinide group than in the placebo group (p<0.001)			
FPG	There was a mean 1.44 mmol/l greater reduction in the repaglinide group compared with the placebo group (p<0.001)			
Post load glucose/PPBG	NE			
Lipid profile	**TC** NE	**LDL** NE	**TG** NE	**HDL** NE
BMI/body weight	**BMI** NE	**Body weight** NS		
AEs	The overall tolerability of repaglinide was similar to placebo excluding hypoglycaemic events Hypoglycaemia 17% of patients in the repaglinide group and 3% in the placebo group reported minor episodes of hypoglycaemia 3 repaglinide patients reported a total of 4 major hypoglycaemic events			

▷ Meglitinides vs sulfonylureas

In head-to-head comparisons with sulfonylureas, metiglinides failed to demonstrate better glucose control and led to a similar number of hypoglycaemic events. No significant differences were observed in terms of lipid profile and body weight reduction.

Table 9.13 Repaglinide vs glimepiride
1 study[84] N=132
Level of evidence 1+

HbA$_{1c}$	NS			
FPG	NS			
Post load glucose/PPBG	PPG levels were significantly lower with repaglinide compared with glimepiride (p<0.01)			
Lipid profile	**TC** NS	**LDL** NS	**TG** NS	**HDL** NS
BMI/body weight	**BMI** NS	**Body weight** NS		
AEs	AE data not reported			

Table 9.14 Repaglinide vs glipizide
1 study[85] N=256
Level of evidence 1+

HbA$_{1c}$	Statistically significant difference between HbA$_{1c}$ changes from baseline in the two treatment groups in favour of repaglinide (0.19% vs 0.78%, difference −0.59%, p<0.05)			
FPG	Statistically significant difference between FPG changes in the two treatment groups in favour of repaglinide (0.5 mmol/l vs 1.3 mmol/l, difference −0.9 mmol/l, p<0.05)			
Post load glucose/PPBG	NE			
Lipid profile	**TC** NS	**LDL** NS	**TG** NS	**HDL** NS
BMI/body weight	**BMI** NE	**Body weight** NS		
AEs	A total of 20 patients in the repaglinide group and nine in the glipizide group reported AEs other than hypoglycaemia. The most common were nausea and fatigue Hypoglycaemia The number of patients experiencing minor hypoglycaemic events was similar in the repaglinide and glipizide groups (15% vs 19% respectively)			

Table 9.15 Repaglinide vs glibenclamide
1 study[86] N=175
Level of evidence 1+

HbA$_{1c}$	NS			
Fasting glucose	Glibenclamide caused a significantly greater decrease than repaglinide (p<0.001)			
PPG peak and 2 hour PPG levels	Repaglinide caused a significantly greater decrease in peak glucose than glibenclamide (p<0.001) AUC 0–2h decreased significantly more among patients receiving repaglinide (p=0.01)			
Lipid profile	**TC** NS	**LDL** NE	**TG** NS	**HDL** NS
BMI/body weight	**BMI** NE	**Body weight** NE		
AEs	Hypoglycaemic events; repaglinide (9%) and glibenclamide (13%)			
CIMT	CIMT regression was observed in 52% of patients receiving repaglinide and in 18% of those receiving glibenclamide (p<0.01)			
Inflammatory markers IL-6 and C-reactive protein	IL-6 and C-reactive protein decreased more in the repaglinide group than in the glibenclamide group (p=0.04 and p=0.02 respectively)			

AUC, area under curve; CIMT, carotid intima-media thickness

> ## Gliclazide modified release vs gliclazide

When a modified-release version of gliclazide was compared with the immediate-release version of gliclazide in people with Type 2 diabetes who had been on diet control or on treatment with oral hypoglycaemic agents:

- both versions were associated with significant reductions in HbA$_{1c}$ (non-significant difference between the two groups). FPG decreased significantly on gliclazide MR but not on gliclazide (non-significant difference between the two groups)
- no clinically significant changes were seen in terms of lipid profile (non-significant difference between the two groups)
- hypoglycaemic events were only reported by patients receiving gliclazide MR (9%) (non-significant difference was reported between the two groups).

Table 9.16 Gliclazide MR vs gliclazide
1 study[94] N=63
Level of evidence 1+

HbA$_{1c}$	NS			
FPG	NS			
Post load glucose/PPBG	NE			
Lipid profile	**TC**	**LDL**	**TG**	**HDL**
	NE	NE	NE	NE
BMI/body weight	**BMI**	**Body weight**		
	NE	NS		
AEs	In the gliclazide MR group, the most common adverse effects reported by patients were abdominal pain (9%) and pharyngitis (9%), while in the gliclazide group the most common adverse effect was neuropathy (14%) Hypoglycaemia Three patients (9.3%) experienced five mild hypoglycaemic episodes in the gliclazide MR treatment group. No suspected hypoglycaemic episodes were observed in the gliclazide treatment group			

> ## Gliclazide MR vs glimepiride

When a modified-release version of gliclazide was compared with glimepiride in people with Type 2 diabetes being treated with diet alone or with either metformin or alpha-glucosidase inhibitors:

- both interventions were equally effective in terms of glycaemic control (alone or in combination with metformin or alpha-glucosidase inhibitors)
- gliclazide MR had a better safety profile than glimepiride.

Table 9.17 Gliclazide MR vs glimepiride
1 study[93]
Level of evidence 1+

HbA$_{1c}$	NS			
FPG	NS			
Post load glucose/PPBG	NE			
Lipid profile	**TC** NS	**LDL** NS	**TG** NS	**HDL** NS
BMI/body weight	**BMI** NE	**Body weight** gliclazide MR: 83.1 to 83.6 kg glimepiride: 83.7 to 84.3 kg*		
AEs	Hypoglycaemia Hypoglycaemia with blood glucose <3 mmo/l occurred significantly less frequently (p=0.003) in the gliclazide MR group (3.7%) compared with the glimepiride group (8.9%) with an odds ration of 2.5 (95% CI, 1.4 to 4.7)			

* Indicates statistical significance tests between groups were not reported/performed

▷ Insulin lispro vs glibenclamide

When insulin lispro was compared with glibenclamide in people with Type 2 diabetes who had been treated with oral antidiabetic (OAD) therapy, but not insulin:

- both regimes produced comparable effects in the control of glycaemia with respect to HbA$_{1c}$. However, treatment with insulin lispro resulted in smaller postprandial blood glucose excursions compared to oral treatment with glibenclamide
- no significant differences were observed between the treatment groups regarding hypoglycaemic episodes and other AEs.

Table 9.18 Insulin lispro vs glibenclamide
1 study[96] N=143
Level of evidence 1+

HbA$_{1c}$	NS			
FPG	NE			
Post load glucose/PPBG	The change in mean overall blood glucose excursions from baseline to endpoint was −1.0±1.5 mmol/l in the insulin lispro-treatment group and −0.3±1.5 mmol/l in the glibenclamide group, (p=0.013)			
Lipid profile	**TC** NE	**LDL** NE	**TG** NE	**HDL** NE
BMI/body weight	**BMI** NE	**Body weight** NS		
AEs	AEs No significant difference between groups Hypoglycaemia No significant difference between groups			

▷ Bedtime NPH + repaglinide vs bedtime NPH + gliclazide

When repaglinide was compared with gliclazide (both drugs in combination with bedtime NPH) in Type 2 diabetes patients inadequately controlled with oral hypoglycaemic therapy:

● both interventions were associated with significant reductions in HbA_{1c} and FPG (non-significant difference between the two groups)

● weight gain during the treatment period was similar in both groups

● no significant differences were observed between the treatment groups regarding hypoglycaemic episodes and other AEs.

Table 9.19 Bedtime NPH + repaglinide vs bedtime BPH + gliclazide 1 study[87] N=80 Level of evidence 1++			
HbA_{1c}	NS		
FPG	NS		
Post load glucose/PPBG	N		
Lipid profile	**TC** NE	**LDL** NE	**TG** NE	**HDL** NE
BMI/body weight	**BMI** NE	**Body weight** NS	
AEs	AEs A total of 70 AEs were recorded throughout the study, 38 in the insulin/gliclazide and 32 in the insulin/repaglinide group. Hypoglycaemia No significant difference between groups		

▷ Nateglinide + metformin vs gliclazide + metformin

Nateglinide in combination with metformin was compared with gliclazide and metformin, to compare the effects on glycaemic control in patients with Type 2 diabetes:

● no significant difference was seen between the groups in terms of HbA_{1c}

● the nateglinide group demonstrated better PPG control.

Table 9.20 Nateglinide + metformin vs gliclazide + metformin
1 study[91] N=262
Level of evidence 1+

		Nateglinide + metformin	Gliclazide + metformin	p-value
HbA$_{1c}$	NS			
FPG	NS			
Post load glucose/PPBG				
	Max PPG excursion (mmol/l)	−0.71±0.22	−0.10±0.23	p=0.037
	30 minute postprandial insulin (pmol/l)	98.9±12.1	32.5±12.56	p<0.001
	2 hour postprandial insulin (pmol/l)	83.9±16.6	39.6±17.8	p=0.047
	2 hour postprandial insulin excursion (pmol/l)	75.5±16.0	30.2±16.6	p=0.033
Lipid profile	**TC** NE	**LDL** NE	**TG** NE	**HDL** NE
BMI/body weight	**BMI** NE	**Body weight** NS		
AEs	Suspected drug-related AEs Nateglinide arm 6.9% Gliclazide arm 7.1% NS			

▷ Glimepiride + metformin vs glimepiride vs metformin

When glimepiride in combination with metformin was compared with monotherapy of each drug in Type 2 diabetes patients inadequately controlled by metformin monotherapy:

- combination treatment was more effective than either drug alone in terms of glycaemic control
- combination therapy was more effective than either drug in reducing TC levels
- metformin alone resulted in a significantly lower BMI than either glimepiride alone, or the combination
- the incidence of hypoglycaemic episodes was significantly higher in the combination treatment group than in either of the monotherapy groups.

Table 9.21 Glimepiride vs metformin vs glimepiride + metformin
1 study[95] N=372
Level of evidence 1++

HbA$_{1c}$	Combination treatment (glimepiride + metformin) was significantly more efficient in reducing HbA$_{1c}$ levels than: glimepiride alone (difference in mean change 1.04% 95% CI 0.81 to 1.27%; p<0.001) metformin alone (difference in mean change 0.92% 95% CI 0.63 to 1.21%; p<0.001) There was no significant difference between metformin or glimepiride monotherapy in terms of HbA$_{1c}$
FPG	Combination treatment was significantly more effective than either monotherapy in reducing FBG (p<0.001) There was no significant difference between metformin or glimepiride monotherapy in terms of FPG
Post load glucose/PPBG	Combination treatment was significantly more effective than either monotherapy in reducing PPBG (p<0.001) Treatment with glimepiride was significantly more effective than metformin in reducing PPBG (p<0.001)

Lipid profile	TC	LDL	TG	HDL
	Combination was significantly more effective than glimepiride alone (p<0.001) in reducing TC levels, although there was no significant difference between the combination and metformin alone	NS	NS	NS

BMI/body weight	BMI	Body weight
	Treatment with metformin resulted in a significantly lower BMI than either glimepiride alone (p<0.001) or the combination treatment (p<0.002); however there was NS difference between the glimepiride and combination treatment groups	NE

AEs	AEs were experienced by 105 patients

	N	(%)
Metformin	22	(29%)
Glimepiride	38	(25%)
G + M	45	(31%)

Hypoglycaemia
The incidence of symptomatic episodes was significantly higher in the combination treatment group than in either of the monotherapy groups (22% of patients vs 11% of patients in the metformin group and 13% of patients in the glimepiride group, p=0.039)
Diarrhoea was more commonly reported in the metformin group than in the other two treatment groups (7% of patients vs 1% of patients in the glimepiride group and 3% of patients in the combination group)

▷ Nateglinide + metformin vs nateglinide vs metformin vs placebo

When nateglinide in combination with metformin was compared with monotherapy of each treatment and placebo in drug naive patients with Type 2 diabetes:

- nateglinide, metformin and combination therapy (nateglinide + metformin), were associated with significant reductions in HbA_{1c}, FPG and PPGE (an additive effect was seen with combination therapy)
- the incidence of GI AEs was higher in patients receiving combination therapy and metformin than in those receiving placebo and nateglinide
- the incidence of hypoglycaemic episodes was higher in the combination treatment group than in either of the monotherapy groups.

Table 9.22 Nateglinide vs metformin vs nateglinide + metformin
1 study[91] N=401
Level of evidence 1+

HbA_{1c}	Changes from baseline			
	Placebo	($\Delta = +0.3\pm0.1\%$)		
	Nateglinide	($\Delta = -0.8\pm0.1\%$)		
	Metformin	($\Delta = -0.8\pm0.1\%$)		
	Combination therapy	($\Delta = -1.6\pm0.1\%$)		
FPG	Changes from baseline			
	Placebo	not change		
	Nateglinide	($\Delta = -1.1\pm0.3$ mmol/l)		
	Metformin	($\Delta = -1.2\pm0.3$ mmol/l)		
	Combination therapy	($\Delta = -2.3\pm0.3$ mmol/l)		
Post load glucose/PPBG	Changes from baseline			
	Placebo	($\Delta = -0.5\pm0.2$ mmol/l)		
	Metformin	($\Delta = -1.0\pm0.2$ mmol/l)		
	Nateglinide	($\Delta = -1.9\pm0.2$ mmol/l)		
	Combination therapy	($\Delta = -2.3\pm0.2$ mmol/l)		
Lipid profile	**TC**	**LDL**	**TG**	**HDL**
	NE	NE	NE	NE
BMI/body weight	**BMI**	**Body weight**		
	NE	NS changes from baseline for combination therapy ($\Delta = +0.2\pm0.4$ kg) placebo ($\Delta = -0.2\pm0.4$ kg)		
AEs	No serious AEs judged to be related to study medication GI The percentage of patients randomised to combination therapy experiencing one or more GI AE (27%) was essentially identical to that of those receiving metformin monotherapy (27.9%), and approximately twofold that of patients receiving placebo and nateglinide monotherapy (14.4% and 16.3% respectively) Incidence of symptomatic hypoglycaemia in patients receiving combination therapy=29% Incidence of confirmed hypoglycaemia in drug naive patients receiving combination therapy 3.4% (with all considered to be mild)			

▷ Nateglinide + insulin glargine vs placebo + insulin glargine

The effect of adding nateglinide to therapy with insulin glargine in adults with Type 2 diabetes previously treated with insulin and with poor blood glucose control.

- Adding nateglinide improved blood glucose control in the early part of the day after breakfast and lunch.
- Adding nateglinide did not provide good blood glucose control overall.

Table 9.23 Nateglinide + insulin vs placebo + insulin glargine 1 study[91] N=55 **Level of evidence 1+**			
HbA$_{1c}$	NS		
Post load glucose/PPBG	Self-monitored blood glucose concentrations (mmol/l) were significantly lower in the nateglinide group only at certain times of the day. **Time** **Difference in mmol/l (95% CI)** **p-value** After breakfast −2.3 (−4.4, 0.2) 0.030 Before lunch −2.5 (−4.6, −0.3) 0.029 After lunch −2.3 (−4.6, −0.4) 0.021		
Lipid profile	**TC** NE	**LDL** NE	**TG** NE	**HDL** NE
BMI/body weight	**BMI** NE	**Body weight** NS		
AEs	NS		

▷ Diet vs sulphonylurea vs insulin

This cohort study investigated the incidence of hypoglycaemia in patients treated with diet alone, sulphonylurea, metformin or insulin monotherapy. The results on metformin are not discussed here as they are considered in a separate question.

Table 9.24 Diet vs sulphonylurea vs insulin 1 study[97] N=5,063 Level of evidence 2+			
HbA$_{1c}$	NE		
FPG	NE		
Post load glucose/PPBG	NE		
Lipid profile	**TC** NE	**LDL** NE	**TG** NE	**HDL** NE
BMI/body weight	**BMI** NE	**Body weight** NE		

AEs	Annual percentage (95% CI) of patients reporting at least one hypoglycaemic episode in relation to therapy		
	Therapy	**Grades 1–4 hypoglycaemia**	**Grades 2–4 hypoglycaemia**
	Diet alone	0.8 (0.6 to 1.0)	0.1 (0.1 to 0.2)
	Sulphonylurea	7.9 (5.1 to 11.9)	1.2 (0.4 to 3.4)
	Basal insulin alone	21.2 (14.6 to 29.8)	3.8 (1.2 to 11.1)
	Basal + prandial insulin	32.6 (21.8 to 45.6)	5.5 (2.0 to 14.0)

Hypoglycaemia was defined on the following scale: 1) transitory symptoms not affecting normal activity 2) temporarily incapacitated but patient able to control symptoms without help 3) incapacitated and required assistance to control symptoms without help 4) required medical attention or glucagon injection

9.3.4   Health economic evidence statements

▷ Sulfonylurea monotherapy

Conventional glucose control, mainly through diet was compared to more intense blood glucose control with insulin or sulfonylureas in the UKPDS. Intensive treatment was cost-saving with the resource use according to the trial protocol. Using standard clinical resource use, intensive treatment had an incremental cost-effectiveness ratio (ICER) of £1,166 per event-free year gained within the trial period (6% discount rate, 1997 cost year).[98]

In a further cost-utility analysis published in 2005 intensive blood glucose control with insulin or sulfonylurea was found to have a cost-effectiveness ratio of £6,028 per QALY gained compared to conventional glucose (2004 cost year, 3.5%).[33]

▷ Combination therapy

Metformin monotherapy (1,500 mg/day) was compared with nateglinide (360 mg/day) plus metformin (1,500 mg/day) in a UK setting. A hypothetical population based on US data was used. The mean baseline HbA$_{1c}$ level was 8.4%. The duration of diabetes was not stated, although a pre-model period of 7 years was included. The resulting cost per QALY was £8,058 (1999 cost year, 3% discount rate).[74]

9.4 Acarbose

9.4.1 Methodological introduction

A Cochrane review[99] and eight RCTs[100–107] compared monotherapy acarbose or other combination OAD drugs, with other OAD drug regimens or placebo. Studies were excluded unless they were of at least 12-weeks duration. Two of the RCTs[100,107] were excluded due to methodological limitations.

The Cochrane review[99] identified 30 RCTs in a search performed in April 2003 which compared acarbose monotherapy with placebo, sulfonylureas, metformin or nateglinide. The additional six RCTs included in this analysis compared acarbose with placebo when both groups were also treated with metformin,[104] with sulphonylureas,[105,106] or with insulin,[103] and there were also comparisons between acarbose and pioglitazone[101] and acarbose and sulfonylurea.[102]

Although a substantial amount of evidence has been found in this area, several different drug combinations and comparisons, differing dosing and titration regimens and the differing populations included in the studies, limit direct comparison between studies. Additionally, some study results may not be generalisable to a UK population of people with Type 2 diabetes. For example, the study by Lin[106] was undertaken in a Chinese population with a mean BMI of 25 kg/m^2.

9.4.2 Health economic methodological introduction

Three papers were identified from the literature search. All three were excluded. One was an analysis of adherence to oral antihyperglycaemic medication conducted in the US. This was not an economic analysis, and the comparison of costs was of patients with diabetes compared to patients with diabetes and cardiovascular disease.[108]

One paper was a cost-effectiveness analysis with an outcome of prevention of progression to Type 2 diabetes, which is outside of the scope of these guidelines.[109]

The final paper identified was a cost-effectiveness analysis. The focus was on quality of life in older patients. Not enough description was given of the treatments, referring only to oral medication with no further details.[110]

9.4.3 Evidence statements

The evidence appraised suggested that acarbose (used as monotherapy or in combination) failed to demonstrate better glycaemic control when compared with other oral agents. Treatment with acarbose did not demonstrate superiority over other oral agents when lipid profile and body weight were evaluated.

Reports of adverse effects were higher in the acarbose groups across all studies.[99,101–106] The main difference between the treatment groups was the high frequency of GI complaints reported by acarbose-treated patients. Flatulence was reported in all acarbose arms ranging from 28.6% to 57.5% of all patients.

Table 9.25 HbA$_{1c}$

Comparison	Study	Change in HbA$_{1c}$ (%)
Acarbose vs placebo	Cochrane systematic review[99] 28 studies N=2,831	−0.77, 95% CI −0.90 to −0.64
Acarbose vs metformin	Cochrane systematic review[99] One study N=62	NS
Acarbose vs sulfonylurea	Cochrane systematic review[99] Eight studies N=596	NS
	One study[102] N=219	Greater reduction in HbA$_{1c}$ in the glimepiride group (2.5±2.2%) compared with the acarbose group (1.8±2.2%, p=0.014)
Acarbose vs pioglitazone	One study[101] N=271	Greater reduction for the patients treated with pioglitazone compared with those treated with acarbose (p<0.001)
Acarbose vs nateglinide	Cochrane systematic review[99] One study N=179	NS
Acarbose + metformin vs placebo + metformin	One study[104] N=83	LSM* difference between the treatment arms of 1.02%, 95% CI 0.543 to 1.497%, p=0.0001
Acarbose + sulfonylurea vs placebo + sulfonylurea	One study[106] N=69	The difference in the mean endpoints between the two treatment groups was −1.05%, 95% CI −1.69 to −0.41, p=0.0018
	One study[105] N=373	LSM difference −0.54%, CI −0.86 to −0.22; p=0.001)
Insulin + acarbose vs insulin + placebo	One study[103] N=112	Comparison between the treatment groups showed a difference of −0.69%, 95% CI −1.18 to −0.20; p=0.008

*Adjusted least square mean
LSM, least square mean; NS, non-significant; PP, postprandial

Table 9.26 Fasting blood glucose

Comparison	Study	Change in FBG (mmol/l)
Acarbose vs placebo	Cochrane systematic review[99] 28 studies N=2,838	−1.09, 95% CI −1.36 to −0.83
Acarbose vs metformin	Cochrane systematic review[99] One study N=62	NS
Acarbose vs sulfonylurea	Cochrane systematic review[99] Eight studies N=596	0.69, 95% CI 0.16 to 1.23
	One study[102] N=219	The reduction was greater in the glimepiride-treated patients (2.6±2.6 mmol/l) than in the acarbose-treated patients (1.4±2.8 mmol/l, p=0.004)
Acarbose vs pioglitazone	One study[101] N=271	The decrease was significantly greater with pioglitazone than acarbose. (−56.41±73.6 vs −22.54±65.86, p=0.001)*
Acarbose vs nateglinide	Cochrane systematic review[99] One study N=175	NS
Acarbose + metformin vs placebo + metformin	One study[104] N=83	LSM** 1.132, 95% CI 0.056 to 2.208; p=0.0395. This was an increase at endpoint in both groups: 0.34±0.42 for acarbose compared to 1.48±0.39 for placebo
Acarbose + sulfonylurea vs placebo + sulfonylurea	One study[106] N=69	NS
	One study[105] N=373	LSM** difference −14.8 mg/dl, 95% CI −27.3 to −2.4, p=0.0195
Insulin + acarbose vs insulin + placebo	One study[103] N=112	NS

* This study evaluated FPG
**Adjusted least square mean

Table 9.27 Post-load blood glucose

Comparison	Study	Change in post-load blood glucose (mmol/l)
Acarbose vs placebo	Cochrane systematic review[99] 22 studies N=2,238	−2.32, 95% CI −2.73 to −1.92.
Acarbose vs metformin	Cochrane systematic review[99] One study N=62	−0.42 95% CI −0.79 to −0.05
Acarbose vs sulfonylurea	Cochrane systematic review[99] Eight studies N=596	NS
	One study[102] N=219	3.1±3.1 mmol/l glimepiride vs 1.7±3.5 mmol/l acarbose, p=0.004 (decreased glucose response to breakfast)
Acarbose vs pioglitazone	One study[101] N=271	NE
Acarbose vs nateglinide	Cochrane systematic review[99]	NE
Acarbose + metformin vs placebo + metformin	One study[104] N=83	NE
Acarbose + sulfonylurea vs placebo + sulfonylurea	One study[106] N=69	−2.49 mmol/l, 95% CI −4.01 to −0.96, p=0.002
	One study[105] N=373	LSM of −33.4 mg/dl, 95% CI −49.2 to −17.7, p=<0.0001
Insulin + acarbose vs insulin + placebo	One study[103] N=112	−34 mg/dl 95% CI −63 to −5, p=0.029) Change in 2 hours PP=NS

Table 9.28 Body mass index/body weight

Comparison	Study	BMI (kg/m^2)	Body weight (kg)
Acarbose vs placebo	Cochrane systematic review[99]	14 studies N=1,430 −0.17, 95% CI −0.25 to −0.08	NS
Acarbose vs metformin	Cochrane systematic review[99]	NE	One study N=62 NS
Acarbose vs sulfonylurea	Cochrane systematic review[99]	Four studies N=230 NS	Five studies N=397 NS
	One study[102] N=219	NE	Acarbose change from baseline: 1.9±3.9 (p=0.001) Glimepiride change from baseline: 0.4±5.2 (NS)
Acarbose vs pioglitazone	One study[101] N=271	NE	Increased with pioglitazone treatment (1.23±5.42) and decreased with acarbose (−2.09±3.58,p<0.001)

continued

Table 9.28 Body mass index/body weight – *continued*

Comparison	Study	BMI (kg/m^2)	Body weight (kg)
Acarbose vs nateglinide	Cochrane systematic review[99]	NE	One study N=169 −0.68 95% −1.30 to −0.06
Acarbose + metformin vs placebo + metformin	One study[104] N=83	NE	NS
Acarbose + sulfonylurea vs placebo + sulfonylurea	One study[106] N=69	NE	NS
	One study[105] N=373	NE	NE
Insulin + acarbose vs insulin + placebo	One study[103] N=112	NE	NS

Table 9.29 Lipid profile

Comparison	Study	TC	LDL	TG	HDL	VLDL
Acarbose vs placebo	Cochrane systematic review[99]	NS	NS	NS	NS	NE
Acarbose vs metformin	Cochrane systematic review[99]	One study N=62 −0.94, 95% CI −1.66 to 0.22	One study N=62 −0.94 95% −1.52 to 0.36	NS	NS	NE
Acarbose vs sulfonylurea	Cochrane systematic review[99]	NS	NS	NS	NS	NE
	One study[102] N=219	NE	NE	NE	NE	NE
Acarbose vs pioglitazone	One study[101] N=271	NS	NS	Greater mean decrease with pioglitazone (p<0.001)	Greater mean increase with pioglitazone (p<0.001)	Greater mean decrease with pioglitazone (p=0.037)
Acarbose vs nateglinide	Cochrane systematic review[99]	NE	NE	NE	NE	NE
Acarbose + metformin vs placebo + metformin	One study[104] N=83	NE	NE	NE	NE	NE
Acarbose + sulfonylurea vs placebo + sulfonylurea	One study[106] N=69	NS	NS	NS	NS	NS
	One study[105] N=373	NS	NE	NS	NS	NE
Insulin + acarbose vs insulin + placebo	One study[103] N=112	NS	NS	NS	NS	NE

Table 9.30 Adverse effects

Comparison	Study	Effect size
Acarbose vs placebo	Cochrane systematic review[99] Four studies N=1,442	Occurrence of AEs: OR=3.37, 95% CI 2.6 to 4.36 Occurrence of GI AEs: OR=3.30, 95% CI 2.31 to 4.71
Acarbose vs metformin	Cochrane systematic review[99] One study N=62	OR=15.00, 95% CI 3.06, 73.58
Acarbose vs sulfonylurea	Cochrane systematic review[99] One study N=145	Occurrence of AEs: OR=3.95, 95% CI 2.00 to 7.80 Occurrence of GI AEs: OR=7.70, 95% CI 3.64 to 16.31
	One study N=219	52% glimepiride vs 81% acarbose, p=0.001.* Hypoglycaemic episodes were experienced by 18% of the glimepiride group and 1.9% of the acarbose group (there were no severe episodes requiring external help)
Acarbose vs pioglitazone	One study[101] N=271	Adverse effects occurred in 10.1% patients receiving pioglitazone, and in 39.7%) patients receiving acarbose**
Acarbose vs nateglinide	Cochrane systematic review[99] One study N=179	Occurrence of AEs: 1.92, 95% CI 1.05 to 3.5 Occurrence of GI effects: OR=3.22, 95% CI 1.66 to 6.24
Acarbose + metformin vs placebo + metformin	One study[104] N=83	75% of patients in the acarbose group reported side effects, compared to 55.8% of placebo patients. The main difference between the treatment groups was the higher frequency of GI complaints (Flatulence: Acarbose= 57.5% Placebo=27.9%)
Acarbose + sulfonylurea vs placebo + sulfonylurea	One study[106] N=69	48.5% of the patients in the acarbose group reported at least one adverse side effect, compared with 12.5% of the placebo group. The incidence of GI side effects was especially high in the acarbose group (flatulence 33% vs 6.3%, abdominal pain 9.1% vs 0.0)
	One study[105] N=373	33.3% of patients in the acarbose arm (reported AEs) versus 16% in the placebo group. Flatulence: reported by 26.2% in the acarbose group compared with 10.6% in the placebo.
Insulin + acarbose vs insulin + placebo	One study[103] N=112	44.6% patients in the acarbose group reported 46 drug-related events and 36.4% patients in the placebo group had 40 drug-related events. Incidence of side effects was similar in the two treatment groups, except for flatulence (acarbose 28.6% placebo 16.4%)

* The AE in glimepiride-treated patients were predominantly hypoglycaemic episodes, whereas GI symptoms prevailed in the acarbose group

** Pioglitazone: including six cases of edema (in five females and one male). Acarbose: mainly abdominal distension/flatulence which was reported by 46 patients

9.5 Oral glucose control therapies; from evidence to recommendations

9.5.1 Metformin

None of the newer evidence altered the priority given to metformin cited in the previous guideline. Although the specific cardioprotective effects of metformin suggested by the UKPDS study were open to challenge from some of the very recent studies, this was not on the basis of strong outcome data. Large observational studies from Canada and Scotland[111,112] appeared to support the widespread advantage of metformin over sulfonylureas, but the A Diabetes Outcome Progression Trial (ADOPT) study did not. The cardioprotective gains shown in the UKPDS and in the Scottish study far outweighed the concerns over lactic acidosis (provided renal function was adequate) in people with mild to moderate hepatic and cardiac disease. Nearly all the data related to overweight people, and there was little to guide metformin use in the normal weight person without extrapolation of the evidence. However, the overwhelming majority of people with Type 2 diabetes are overweight; in making this judgement however attention has to be paid to differences between ethnic groups.

The studies confirmed the glucose-lowering benefits of metformin in combination with all other available glucose-lowering medications. The widespread use of the previous recommendations in regard of levels of serum creatinine for reduction and discontinuing therapy was acknowledged. The complete substitution of estimated glomerular filtration rate (eGFR) for serum creatinine is not possible because of uncertainty surrounding methods of eGFR calculation in many people with Type 2 diabetes.

An evidence call on the use of extended-release metformin preparations did not find that their use in unselected patients reduced GI side effects. Differences in cost, and lack of other documented benefit, led to the conclusion that these therapies should be used only where intolerance to the immediate-release preparation had been documented.

9.5.2 Insulin secretagogues

Insulin secretagogues include the sulfonylureas and the rapid-acting insulin secretagogues (nateglinide and repaglinide).

The evidence base for the insulin secretagogues was more extensive than ascertained for the parent guideline. However, in many of the papers in which they are compared to other drugs they were being used as the comparator therapy rather than the investigated therapy. New evidence did not lead to new conclusions about the role of these drugs in clinical management, either from the point of view of efficacy or safety. Sulfonylureas proved as efficacious as newer comparator therapies in reducing surrogate outcomes (principally HbA$_{1c}$) highlighting that they still have a role in modern management of Type 2 diabetes. In the ADOPT study[54] the sulfonylurea glibenclamide controlled HbA$_{1c}$ as effectively as rosiglitazone or metformin as monotherapy for the first 3 years, but persistence of glucose control after this time was worse. Cardiovascular outcomes were, if anything, better with the sulfonylurea.

There was little new evidence on comparative hypoglycaemia within the class, although the tighter blood glucose targets achieved in modern practice was leading to an overall increase in risk. With the relative demise in use of glibenclamide in the UK, hypoglycaemia was not regarded as a problem for most people, though sulfonylureas were regarded as a problem in some occupations (e.g. vocational drivers).

Where medication adherence is a concern the case for the general use of once daily or long-acting sulfonylurea preparations was supported.

The rapid-acting insulin secretagogues (meglitinides) also appeared to be efficacious in people with Type 2 diabetes, though the evidence for comparability of nateglinide to sulfonylureas was less certain. While the flexible use of these drugs in mealtime regimens appeared appealing for some people with diabetes, the multiple dosing requirements had inhibited uptake in clinical practice. These drugs are more expensive than sulfonylureas. Accordingly the GDG saw no reason to make general recommendation for their use in preference to the sulfonylureas, or to change the previous recommendations.

9.5.3 α-glucosidase inhibitors

The newer evidence did not add significantly to the previous understanding of the role of α-glucosidase inhibitors in the management of Type 2 diabetes, except in so far as the evidence suggested that the efficacy and intolerance problems were similar in oriental ethnic groups to Europids. Lower glucose-lowering efficacy, a higher rate of intolerance and dropout from therapy, and relative expense compared to generic metformin and sulfonylureas were noted. However, hypoglycaemia is not a problem when this drug is used as monotherapy, though through glucose lowering it may enhance the hypoglycaemic potential of other medications.

ORAL GLUCOSE CONTROL THERAPIES; RECOMMENDATIONS

For oral agent combination therapy with insulin please refer to chapter 11.

Metformin

R26   Start metformin treatment in a person who is overweight or obese (tailoring the assessment of body weight associated risk according to ethnic group*) and whose blood glucose is inadequately controlled (see recommendation 16) by lifestyle interventions (nutrition and exercise) alone.

R27   Consider metformin as an option for first-line glucose-lowering therapy for a person who is not overweight.

R28   Continue with metformin if blood glucose control remains or becomes inadequate (see recommendation 16) and another oral glucose-lowering medication (usually a sulfonylurea) is added.

R29   Step up metformin therapy gradually over weeks to minimise risk of gastrointestinal side effects. Consider a trial of extended absorption metformin tablets where gastrointestinal tolerability prevents continuation of metformin therapy.

R30   Review the dose of metformin if the serum creatinine exceeds 130 micromol/l or the eGFR is below 45 ml/minute/1.73 m^2.

---

* Please see the NICE Obesity guideline (CG43) www.nice.org.uk/guidance/index.isp?action= byID86=11000

- Stop the metformin if the serum creatinine exceeds 150 micromol/l or the eGFR is below 30 ml/minute/1.73 m^2.
- Prescribe metformin with caution for those at risk of a sudden deterioration in kidney function and those at risk of eGFR falling below 45 ml/minute/1.73 m^2.

R31   The benefits of metformin therapy should be discussed with a person with mild to moderate liver dysfunction or cardiac impairment so that:
- due consideration can be given to the cardiovascular-protective effects of the drug
- an informed decision can be made on whether to continue or stop the metformin.

Insulin secretagogues

R32   Consider a sulfonylurea as an option for first-line glucose lowering-therapy if:
- the person is not overweight
- the person does not tolerate or is contraindicated
- a rapid response to therapy is required because of hyperglycaemic symptoms.

R33   Add a sulfonylurea as second-line therapy when blood glucose control remains, or becomes, inadequate (see recommendation 16) with metformin.

R34   Continue with a sulfonylurea if blood glucose control remains, or becomes, inadequate (see recommendation 16) and another oral glucose-lowering medication is added.

R35   Prescribe a sulfonylurea with a low acquisition cost (but not glibenclamide) when an insulin secretagogue is indicated (see recommendation 32 and 33).

R36   When drug concordance is a problem, offer a once daily, long-acting sulfonylurea.

R37   Educate a person being treated with an insulin secretagogue, particularly if renally impaired, about the risk of hypoglycaemia.

Rapid-acting insulin secretagogues

R38   Consider offering a rapid-acting insulin secretagogue to a person with an erratic lifestyle.

Acarbose

R39   Consider acarbose for a person unable to use other oral glucose-lowering medications.

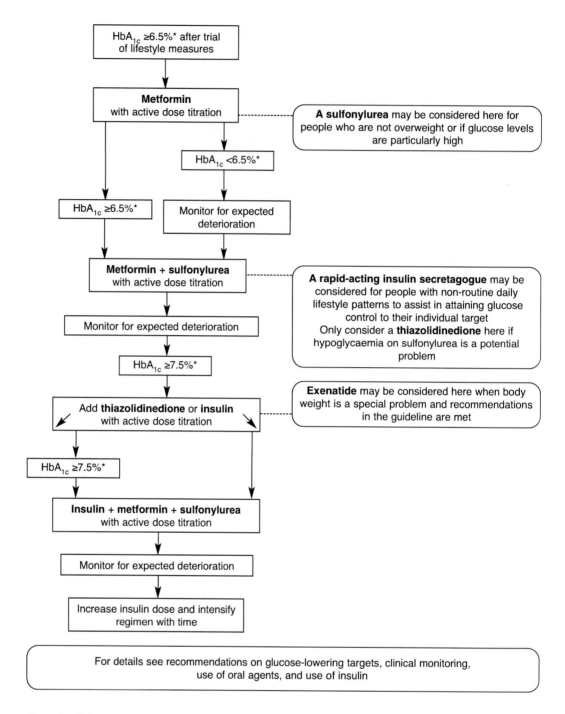

Figure 9.1 Scheme for the pharmacotherapy of glucose lowering in people with Type 2 diabetes
For details see recommendations on glucose lowering targets, clinical monitoring, use of oral agents, and use of insulin
* or as individually agreed

10 Oral glucose control therapies (2): other oral agents and exenatide

10.1 Clinical introduction

Maintenance of glucose control to target levels is achieved in only very few people with Type 2 diabetes for more than a few months using lifestyle measures, and as described in the previous chapter metformin and sulfonylureas are then generally used to assist in achieving glucose control targets.

However, as also discussed above, glucose control continues to deteriorate with time in most people with Type 2 diabetes, due to progressive failure of insulin secretion.[43–45] Accordingly other therapies need to be added with time, until such time as only exogenous insulin replacement will suffice. Other therapies may also be useful where metformin and sulfonylureas are contraindicated or not tolerated.

The newer oral agent therapies and exenatide are inevitably more expensive than the older ones and evidence of efficacy and side effects less well documented or more controversial. In the case of one class of drugs, the gliptins (GLP-1 enhancers), licensing during the finalisation of the guideline, and a paucity of published evidence at the time, has meant deferral of consideration of their role to a future guideline update.

The clinical questions concern the order with which these oral glucose-lowering medications should be introduced and added to one another in different groups of people with Type 2 diabetes. Because such people vary in attributes (such as body weight and insulin sensitivity) which can affect choice of medication, and because some medication side effects can have consequences for aspects of daily living (such as driving motor vehicles), blanket recommendations cannot be made for everyone with Type 2 diabetes.

10.2 Thiazolidinediones (glitazones)

10.2.1 Methodological introduction

A NICE technology appraisal (TA)[113] previously reviewed the evidence available up to April 2002 and made recommendations on the use of the glitazones (pioglitazone and rosiglitazone) in Type 2 diabetes. This guideline updates the appraisal and the GDG considered whether the appraisal recommendations should be changed in the light of new evidence.

Recommendations from the 2003 NICE TA:

'For people with Type 2 diabetes, the use of a glitazone as second-line therapy added to either metformin or a sulfonylurea – as an alternative to treatment with a combination of metformin and a sulfonylurea – is not recommended except for those who are unable to take metformin and a sulfonylurea in combination because of intolerance or a contraindication to one of the drugs. In this instance, the glitazone should replace in the combination the drug that is poorly tolerated or contraindicated.

The effectiveness of glitazone combination therapy should be monitored against treatment targets for glycaemic control (usually in terms of haemoglobin A_{1c} (HbA_{1c}

level) and for other cardiovascular risk factors, including lipid profile. The target HbA$_{1c}$ level should be set between 6.5% and 7.5%, depending on other risk factors.'

▷ Rosiglitazone

Rosiglitazone is now licensed for use as monotherapy, combination therapy with metformin or a sulfonylurea, or as part of triple therapy with metformin and a sulfonylurea in the UK. Combination therapy with insulin is not licensed at present. As from January 2008 the European Medicines Agency (EMEA)[114] states that* 'rosiglitazone is indicated in the treatment of Type 2 diabetes mellitus:

- as monotherapy in patients (particularly overweight patients) inadequately controlled by diet and exercise for whom metformin is inappropriate because of contraindications or intolerance
- as dual oral therapy in combination with:
  - metformin in patients (particularly overweight patients) with insufficient glycaemic control despite maximal tolerated dose of monotherapy with metformin
  - a sulfonylurea, only in patients who show intolerance to metformin or for whom metformin is contraindicated, with insufficient glycaemic control despite monotherapy with a sulfonylurea
- as triple oral therapy in combination with metformin and a sulfonylurea, in patients (particularly overweight patients) with insufficient glycaemic control despite dual oral therapy.'
- Rosiglitazone is also available in two combination tablet formats (with metformin and also with glimepiride).

Studies reporting cardiovascular outcomes

A recent meta-analysis studying rosiglitazone's cardiovascular (CV) safety was identified.[115] This meta-analysis is based on 42 clinical trials of rosiglitazone, as compared either with other therapies for Type 2 diabetes or with placebo. The prespecified primary endpoints of interest were MI and death from CV causes. The meta-analysis includes nearly 30 trials for which the only available source was a clinical trial registry maintained by GlaxoSmithKline (GSK) since 2004.

A clinical trial reporting an unplanned interim analysis of the CV endpoints of the Rosiglitazone Evaluated for Cardiac Outcomes and Regulation of Glycaemia in Diabetes (RECORD) study was also identified.[116] The primary endpoint of the RECORD trial consists of an aggregate of time to first hospitalisation for a CV event or death from CV causes.

A further review of meta-analyses looking at the glitazones CV safety was undertaken in order to clarify the concerns in relation to the apparent risk of MI in patients treated with rosiglitazone. Five meta-analyses[117–121] and one Cochrane systematic review[122] were identified. Among the five meta-analyses, three were looking at rosiglitazone,[118,119,121] one at pioglitazone[117] and one at both glitazones agents.[120] EMEA, US Food and Drug Administration (FDA), and the Medicines

---

* The European Medicines Agency (EMEA) have issued recent updates for rosiglitazone contained in the 'Update Summary of Product Characteristics' (SPC) dated: (a) 30 May 2007 to inform prescribers about new safety information concerning bone fractures following analysis of a long-term efficacy and safety study (ADOPT); (b) 21 November 2007 removing the contraindication for the use of rosiglitazone in combination with insulin with a warning regarding the risk of this combination; (c) 24 January 2008 to inform prescribers that the use of rosiglitazone in patients with IHD and/or peripheral arterial disease is not recommended. A new contraindication was also adopted stating that rosiglitazone must not be used in patients with acute coronary syndrome, such as angina or some types of MI.

and Healthcare products Regulatory Agency (MHRA) statements on glitazones were also reviewed along with an independent FDA meta-analysis on rosiglitazone presented at the FDA joint advisory committee on 30 July 2007.

Studies reporting surrogate outcomes

Seventeen RCTs were identified which compared rosiglitazone as monotherapy or in combination with other oral antidiabetic agents, with other oral antidiabetic agents and/or placebo.[54,61,62,123–136]

One RCT was not considered as part of the evidence due to methodological limitations.[61] Two studies comparing the combination of rosiglitazone and insulin therapy with other glucose-lowering medications were excluded because this combination is not currently licensed in the UK.[137,138]

Two additional studies looking at the addition of insulin glargine or rosiglitazone to the combination therapy of sulfonylurea plus metformin in insulin-naive patients were also identified.[139,140]

Studies were only included if sample sizes were equal to, or more than, 300; unless this meant the omission of a particular comparison.

Only one small study[131] (N=95) was identified which compared metformin and rosiglitazone with metformin and a sulfonylurea. Such a comparison is useful in the consideration of whether rosiglitazone could displace sulfonylureas second line (added to metformin).

Three studies were found looking at the newer rosiglitazone fixed-dose combination (FDC) tablet of rosiglitazone combined with metformin.[62,134,135] No study was found for the fixed-dose combination of rosiglitazone and glimepiride.

▷ Pioglitazone

Pioglitazone is now licensed for use as monotherapy, combination therapy with metformin or a sulfonylurea, as part of triple therapy with metformin and a sulfonylurea, or in combination therapy with insulin. As from September 2007 the EMEA[114] states that, 'pioglitazone is indicated in the treatment of Type 2 diabetes mellitus:

* as monotherapy in patients (particularly overweight patients) inadequately controlled by diet and exercise for whom metformin is inappropriate because of contraindications or intolerance
* as dual oral therapy in combination with:
  – metformin in patients (particularly overweight patients) with insufficient glycaemic control despite maximal tolerated dose of monotherapy with metformin
  – a sulfonylurea, only in patients who show intolerance to metformin or for whom metformin is contraindicated, with insufficient glycaemic control despite maximal tolerated dose of monotherapy with a sulfonylurea
* as triple oral therapy in combination with:
  – metformin and a sulfonylurea, in patients (particularly overweight patients) with insufficient glycaemic control despite dual oral therapy
* pioglitazone is also indicated for combination with insulin in Type 2 diabetes mellitus patients with insufficient glycaemic control on insulin for whom metformin is inappropriate because of contraindications or intolerance.'

A Cochrane review[141] was identified which searched for pioglitazone RCTs of at least 24-weeks duration published up until August 2006. The review identified 22 studies including comparisons of pioglitazone monotherapy with placebo, pioglitazone monotherapy with any other OAD medication, and pioglitazone in combination with any other OAD medication or insulin, compared with any other OAD medication or insulin.

Most studies were of 6-months duration and investigated HbA_{1c} and lipid parameters as primary outcomes. Only one study of mean follow-up duration 34.5 months included mortality and morbidity outcomes within composite endpoints.[142] There was some controversy surrounding the results of this study however, in particular due to debate as to whether the main secondary endpoint was specified a-priori or whether this was the result of a post hoc analysis.[143,144]

Due to study heterogeneity, it was only possible to perform meta-analysis for the adverse event (AE) outcome 'oedema'.

The Cochrane systematic review noted at the moment of its publication, that there were five ongoing studies (Action to Control Cardiovascular Risk in Diabetes (ACCORD), Bypass Angio-plasty Revascularization Investigation 2 Diabetes (BARI-2D), Carotid Intima-media Thickness in Atherosclerosis using Pioglitazone (CHICAGO) study, Pioglitazone Effect on Regression and Intravascular Sonographic Coronary Obstruction Prospective Evaluation (PERISCOPE), and Peroxisome Proliferator-activated Receptor study (PPAR)) which, according to the review, may contribute important information to future understanding of the role of pioglitazone in Type 2 diabetes.

Seven studies which compared pioglitazone as monotherapy or in combination with other OAD agents, with other OAD agents and/or placebo were identified in the re-runs.[145–151] One RCT was not considered as part of the evidence due to methodological limitations.[149]

Two of the studies identified by the re-runs were substudies of the Prospective Pioglitazone Clinical Trial In Macrovascular Events (PROactive) trial which assessed the effects of pioglitazone on mortality and macrovascular morbidity in patients with Type 2 diabetes and a previous MI or previous stroke.[150,152] Three other pioglitazone-based studies were identified as relevant from the re-runs.[145,146,148]

As noted in the rosiglitazone section a further review of meta-analyses published up to December 2007 looking at the glitazones CV safety was undertaken. In relation to pioglitazone two meta-analyses were identified as relevant: a meta-analysis analysing pioglitazone studies[117] and one looking at both glitazones agents.[120]

▷ Thiazolidinediones and the risk of oedema

One meta-analysis[153] was identified assessing the overall risk for developing oedema secondary to glitazones (rosiglitazone and pioglitazone).

10.2.2 Health economic methodological introduction

The 2003 TA found no published economic studies on either pioglitazone or rosiglitazone and the economic evidence was based on the manufacturer submitted economic evaluations. The indications included were pioglitazone and rosiglitazone in oral combination treatment with either metformin or a sulfonylurea.[154]

The economic model submitted for pioglitazone was reviewed for the original 2001 TA.[155] The model compared pioglitazone combination therapy (added to either sulfonylureas or metformin) compared with other combination therapies or changing to insulin. The key results were removed from the 2004 TA because they were submitted in confidence.

The model submitted for rosiglitazone compared rosiglitazone plus a sulfonylurea, or metformin to other CTs or changing to insulin.

Seven other papers were identified of which only one was considered relevant. Beale et al.[156] conducted a cost-effectiveness analysis of rosiglitazone in a population of obese and overweight Type 2 diabetes patients in the UK.

In the re-run of the literature search a further paper was identified comparing pioglitazone with rosiglitazone in the UK.[157]

An economic model was constructed based upon the UKPDS outcomes model to inform the GDG deliberations with regard to choice of glitazones or exenatide as third-line therapy in comparison to other third-line options. This is presented in appendix C available at www.rcplondon.ac.uk/pubs/brochure.aspx?e=247

10.2.3 Evidence statements

▷ Rosiglitazone

Cardiovascular outcomes

One meta-analysis[115] concluded that rosiglitazone was associated with a significant increase in the risk of MI and a borderline significant finding for death from CV causes (see tables 10.1 and 10.2).*

Table 10.1 Rosiglitazone meta-analysis: myocardial infarction data

MI	Rosiglitazone group	Control group	Odds ratio	p value
Small trials	44/10,280	22/6,105	1.45 95 CI% 0.88 to 2.39	0.15
DREAM	15/2,635	9/2,634	1.65 95 CI% 0.74 to 3.68	0.22
ADOPT	27/1,456	41/2,895	1.33 95 CI% 0.80 to 2.21	0.27
Overall	86	72	1.43 95 CI% 1.03 to 1.98	0.03

Table 10.2 Rosiglitazone meta-analysis: death from cardiovascular causes data

Death from CV causes	Rosiglitazone group	Control group	Odds ratio	p value
Small trials	25/6,557	7/3,700	2.40 95 CI% 1.17 to 4.91	0.02
DREAM	12/2,365	10/2,634	1.20 95 CI% 0.52 to 2.78	0.67
ADOPT	2/1,456	5/2,854	0.80 95 CI% 0.17 to 3.86	0.78
Overall	39	22	1.64 95 CI% 0.98 to 2.74	0.06

* Another pharma-sponsored meta-analysis showed a similar higher risk of MI for rosiglitazone (odds ratio, 1.31; 95% CI 1.01 to >1.70). This meta-analysis was submitted to the US Food and Drug Administration (FDA) in 2006.

Findings from an interim report of the RECORD study*[116] were inconclusive regarding the effect of rosiglitazone on the overall risk of hospitalisation or death from CV causes. The report concluded that rosiglitazone was associated with a significant increase in the risk of congestive heart failure (CHF) (see table 10.3).

Table 10.3 RECORD study: 3.75 years results				
Endpoint	**RSG group**	**Control group**	**HR**	**p**
Hospitalisation or death from CV events	217	202	1.08 95% CI 0.89 to 1.31	0.43
Death from CV events	29	35	0.83 95% CI 0.51 to 1.36	0.46
MI	43	37	1.16 95% CI 0.75 to 1.81	0.50
CHF	38	17	2.24 95% CI 1.27 to 3.97	0.006

RSG, rosiglitazone

Overall, the interim results of the RECORD trial do not provide any assurance of the safety of treatment with rosiglitazone in terms of the risk of myocardial ischaemic events.

Studies identified as part of the further review of the evidence published up to December 2007 (rosiglitazone and pioglitazone – meta-analyses and systematic reviews)

None of the 18 rosiglitazone trials analysed by the Cochrane systematic review[122] included mortality or morbidity as a primary or secondary endpoint. The review stated that active glucose-lowering agents like metformin, glibenclamide, or glimepiride resulted in similar reductions of HbA_{1c} compared to rosiglitazone treatment. The only outcome that could be subjected to meta-analysis was oedema whose incidence was significantly raised in patients receiving rosiglitazone (OR 2.27, 95% CI 1.83 to 2.81). The systematic review concluded that new studies should focus on patient-oriented outcomes to clarify the benefit–risk ration of rosiglitazone therapy.

Three of the four rosiglitazone meta-analyses reported a statistically significant increase in the RR of myocardial ischaemic events among patients taking rosiglitazone (see table 10.4). In addition, the meta-analysis by Singh[119] concluded that among patients with Type 2 diabetes, rosiglitazone use for at least 12 months is associated with a significantly increased risk of heart failure, without a significantly increased risk of CV mortality.

---

* The RECORD trial is scheduled to end when there is a median of 6 years of follow-up; the mean follow-up reported in the interim analysis is 3.75 years.

Table 10.4 Rosiglitazone meta-analyses (June–December 2007)

Meta-analysis	Event	Rosiglitazone	Control	Odds/hazard ratio	p value
GSK (2007)[412]	MI	171/8,604	85/5633	1.31 95% CI 1.01 to 1.72	<0.05
FDA (2007)[413]	Any ischemia	171/8,604	85/5633	1.4 95% CI 1.1 to 1.8	0.02
Singh (2007)[119]	MI	94/6,421	83/7,870	1.42 95% CI 1.06 to 1.91	0.02

One additional meta-analysis on rosiglitazone[118] reanalysed the data set of 42 trials considered originally by Nissen and Wolski[115] by using various modelling and weighting statistical methods (e.g. inclusion of trials with zero events). The authors concluded that the risk for MI and death from CV disease for diabetic patients taking rosiglitazone is uncertain. They also advocate for new long-term patient-oriented outcome studies on rosiglitazone to clarify its safety.

A meta-analysis of 19 pioglitazone trials[117] (with the PROactive study being the largest study included) reported that treatment with pioglitazone was associated with a significantly lower risk of death, MI, or stroke. Pioglitazone was also associated with a significantly higher risk of serious heart failure (see table 10.5).

Table 10.5 Pioglitazone meta-analyses (June–December 2007)

Meta-analysis	Event	Pioglitazone	Control	Odds/hazard ratio	p value
Lincoff (2007)[117]	Death/MI/stroke	375/8,554	450/7,836	0.82 95% CI 0.72 to 0.94	0.005
	Death/MI	309/8,554	357/7,836	0.85 95% CI 0.73 to 0.99	0.04
	Serious heart failure	200/8,554	139/7,836	1.41 95% CI 1.14 to 1.76	0.002

A further meta-analysis[120] looking at the risk of CHF and CV death in patient with pre-diabetes and Type 2 diabetes treated with glitazones reported a significantly higher risk of developing heart failure in those treated with rosiglitazone or pioglitazone compared with controls (RR 1.72 95% CI 1.21 to 2.42, p=0.002). By contrast, the study reported that the risk of CV death was not increased with either of the two glitazones.

▷ Glycaemic control

Head-to-head comparisons

Two studies comparing different monotherapies concluded that glycaemic control (HbA$_{1c}$ and FPG values) was similar when rosiglitazone was compared with glibenclamide.[128,129] A third study evaluating monotherapies with rosiglitazone, glibenclamide and metformin in a 4-year clinical trial, concluded that in the long term, rosiglitazone-treated patients experienced a significantly longer durability in terms of reduction of HbA$_{1c}$ and FPG levels.[54]

Combination therapy

Rosiglitazone used in combination with metformin, a sulfonylurea, repaglinide or insulin, significantly improved glycaemic values (HbA$_{1c}$ and FPG) compared to these agents or rosiglitazone used as monotherapy (with or without placebo). This was also true in cases where the monotherapy was uptitrated.

Other studies comparing the addition of rosiglitazone to either metformin or a sulfonylurea with the combination of metformin and a sulfonylurea failed to demonstrate significant between-treatment differences in terms of glycaemic control (HbA$_{1c}$ and FPG).

Triple therapy

Two studies[139,140] compared the addition of rosiglitazone to the combination of sulfonylurea and metformin with the addition of insulin glargine. HbA$_{1c}$ improvements from baseline were similar in both groups with no significant difference between the groups. However, one study[139] found that when baseline HbA$_{1c}$ was more than 9.5%, the reduction of HbA$_{1c}$ with insulin glargine was significantly greater than with rosiglitazone. Both studies revealed significantly greater reductions in FPG levels in the insulin glargine group.

Fixed-dose combination

Fixed-dose combination of rosiglitazone and metformin produced significantly greater reductions in HbA$_{1c}$ and FPG values when compared to rosiglitazone and metformin used as monotherapies. This was also true in cases where the monotherapy was uptitrated.[62,134,135]

▷ Rosiglitazone vs pioglitazone

Only one study compared metformin used in combination with rosiglitazone with treatment with metformin and pioglitazone. The study did not find significant differences between the groups in terms of HbA$_{1c}$ and FPG values.[133]

Table 10.6 HbA$_{1c}$ outcomes

Comparison	Study	Change in HbA$_{1c}$ %
Rosiglitazone vs repaglinide vs repaglinide & rosiglitazone	One study[125] N=252 1+	Greater reduction for combination therapy (−1.43%) than for repaglinide monotherapy (−0.17%) or rosiglitazone (−0.56%) (p<0.001 for combination vs either monotherapy). p≤0.001 for combination vs either monotherapy
Rosiglitazone vs glibenclamide	One study[128] N=203 1	Comparable at endpoint*
	One study[129] N=598 1+	NS
Rosiglitazone vs glibenclamide vs metformin	One study[54] N=4,360	After 6 months, the rate of increase in HbA$_{1c}$ was greatest in the glibenclamide group, which had annual increases of 0.24%, intermediate in the metformin group, which had annual increases of 0.14%; and least in the rosiglitazone group, which had increases of 0.07%, (p<0.001)
Rosiglitazone + sulfonylurea vs placebo + sulfonylurea	One study[124] N=227 1+	The HbA$_{1c}$ reduction with RSG + SU was significantly different from uptitrated SU alone (−0.79%, p<0.0001)
Rosiglitazone + sulfonylurea vs sulfonylurea	One study[127] N=348 1+	The RSG and SU group showed a decrease in HbA$_{1c}$ 9.1% to 7.9%, mean change −1.1, 95% CI −1.37 to −0.89, from baseline. HbA$_{1c}$ increased slightly in the control group. The difference between the treatment groups was significant, (p=0.0001)
Rosiglitazone + gliclazide vs gliclazide uptitration	One study[132] N=471 1+	HbA$_{1c}$ was reduced by ≥0.7% 65% of patients in the combination treatment group compared to 21% in the uptitrated gliclazide group, (p<0.0001)
Rosiglitazone + glibenclamide vs glibenclamide uptitration	One study[130] N=340 1+	Combination therapy reduced HbA$_{1c}$ by 0.81% compared with glibenclamide monotherapy, (p<0.0001)
Rosiglitazone + metformin vs glimepiride + metformin	One study[131] N=95 1+	NS
	One study[123] N=99 1+	NS
Rosiglitazone + metformin vs glibenclamide + metformin	One study[126] N=389 1+	NS
Rosiglitazone + metformin or sulfonylurea vs metformin + sulfonylurea	One study[136] N=1,122 1+	NS

continued

Table 10.6 HbA$_{1c}$ outcomes – *continued*

Comparison	Study	Change in HbA$_{1c}$ %
Rosiglitazone + sulfonylurea + metformin vs insulin glargine + sulfonylurea + metformin	One study[139] N=217 1+	Improvements from baseline were similar in both groups (−1.66% vs −1.51% for glargine and rosiglitazone respectively) with no significant difference between the groups, (p=0.14) In patients with HbA$_{1c}$ glargine resulted in significantly greater A$_{1C}$ reduction compared with rosiglitazone, (p<0.05)
Insulin glargine + sulfonylurea + metformin vs rosiglitazone + sulfonylurea + metformin	One study[140]	NS
Rosiglitazone/metformin (FDC) vs metformin uptitrated	One study[62] N=569 1++	The treatment difference was −0.22% (95% CI −0.36 to −0.09, p=0.001) in favour of the FDC
Rosiglitazone/metformin (FDC) vs metformin monotherapy	One study[135] N=526	At week 32 there was a reduction from baseline in mean HbA$_{1c}$ in the RSG/MET group from 7.2±0.6 to 6.7±0.8% compared with 7.2±0.6 to 6.8±0.9% in the MET group, (p=0.0357)
Rosiglitazone/metformin (FDC) vs rosiglitazone vs metformin	One study[134] N=468 1+	At week 32, reductions in HbA$_{1c}$ were observed in all the treatment groups. The greatest mean reduction, 2.3%, was observed in the RSG/MET group from a baseline of 8.9±1.1% to 6.6±1.0% at study end. This reduction was significantly greater when compared with the 1.8% reduction in the MET group (p=0.0008) and 1.6% in the RSG group (p<0.0001)
Metformin + pioglitazone 15 mg OD vs metformin + rosiglitazone 4 mg OD	One study[133] N=96 1+	NS

*Significance tests not performed
MET, metformin; RSG, rosiglitazone; SU, sulfonylurea

Table 10.7 Fasting plasma glucose/fasting blood glucose outcomes

Comparison	Study	Change in FPG/FBG
Rosiglitazone vs repaglinide vs repaglinide and rosiglitazone	One study[125] N=252 1+	Greater for combination therapy (−5.2 mmol/l, −94 mg/dl) than for repaglinide monotherapy (−3.0 mmol/l, −54 mg/dl) or rosiglitazone monotherapy (−3.7 mmol/l, −67 mg/dl) p≤0.001 for combination vs either monotherapy
Rosiglitazone vs glibenclamide	One study[128] N=203 1+	Mean FPG decreased from 236.4 to 161.1 mg/dl for rosiglitazone and from 245.5 to 188.3 mg/dl for glibenclamide*
	One study[129] N=598	The difference (0.6 mmol/l) between the mean FPG reduction with rosiglitazone 8 mg/d (−2.3 mmol/l) and glibenclamide (−1.7 mmol/l) was statistically significant (95% CI −15.4 to −0.6, p=0.03)

continued

Table 10.7 Fasting plasma glucose/fasting blood glucose outcomes – *continued*

Comparison	Study	Change in FPG/FBG
Rosiglitazone vs glibenclamide vs metformin	One study[54] N=4,360	After 6 months, the rate of increase in FPG levels was greatest in the glibenclamide group, which had annual increases of 0.31 mmol/l; intermediate in the metformin group, which had annual increases of 0.15 mmol/l; and least in the rosiglitazone group, which had increases of 0.04 mmol/l, (p<0.001)
Rosiglitazone + sulfonylurea vs placebo + sulfonylurea	One study N=227 1+	FPG was reduced with RSG + SU but increased with uptitrated SU alone The difference between treatment groups was statistically significant (−2.09 mmol/l, p<0.0001)
Rosiglitazone + sulfonylurea vs sulfonylurea	One study N=348 1+	The RSG and SU group showed a decrease in mean FPG (199 to 166 mg/dl, mean change −38.4, 95% CI −47.1 to −19.7) from baseline. Mean FPG increased slightly in the control group. The difference between the treatment groups was significant (p=0.0001)
Rosiglitazone + gliclazide vs gliclazide uptitration	One study[132] N=471 1+	FPG was reduced by 3.0 mmol/l (p=0.0001) in the rosiglitazone plus gliclazide group compared to the uptitrated gliclazide group after 26 weeks
Rosiglitazone + glibenclamide vs glibenclamide uptitration	One study[130] N=340 1+	Combination therapy reduced FPG by 2.4 mmol/l compared with glibenclamide monotherapy (p<0.0001)
Rosiglitazone + metformin vs metformin + glimepiride	One study[131] N=95 1+	NS
	One study[123] N=99 1+	NS
Rosiglitazone + metformin vs glibenclamide + metformin	One study[126] N=389 1+	NS
Rosiglitazone + metformin or sulfonylurea vs metformin + sulfonylurea	One study[136] N=1,122 1+	NS
Rosiglitazone + sulfonylurea + metformin vs insulin glargine + sulfonylurea + metformin	One study[139] N=217 1+	FPG decreased significantly from baseline to endpoint in both groups; however, greater reductions occurred in the insulin glargine group than in the rosiglitazone group (−3.60±0.23 vs −2.57±0.22 mmol/l) p=0.001
Insulin glargine + sulfonylurea + metformin vs rosiglitazone + sulfonylurea + metformin	One study[140]	Patients in the glargine group experimented a significantly greater reduction in FPG levels when compared with the rosiglitazone group (glargine −3.60±0.23 mmol/l; rosiglitazone −2.57±0.22 mmol/l p=0.001)
Rosiglitazone/metformin (FDC) vs metformin uptitrated	One study[62] N=569 1++	The treatment difference was −18.3 mg/dl (95% CI −23.5 to −13.2; p<0.0001) in favour of the FDC

continued

Table 10.7 Fasting plasma glucose/fasting blood glucose outcomes – *continued*

Comparison	Study	Change in FPG/FBG
Rosiglitazone/metformin (FDC) vs metformin monotherapy	One study[135] N=526	At week 32 the reduction in FPG from baseline was greater in the RSG/MET group. The proportion of participants achieving a FPG target of <7.0 mmol/l at week 32 was 56% in the RSG/MET group compared with 38% in the MET group (odds ratio = 2.33, p<0.0001)
Rosiglitazone/metformin (FDC) vs rosiglitazone vs metformin	One study[134] N=468 1+	At week 32 the greatest mean decrease in FPG was seen with RSG/MET. This difference in FPG reduction was clinically and statistically significant compared with the 2.8 mmol/l reduction in the MET group (p<0.0001) and the 2.6 mmol/l reduction in the RSG (p< 0.0001)
Metformin + pioglitazone 15 mg OD vs metformin + rosiglitazone 4 mg OD	One study[133] N=96 1+	NS

* Significance testing not performed

Lipid profile

Overall, treatment with rosiglitazone (used as monotherapy, dual therapy, fixed-dose combination or triple therapy) was associated with significantly larger increases in total cholesterol (TC) and low-density lipoprotein cholesterol (LDL-C) compared to other therapies.* In addition, rosiglitazone was associated with a significantly greater use of lipid-lowering therapy.

The study comparing rosiglitazone and pioglitazone showed that patients in the pioglitazone add-on to metformin group experienced significant reductions (p≤0.05) in TC, low-density lipoprotein (LDL) and triglyceride (TG) levels when compared to those receiving rosiglitazone + metformin. High-density lipoprotein (HDL) levels were significantly higher (p≤0.05) in patients treated with pioglitazone + metformin when compared to patients in the rosiglitazone add-on to metformin group.

Table 10.8 Lipid profile outcomes* (changes from baseline)

Comparison	Study	TC	LDL	TG	HDL
Rosiglitazone vs repaglinide vs repaglinide and rosiglitazone	One study[125] N=252 1+	+8% +1% +5%	+9% +1% +6%	−8% +4% −4%	+7% 0% +7%
Rosiglitazone vs glibenclamide	One study[128] N=203 1+	NE	+7.7 mg/dl −8.9 mg/dl	−2.8 mg/dl −13.8 mg/dl	+7.7 mg/dl
	One study[129] N=598 1+	+0.7 mmol/l −0.1 mmol/l	+0.4 mmol/l −0.1 mmol/l	NS	+0.17 mmol/l −0.08 mmol/l

continued

* For TGs and HDL-C no clear pattern emerged.

Table 10.8 Lipid profile outcomes* (changes from baseline) – *continued*

Comparison	Study	TC	LDL	TG	HDL
Rosiglitazone vs glibenclamide vs metformin	One study[54] N=4,360	Not reported	RSG 104 mg/dl GLI 99.3 mg/dl MET 96.5 mg/dl	RSG 163.5 mg/dl GLI 171.7 mg/dl MET 166.5 mg/dl	RSG 51.8 mg/dl GLI 48.9 mg/dl MET 50.5 mg/dl
Rosiglitazone + sulfonylurea vs placebo + sulfonylurea	One study[124] N=227	+6.2% −1.7%	+3.3% −1.3%	+9.5% −5.4%	+2.7% +1.6%
Rosiglitazone + sulfonylurea vs sulfonylurea	One study[127] N=348 1+	+14 mg/dl −2 mg/dl	+5 mg/dl −5 mg/dl	NE	+4 mg/dl +2 mg/dl
Rosiglitazone + gliclazide vs gliclazide uptitration	One study[132] N=471	+8.8% +1.2%	+10.9% 0%	+7.7% +3.5%	+6.8% 0%
Rosiglitazone + glibenclamide vs glibenclamide uptitration	One study[130] N=340 1+	+7.7% −5%	+7.0% −6.7%	−5.8% −1.9%	+15.8% +14.6%
Rosiglitazone + metformin vs metformin + glimepiride	One study[131] N=95 1+	NE	NE	NE	NE
	One study[123] N=99 1+	+7 mg/dl (R+M) −15 mg/dl (M+G)	+4 mg/dl (R+M) −16 mg/dl (M+G)	−57 mg/dl (R+M) −41 mg/dl (M+G)	0 mg/dl (R+M) +1 mg/dl (M+G)
Rosiglitazone/metformin (FDC) vs metformin uptitrated	One study[62] N=569 1++	FDC −0.1% MET −10.7%	FDC +3.4% MET +14.5%	FDC −1.2% MET −8.5%	FDC +4.1% MET −1.3%
Rosiglitazone/metformin (FDC) vs metformin monotherapy	One study[135] N= 526	FDC +4.1% MET −5.9%	FDC +2.8% MET −8.8%	FDC +1.9% MET −6.2%	FDC +7.9% MET +2.6%
Rosiglitazone/metformin (FDC) vs rosiglitazone vs metformin	One study[134] N=468 1+	FDC −2.2% RSG +5.3% (p=0.0006 vs FDC) MET −9% (p=0.009 vs FDC)	FDC −0.2% RSG +4.5% (p=0.16 vs FDC) MET −10.7% (p=0.016 vs FDC)	FDC −18.7% RSG −4.8% (p=0.005 vs FDC) MET −15.4% (p=0.5 vs FDC)	FDC +5.8% RSG +3.1% (p=0.25 vs FDC) MET 0% (p=0.01 vs FDC)

continued

Table 10.8 Lipid profile outcomes* (changes from baseline) – *continued*

Comparison	Study	TC	LDL	TG	HDL
Rosiglitazone + SU or metformin vs metformin + SU	One study[136] N=1,122 1+	RSG + M vs M + SU Difference 0.53 mmol/l p<0.001 RSG+ SU vs SU + M Difference 0.56 mmol/l p=0.001	RSG + M vs M + SU Difference 0.30 mmol/l p no reported RSG+ SU vs SU + M Difference 0.48 mmol/l p no reported	RSG + M vs M + SU Difference 0.26 mmol/l p=0.16 RSG+ SU vs SU + M Difference 0.06 NS	RSG + M vs M + SU Difference 0.06 mmol/l p=0.001 RSG+ SU vs SU + M Difference 0.01 NS
Rosiglitazone + sulfonylurea + metformin vs insulin glargine + sulfonylurea + metformin	One study[139] N=217 1+	Insulin glargine: (196 to 186 mg/dl vs rosiglitazone: 196 to 215 mg/dl (−4.4 vs +10.1%) respectively p=0.0001)	Insulin glargine: (117 to 115 mg/dl vs rosiglitazone 106 to 120 mg/dl (−1.4 vs +13.1%) respectively p=0.0004)	Insulin glargine: (217 to 176 mg/dl vs rosiglitazone 241 to 252 mg/dl (−19.0 vs +4.6%) respectively p=0.0011)	Insulin glargine: unchanged but increased with rosiglitazone (+4.4%, p=0.0407)
Metformin + pioglitazone 15 mg OD vs metformin + rosiglitazone 4 mg OD	One study[133] N=96 1+	−0.49 mmol/l +0.21 mmol/l	−0.20 mmol/l +0.08 mmol/l	−0.48 mmol/l −0.03 mmol/l	+0.10 mmol/l −0.03 mmol/l

* Significance testing not performed

Body weight/body mass index

Across most of the studies treatment with rosiglitazone was associated with a significant increase in body weight/BMI.

Table 10.9 Weight/body mass index

Comparison	Study	Change in weight/BMI
Rosiglitazone vs repaglinide vs repaglinide and rosiglitazone	One study[125] N=252 1+	Mean change +2.3 kg +1.6 kg +4.4 kg*
Rosiglitazone vs glibenclamide	One study[128] N=203 1+	Mean body weight increased by 3.4 kg with glibenclamide and by 5 kg with rosiglitazone*
	One study[129] N=598 1+	Mean body weight increased by 1.9 kg with glibenclamide and by 2.9 kg with rosiglitazone

continued

Table 10.9 Weight/body mass index – *continued*

Comparison	Study	Change in weight/BMI
Rosiglitazone vs glibenclamide vs metformin	One study[54] N=4,360	Over a period of 5 years, the mean weight increased in the rosiglitazone group (change from baseline, 4.8 kg; 95% CI 4.3 to 5.3) but decreased in the metformin group (−2.9 95% CI −3.4 to −2.3 kg). In the glibenclamide group, weight gain occurred in the first year (1.6 kg; 95% CI 1.0 to 2.2), then remained stable. p values were significant for the treatment differences (RSG vs MET and RSG vs GLI)
Rosiglitazone + sulfonylurea vs placebo + sulfonylurea	One study[124] N=227 1+	Body weight increased by 4.3 kg with RSG + SU compared with a decrease of 1.2 kg with uptitrated SU alone*
Rosiglitazone + sulfonylurea vs sulfonylurea	One study[127] N=348 1+	NE
Rosiglitazone + gliclazide vs gliclazide uptitration	One study[132] N=471 1+	A significant increase in body weight was observed in patients receiving rosiglitazone plus gliclazide versus uptitrated gliclazide (3.4 kg, p=0.0001)
Rosiglitazone + libenclamide vs glibenclamide uptitration	One study[130] N=340 1+	Treatment with rosiglitazone + glibenclamide increased body weight by a mean of 3.1 kg. There was a small and non-significant increase in body weight of 0.14 kg compared with baseline in the uptitrated glibenclamide group*
Rosiglitazone + metformin vs metformin + glimepiride	One study[131] N=95 1+	NS (BMI)
	One study[123] N=99 1+	NS (BMI)
Rosiglitazone + metformin vs glibenclamide + metformin	One study[126] N=389 1+	At trial end, there were comparable increases in body weight in both treatment groups compared with baseline, with a mean weight gain of 1.94±4.63 kg with RSG + MET compared with 1.50±3.53 kg with GLY + MET
Rosiglitazone/metformin (FDC) vs metformin uptitrated	One study[62] N=569 1++	There was a mean (SE) increase from baseline in weight in the RSG/MET group (1.3 (0.22) kg) and a mean decrease in the MET group (-0.9 (0.26) kg)*
Rosiglitazone/metformin (FDC) vs metformin monotherapy	One study[135] N=526	Patients receiving RSG/MET experienced weight gain (0.01±0.3 kg) compared with a decrease of 1.9±0.3 kg in the MET group (p<0.0001 for difference)
Rosiglitazone/metformin (FDC) vs rosiglitazone vs metformin	One study[134] N=468 1+	Mean weight was reduced −2.9±4.4 kg with MET and increased 1.5±5.9 kg with RSG. There was no overall change in mean body weight with RSG/MET. Significant treatment differences in weight between RSG/MET and MET (p<0.001) and RSG/MET and RSG (p=0.01) were observed

continued

Table 10.9 Weight/body mass index – *continued*

Comparison	Study	Change in weight/BMI
Rosiglitazone + SU or metformin vs metformin + SU	One study[136] N=1,122 1+	Increases in body weight were observed in both arms of the metformin stratum; however, this increase was greater with rosiglitazone (+2.3 kg) than sulfonylurea (1.1 kg), p=0.003 In the sulfonylurea stratum there was a significant increase in body weight with rosiglitazone (+3.4 kg) compared with a slight decrease with metformin (–0.9 kg) p<0.001
Rosiglitazone + sulfonylurea + metformin vs insulin glargine + sulfonylurea + metformin	One study[139] N=217 1+	Rosiglitazone-treated patients gained more weight (3.0±0.4 kg) than those on insulin glargine (1.7±0.4 kg) (p=0.02)
Metformin + pioglitazone 15 mg OD vs metformin + rosiglitazone 4 mg OD	One study[133] N=96 1+	NS

* Significance testing not performed

Quality of life

When the addition of rosiglitazone to the combination of sulfonylurea and metformin (triple therapy) was compared to the addition of insulin glargine, significantly greater improvements were reported across several health-related quality of life outcomes (e.g. symptom score, mood symptoms, perception of general health) by patients in the glargine group compared to those in the rosiglitazone group.

Adverse events

Apart from the CV data described earlier in this chapter, the evidence appraised suggested that patients treated with rosiglitazone experienced a significantly higher incidence of oedema and anaemia. Similarly, rosiglitazone was associated with a significant risk of distal fractures in women patients.

Table 10.10 Adverse events

Comparison	Study	Change in AE
Rosiglitazone vs repaglinide vs repaglinide and rosiglitazone	One study[125] N=252 1+	Minor hypoglycaemia NS
Rosiglitazone vs glibenclamide	One study[128] N=203 1+	The absolute number and percentage of patients with at least one AE was similar between the two groups* Rosiglitazone-treated patients had more reports of oedema and anaemia (6.7% each) than patients in the glibenclamide group (1 and 2%)* Signs and symptom of hypoglycaemia were reported more commonly in glibenclamide-treated patients (7.1%) than in rosiglitazone-treated patients (1.9%)*

continued

Table 10.10 Adverse events – *continued*

Comparison	Study	Change in AE
	One study[129] N=598 1+	The most commonly reported AE was hypoglycaemia, which occurred in 25 patients (12.1%). Oedema was more common with rosiglitazone 8 mg/d (17 patients, 8.9%) than with rosiglitazone 4 mg/d (7 patients, 3.5%) or glibenclamide (4 patients, 1.9%) Small dose-dependant and statistically significant reductions in haemoglobin and haematocrit were observed in the rosiglitazone 4 mg/d (0.48 g/dl and 1.92% respectively) and rosiglitazone 8 mg/d (0.98 g/dl and 3.33% respectively) groups
Rosiglitazone vs glibenclamide vs metformin	One study[54] N=4,360	CV events: CV events were reported in 62 patients in the rosiglitazone group, 58 in the metformin group, and 41 in the glibenclamide group For all investigator reported CHF events, 22 occurred in the rosiglitazone group (1.5%), 19 in the metformin group (1.3%), and nine in the glibenclamide group (0.6%). The hazard ratio for CHF in the rosiglitazone group, as compared with the metformin group, was 1.22 (95% CI 0.66 to 2.26, p=0.52); the hazard ratio for the rosiglitazone group, as compared with the glibenclamide group, was 2.20 (95% CI, 1.01 to 4.79; p=0.05) Anaemia: Treatment with rosiglitazone was associated with a significantly decreased hematocrit, as compared with both metformin and glibenclamide (p<0.001 for both comparisons) Fractures: A higher rate of fractures was seen in the group receiving rosiglitazone More women in the rosiglitazone group had upper limb fractures involving the humerus and hand. Lower limb fractures were primarily increased in the foot GI: Rosiglitazone was less frequently associated with GI side effects than was metformin (p<0.001) Hypos: Fewer patients in the rosiglitazone group than in the glibenclamide group had hypoglycaemia (p<0.001)
Rosiglitazone + sulfonylurea vs placebo + sulfonylurea	One study[124] N=227 1+	Oedema was more frequent with RSG + SU (23 vs 9%)* There was no difference in the incidence of CHF between groups* The incidence of symptomatic hypoglycaemia was similar in the two treatment groups*
Rosiglitazone + sulfonylurea vs sulfonylurea	One study[127] N=348 1+	Hypoglycaemia occurred in 19 cases in the RSG and SU group and two in the SU alone group (p<0.001)

continued

Table 10.10 Adverse events – *continued*

Comparison	Study	Change in AE
Rosiglitazone + gliclazide vs gliclazide uptitration	One study[132] N=471 1+	The % of patients reporting on-therapy AEs in the rosiglitazone + gliclazide group (71%) was higher than in the uptitrated gliclazide group (59%)* Incidence of hypoglycaemia was 6% total; 1% severe in the rosiglitazone + gliclazide group and 2% total; 0.4% severe in the uptitrated gliclazide group* More patients in the combination group experienced oedema (11% vs 3%)*
Rosiglitazone + libenclamide vs glibenclamide uptitration	One study[130] N=340 1+	Incidence of hypoglycaemia was 18.5% in the rosiglitazone + glibenclamide group and 4.1% in the uptitrated glibenclamide group Incidence of oedema was 9.5% in the rosiglitazone + glibenclamide group and 2.5% in the uptitrated glibenclamide group*
Rosiglitazone + metformin vs metformin + glimepiride	One study[131] N=95 1+	Between group difference in terms of patients who had adverse effects: NS
Rosiglitazone + metformin vs glibenclamide + metformin	One study[126] N=389 1+	There was one death due to a serious AE (acute MI), which occurred in the RSG + MET group and was judged unlikely to be related to study medication The incidence of hypoglycaemia was 12.4% (23/124) with GLY + MET compared with 1.0% (2/133) of patients with RSG + MET Peripheral oedema was reported by 5.4% (11/133) of patients with RSG + MET compared with 2.2% (4/124) with GLY + MET The incidence of anaemia was 4.4% (9/133) and 1.1% (2/124) with RSG + MET and GLY + MET respectively
Rosiglitazone/metformin (FDC) vs metformin uptitrated	One study[62] N=569 1++	GI disorders were the most common leading to withdrawal in 5% of the MET group and 3% in the RSG/MET group 1% of patients in the RSG/MET group and 0.4% in the MET group reported on-therapy hypoglycaemia The incidence of diarrhoea was 14% in the MET group and 6% with RSG/MET. This was 9% and 6% for abdominal pain respectively Oedema was reported in 3% who received RSG/MET and in 1% in the MET group*

continued

Table 10.10 Adverse events – *continued*

Comparison	Study	Change in AE
Rosiglitazone/metformin (FDC) vs metformin monotherapy	One study[135] N=526	The overall proportion of participants with GI AEs was similar in both groups (33%); however, there was a reduced incidence of diarrhoea (8 vs 18%) in the RSG/MET group compared with the MET group Hypoglycaemia was reported in 17 participants (7%) in the RSG/MET group compared with 10 participants (4%) in the MET group. Six participants (2%) in the RSG/MET group vs none in the MET group had oedema Four participants (2%) in the RSG/MET vs none in the MET group had ischaemic events (two cases of angina pectoris, one myocardial ischemia, and one MI and coronary artery insufficiency) There were greater reductions in mean haemoglobin a haematocrit over 32 weeks in the RSG/MET group (Hb -0.75 ± 0.007 g/dl, Hct $-0.02\pm0.002\%$) compared with the MET group (Hb -0.34 ± 0.07 g/dl, Hct $-0.01\pm0.002\%$). The difference between the groups was significant for both parameters ($p<0.0001$)
Rosiglitazone/metformin (FDC) vs rosiglitazone vs metformin	One study[134] N=468 1+	Five events of IHD were reported. One in the RSG/MET group, two in the MET group and two in the RSG group Oedema was comparable between the RSG/MET (6%) and RSG groups (7%), but lower in the MET group (3%) There were no reports of CHF or pulmonary oedema The incidence of GI AE was similar with RSG/MET (47%) and MET (51%), but was less frequent with RSG (37%) Self-reported hypoglycaemic symptoms were similar across treatment groups (12% RSG/MET; 9% MET; 8% RSG)
Rosiglitazone + SU or metformin vs metformin + SU	One study[136] N=1,122 1+	Not reported
Rosiglitazone + sulfonylurea + metformin vs insulin glargine + sulfonylurea + metformin	One study[139] N=217 1+	AE possibly related to the study medication occurred significantly more among patients on rosiglitazone than on insulin glargine (28.6 vs 6.7% respectively, $p<0.0001$) Peripheral oedema occurred only in the rosiglitazone group, whereas no patient on insulin glargine reported oedema (12.5 vs 0% respectively, $p<0.001$) Hypoglycaemia: Confirmed hypoglycaemic events at plasma glucose <3.9 mmol/l were slightly greater with insulin glargine (N=57) (rosiglitazone, N=47, $p=0.0528$). Confirmed symptomatic hypoglycaemic events at plasma glucose <2.8 mol/l were greater in the insulin glargine-treated group (insulin glargine, N=26; rosiglitazone, N=14, $p<0.0165$) More patients in the insulin glargine group had confirmed nocturnal hypoglycaemia of <3.9 mmol/l (insulin glargine, N=29; rosiglitazone, N=12; $p=0.02$) and <2.8 mmol/l (insulin glargine, N=10; rosiglitazone, N=3; $p<0.05$) than in the rosiglitazone group. The calculated average rate per patient-year of a confirmed hypoglycaemic event (defined as <70 mg/dl), after adjusting for BMI, was 7.7 (95% CI 5.4 to 10.8) and 3.4 (2.3 to 5.0) events for insulin glargine and rosiglitazone respectively ($p=0.0073$)

continued

Table 10.10 Adverse events – *continued*		
Comparison	**Study**	**Change in AE**
Metformin + pioglitazone 15 mg OD vs metformin + rosiglitazone 4 mg OD	One study[133] N=96 1+	No CV events reported In the pioglitazone arm, two patients has AST and ALT values that increased to 1.5 times the upper limit of normal (<40 U/l), but these values normalised after 15 days

*Significance tests not performed

▷ Pioglitazone

*Cardiovascular outcomes**

The systematic review[141] found only one study[158] evaluating mortality and morbidity as endpoints outcomes. As the primary composite endpoint, the PROactive study explored the incidence of the following outcomes from the time of randomisation.

- All-cause mortality.
- Non-fatal MI (including silent MI).
- Stroke.
- Acute coronary syndrome (ACS).
- Endovascular or surgical intervention on the coronary or leg arteries, or amputation above the ankle.

The study concluded that for this composite endpoint there were no statistically significant differences between the pioglitazone and placebo group: the hazard ratio (HR) was 0.90 (95% CI 0.80 to 1.02, p=0.095). In the same vein, the individual components of the primary composite endpoint did not disclose statistically significant differences between intervention and control groups. **Level 1++**

Of all secondary endpoints only the so-called 'main' secondary endpoint 'time to the first event of the composite endpoint of death from any cause, MI (excluding silent MI) and stroke' indicated a statistical significant difference between pioglitazone and placebo (HR 0.84, 95% CI 0.72 to 0.98, p=0.027). **Level 1++**

A subgroup analysis** of the PROactive study[150] was identified by the re-runs. It analysed the effect of pioglitazone on recurrent MI in 2,445 patients with Type 2 diabetes and previous MI. The study found no significant differences in the primary or main secondary endpoints defined in the main PROactive study,*** and the individual endpoints of the primary composite. In addition, the subgroup analysis suggest that patients treated with pioglitazone had a statistically significant beneficial effect on the pre-specified endpoint of fatal and non-fatal MI (28% risk reduction (RR), p=0.045) and ACS (37% RR; p=0.035) compared to those treated with placebo. **Level 1+**

---

* See rosiglitazone section for further evidence published up to December 2007.
** The main limitation of this analysis is that it includes both pre-specified and post-hoc endpoints. It is an analysis of a subgroup of a larger study, and randomisation was not stratified by history of MI.
*** Primary endpoint: time to death, non-fatal MI, ACS, cardiac intervention (PCI/CABG), stroke, leg amputation, revascularisation in the leg. Secondary endpoint: time to the first event of the composite endpoint of death from any cause, MI (excluding silent MI), and stroke. Individual components of the primary endpoint and CV mortality were specified as secondary outcomes.

This study also showed that the incidence of CHF was significantly higher in patients receiving pioglitazone as compared to placebo-treated individuals (13.5 vs 9.6%, p=0.003). The incidence of serious CHF (requiring hospitalisation) was also significantly higher in the pioglitazone group (7.5% vs 5.2%, p=0.022). **Level 1+**

Another subgroup analysis* of the PROactive study[152] was also identified by the re-runs. This analysis evaluated outcomes stratified for patients who entered the study with (N=984) and without previous stroke (N=4,254). In the patients with previous stroke, there were no significant differences in the primary or main secondary endpoints as defined in the main PROactive analysis, but there was a trend of benefit (HR 0.78, 95% CI 0.60 to 1.02, p=0.0670) for the primary endpoint. In patients with no previous stroke, there were no significant differences between pioglitazone and placebo for any of the endpoints defined in the main PROactive analysis. **Level 1+**

▷ Surrogate outcomes

HbA$_{1c}$

The systematic review concluded that active glucose-lowering compounds like metformin, glibenclamide, gliclazide or glimepiride resulted in similar reductions of HbA$_{1c}$ compared to pioglitazone treatment. (Due to heterogeneity this outcome could not be subjected to meta-analysis.) **Level 1++**

A head-to-head RCT[151] comparing pioglitazone monotherapy with glimepiride monotherapy reported no significant difference in the HbA$_{1c}$ values between the two treatment groups until week 48. By the end of the study (week 72) there was an absolute difference between the two treatment groups of 0.32% favouring pioglitazone-treated patients (p=0.002). **Level 1+**

A 2-year follow-up study[148] reported no significant differences in terms of HbA$_{1c}$ when patients receiving metformin and pioglitazone were compared with those treated with metformin + gliclazide. **Level 1+**

A study comparing the addition of different doses of pioglitazone (30 and 45 mg) to stable insulin therapy in patients with poorly controlled Type 2 diabetes[146] found that mean HbA$_{1c}$ levels decreased significantly from baseline to week 24 in both groups: 1.2 from 9.9% and 1.5 from 9.7% in the pioglitazone 30- and 45-mg groups respectively (p<0.0001 for each relative to baseline; p=0.011, 30 vs 45 mg). **Level 1+**

One RCT comparing the currently licensed combination of pioglitazone and insulin with insulin plus placebo[145] found that after 6 months there was a significantly higher decrease in HbA$_{1c}$ levels in patients treated with insulin and pioglitazone (difference –0.55; p<0.002).** **Level 1+**

---

* The main limitation of this analysis is that it includes both pre-specified and post-hoc endpoints It is an analysis of a subgroup of a larger study, and randomisation was not stratified by history of MI.
** At baseline the mean HbA$_{1c}$ value for the PIO+INS group was 8.85%. This improved to 8.11% at endpoint (p<0.002). In the PLB+INS group, the mean HbA$_{1c}$ value at baseline (8.79%) was unchanged at endpoint (8.66%).

Fasting plasma glucose

A 2-year follow-up study[148] showed a statistically significant difference in FPG between the pioglitazone add-on to metformin group and the gliclazide add-on to metformin group at week 104 (–1.8 vs –1.1 mmol/l, p<0.001). **Level 1+**

The study comparing the addition of different doses of pioglitazone (30 and 45 mg) to stable insulin therapy in patients with poorly controlled Type 2 diabetes did not find significant differences in the decrease of FPG levels from baseline between the two groups.[146] **Level 1+**

One RCT comparing the combination of pioglitazone and insulin with insulin plus placebo[145] reported at 6 months a significant difference in terms of FPG favouring the pioglitazone + insulin combination (difference 1.80 mmol/l, p<0.002). **Level 1+**

Lipid profile

An RCT[151] comparing pioglitazone monotherapy with glimepiride monotherapy reported that by the end of the study (week 72) pioglitazone-treated patients showed significantly higher HDL levels (difference 0.16 mmol/l, p<0.001).

A 2-year follow-up study[148] reported a statistically significant percentage difference between the pioglitazone add-on to metformin group and the gliclazide add-on to metformin from baseline to last value for TG (–23% vs –7%, p<0.001), HDL-C (22% vs 7%, p<0.001) and LDL-C (2 vs –6%, p<0.001). **Level 1+**

The study comparing the addition of different doses of pioglitazone (30 and 45 mg) to stable insulin therapy in patients with poorly controlled Type 2 diabetes did not find significant differences in terms of lipid profile between the two groups. **Level 1+**

The RCT comparing the combination of pioglitazone and insulin with insulin plus placebo did not find significant differences in LDL and TG levels. However, after 6 months patients receiving pioglitazone and insulin had significantly higher levels of HDL (difference 0.13, p<0.002).*[145] **Level 1+**

Body weight

According to the systematic review, 15 studies evaluated body weight and observed an increase up to 3.9 kg after pioglitazone treatment, seven studies described a rise in BMI up to 1.5 kg/m^2. (Due to heterogeneity this outcome could not be subjected to meta-analysis.) **Level 1++**

A 2-year follow-up study[148] reported a mean increase from baseline of 2.5 kg in the pioglitazone add-on to metformin group and 1.2 kg in the gliclazide add-on to metformin at week 104. **Level 1+**

A study comparing the addition of different doses of pioglitazone (30 and 45 mg) to stable insulin therapy reported that a statistically significant dose response for weight gain was observed at all time points. A mean increase in mean body weight was observed in both

---

* The mean HDL level of the PIO + INS group at baseline (1.23 mmol/l) increased significantly at endpoint (1.35 mmol/l, p<0.002). The mean HDL level of the PLB + INS group at baseline (1.24 mmol/l) was unchanged at endpoint (1.21 mmol/l).

treatment groups: 2.94 and 3.38 kg in the 30- and 45-mg groups respectively, (p<0.001 for both groups).[146] **Level 1+**

A study comparing the combination of pioglitazone and insulin with insulin plus placebo reported a mean increase in body weight with PIO + INS of 4.05 kg, and a mean increase with PLB + INS of 0.20 kg.[145] **Level 1+**

Adverse events

The review concluded that the percentage of overall and serious AEs was comparable between intervention and control groups. The review also noted a somewhat higher discontinuation rate following pioglitazone administration especially in comparison to monotherapy with other OAD drugs. However, true numbers were difficult to evaluate due to study protocols defining withdrawals because of lack of efficacy as a serious AE. **Level 1++**

Oedema

The systematic review found that specific AE oedema was evaluated in 18 of the 22 studies. Overall, 11,565 participants provided data on the occurrence of oedema. The total number of events was 842 in the pioglitazone and 430 in the control groups. Pooling of the 18 studies revealed a RR of 2.86 (95% CI 2.14 to 3.18, p<0.00001). **Level 1++**

Hypoglycaemia

The systematic review found data on hypoglycaemic episodes in 11 of the 22 included studies. The review concluded that compared to active monotherapy control, pioglitazone treatment resulted in somewhat lower rates of hypoglycaemia. However, if pioglitazone was combined with insulin more hypoglycaemic incidents happened.

The review highlighted that the biggest trial[158] which compared pioglitazone versus placebo in combination with a variety of other glucose-lowering drugs reported hypoglycaemia rates of 27.9% after pioglitazone and 20.1% after placebo combinations. Severe hypoglycaemic events were rarely reported.

(Due to heterogeneity hypoglycaemia could not be subjected to meta-analysis.) **Level 1++**

Other adverse events

The review found six studies reporting a more pronounced (sometimes dose related) decrease of haemoglobin after pioglitazone intake in comparison to other active compounds or placebo. Haemoglobin reductions ranged between 0.5 and 0.75 g/dl. **Level 1++**

The 2-year follow-up study[148] reported that there were more symptoms of hypoglycaemia (11.5% vs 2.2%) and GI disorders (5.1% vs 3.8%) in the gliclazide group but less aggravated CHF (0.6% vs 1.6%) and oedema (3.5% vs 7.6%) than in the pioglitazone group. **Level 1+**

A study comparing the addition of different doses of pioglitazone (30 and 45 mg) to stable insulin therapy reported that in both groups, hypoglycaemia was the most commonly reported drug-related AE (37 and 43% of patients respectively), followed by lower limb oedema (13 and

12%), weight gain (7 and 13%) and aggravated oedema in patients with oedema at baseline (4 and 3%). Frequency of CV AEs related to study group was low and comparable between groups (1.2 and 0.6% for the 30- and 45-mg groups respectively). Drug-related CHF was reported for three patients receiving pioglitazone 30 mg (one possibly related and two probably related) and one patient receiving 45 mg (possibly related).[146] **Level 1+**

A study comparing the combination of pioglitazone and insulin with insulin plus placebo[145] showed that there were 90 (63.4%) reported incidences of subjective hypoglycaemic episodes for PIO + INS and 75 (51.0%) for PLB + INS (p<0.05). There was no difference between the treatment groups for clinical hypoglycaemia. The study also reported 20 cases of oedema with PIO + INS and five cases with PLB + INS. No CV events reported. **Level 1+**

Glitazones and the risk of oedema

A meta-analysis[153] revealed a twofold increase in the RR of oedema secondary to thiazolidinedione therapy compared to placebo, oral antihyperglycaemic agents, or insulin. The pooled odds ratio was 2.26 (95% CI 2.02 to 2.53, p<0.00001) the increased risk of oedema was present in both monotherapy and combination therapy studies. **Level 1+**

The same meta-analysis suggested that rosiglitazone was associated with a more pronounced risk for oedema than pioglitazone. The calculated adjusted indirect comparison of rosiglitazone to pioglitazone based on all included studies yielded an approximate threefold higher risk of oedema with rosiglitazone, (2.74 (2.33 to 3.14)). When only placebo controlled studies of pioglitazone (1.18 (0.61 to 2.28), p<0.063) and rosiglitazone (3.58 (2.11 to 6.10), p<0.00001) were considered, the risk was still greater with rosiglitazone. The calculated adjusted indirect comparison of rosiglitazone to pioglitazone using only placebo controlled trials was 3.03 (2.15 to 3.91). The omission of all open-label trials also pointed towards an increased risk with rosiglitazone (3.64 (2.56 to 5.17)), over pioglitazone (2.18 (1.72 to 2.75), p<0.00001). **Level 1+**

10.2.4 Health economics evidence statements

The submission for the TA[154] looked at adding rosiglitazone to sulfonylurea or metformin compared with other CTs or changing to insulin. The efficacy data was unreported in the TA because it was submitted as commercial in confidence.

For patients who failed on metformin monotherapy:

- metformin plus a sulfonylurea compared to metformin plus rosiglitazone, led to an ICER of £9,972 per QALY
- metformin plus sulfonylurea, and when this combination failed, metformin plus rosiglitazone compared to metformin plus rosiglitazone started straight after metformin monotherapy failure, led to an ICER of £11,857 per QALY.

In the TA[154] sensitivity analysis was included that appears to have been conducted by the TA group. The sensitivity analysis indicated that some of the scenarios were very sensitive to changes in key effectiveness variables. Small changes in the effect of rosiglitazone on β-cell function and insulin sensitivity induced large changes in the cost per QALY ratios. When the impact of rosiglitazone on insulin sensitivity and β-cell function was varied, in the comparison of metformin plus a sulfonylurea and metformin plus rosiglitazone, rosiglitazone was dominated by the sulfonylurea in combination therapy (metformin plus sulfonylurea is more effective and less expensive).

The NICE 2003 guidance[113] found that in patients in whom monotherapy with either metformin or a sulfonylurea had failed, the use of combination therapy with a glitazone and either metformin or a sulfonylurea was not likely to be cost-effective when compared with the combination of metformin and a sulfonylurea.

Metformin plus sulfonylurea was compared with metformin plus rosiglitazone in patients who had failed on metformin alone in the cost-effectiveness analysis conducted by Beale et al.[156]

Table 10.11 Incremental cost-effectiveness ratios rounded to nearest £100		
Patient group	Incremental cost per life year gained	Incremental cost per QALY
Obese	£21,300	£16,700
Overweight	£20,000	£11,600

The baseline results showed the combination of metformin plus rosiglitazone to be cost-effective compared to metformin plus sulfonylurea. Sensitivity analysis was performed on the threshold level of HbA$_{1c}$ at which patients were switched, the discount rate, and the mean BMI at diagnosis. Varying these parameters had little effect on the cost-effectiveness ratio. The effectiveness of rosiglitazone was not varied even though the data was taken from a variety of sources and were not necessarily from studies looking at rosiglitazone in combination with metformin.

In the Tilden et al.[157] analysis the glitazones were given after failure on metformin monotherapy. The study was based on a RCT which found no difference in the treatments on change in HbA$_{1c}$ or BMI. Pioglitazone was found to reduce TC: HDL, whereas rosiglitazone was found to increase this ratio. The analysis found that pioglitazone was more effective and cheaper than rosiglitazone. The results were insensitive to changes in key variables and pioglitazone remained dominant.

In contrast to these earlier analyses, the glitazones were appraised as a third-line treatment in patients who were not controlled on metformin plus sulfonylurea. Details are given in appendix C available at www.rcplondon.ac.uk/pubs/brochure.aspx?e=247.

As a broad summary of our results:
- rosiglitazone was consistently dominated by human insulin (both less effective and more expensive)
- pioglitazone was dominated in the base case, but was found cost-effective when some patient characteristics were changed (initial TC and initial systolic blood pressure (SBP))
- pioglitazone was estimated to yield a greater QALY gain at lower cost than rosiglitazone
- adjusting the initial SBP to reflect increased CV risk led to both glitazones being dominated by human insulin.

10.3 Gliptins (GLP-1 enhancers): dipeptidyl peptidase 4 inhibitors (DPP-4 inhibitors)

The GDG considered including sitagliptin and insulin detemir in this guideline; however, they were advised by NICE not to do so. NICE is undertaking a rapid update of recommendations in this guideline on second- and third-line drugs for managing blood glucose, which will cover these drugs. The updated guideline will be published early in 2009. For more information see www.nice.org.uk and search for 'Type 2 diabetes newer agents'.

10.4 Exenatide: GLP-1 mimetics

10.4.1 Methodological introduction

There were eight studies identified in this area, all were RCTs. Three were large, multicentre studies which compared doses of 5 μg and 10 μg exenatide with placebo for participants taking differing OAD treatments.[159–161]

These three studies had an extension open-label phase; this included those who had originally been randomised to have the exenatide treatment, they were invited to continue into this phase of the study. This drug is recently licensed; therefore this extension phase has been included as relevant, though there were methodological issues with it.[162]

One paper compared four differing doses of exenatide (2.5 μg, 5 μg, 7.5 μg and 10 μg) with placebo for participants treated with diet/exercise or a stable dose of metformin.[163]

There were two papers which compared exenatide with insulin glargine,[164,165] these studies by necessity are open-label; the other appraised studies were triple-blinded.

An open-label, non-inferiority RCT compared exenatide (5 μg bid for 4 weeks and 10 μg thereafter) with biphasic insulin aspart (twice daily doses titrated for optimal control).[166]

Finally, one paper compared the addition of exenatide to a glitazone with treatment with glitazone and placebo.[167]

It should be noted that the four triple-blinded studies were undertaken prior to exenatide gaining a therapeutic licence in the US.

Exenatide is indicated for treatment of Type 2 diabetes mellitus in combination with metformin and/or sulphonylureas in patients who have not achieved adequate glycaemic control on maximally tolerated doses of these oral therapies.[168]

10.4.2 Health economic methodological introduction

One published analysis was identified by Ray et al.[169] which compared exenatide to insulin glargine in patients who had failed on metformin and sulfonylurea. The analysis was set in the UK but no perspective was given.

An economic model was constructed based upon the UKPDS outcomes model to inform the GDG deliberations with regard to choice of glitazones or exenatide as third-line therapy in comparison to other third-line options. This is presented in appendix C available at www.rcplondon.ac.uk/pubs/brochure.aspx?e=247

10.4.3 Evidence statements

▷ Exenatide 5 μg and 10 μg compared with placebo

Three studies, all multicentre and triple-blinded based in the US used this comparison, total N=1,446.[159–161] For participants treated with sulfonylureas (N=377), those treated with metformin (N=336), and those treated with both (N=733), exenatide caused significant reductions in HbA_{1c}, FPG (at the higher 10 μg dose), postprandial glucose and body weight. Level 1++

Table 10.12 Exenatide 5 μg and 10 μg compared with placebo

	Sulfonylurea-treated participants[159]		Metformin-treated participants[160]		Metformin- and sulfonylurea-treated participants[161]	
	5 μg	10 μg	5 μg	10 μg	5 μg	10 μg
HbA_{1c}	−0.46±0.12% vs placebo 0.12±0.09% p≤0.0002	−0.86±0.11% vs placebo 0.12±0.09% p≤0.0002	Decrease compared with placebo p<0.001	Decrease compared with placebo p<0.001	−0.55±0.07% vs placebo 0.23±0.07% p<0.0001	−0.77±0.08% vs placebo 0.23±0.07% p<0.0001
Baseline HbA_{1c} >7%	N=31 reached ≤7% vs N=9 for placebo p<0.0001	N=41 reached ≤7% vs N=9 for placebo p<0.0001	N=27 reached ≤7% vs N=11 for placebo p<0.01	N=41 reached ≤7% vs N=11 for placebo p<0.01	24% reached ≤7% vs 7% for placebo p<0.0001	30% reached ≤7% vs 7% for placebo p<0.0001
Baseline HbA_{1c} >9%	−0.58±0.24% vs placebo 0.13±0.17% p<0.05	−1.22±0.19% vs placebo 0.13±0.17% p<0.05			Significant decreases compared with an increase with placebo p≤0.0002	Significant decreases compared with an increase with placebo p≤0.0002
Baseline HbA_{1c} ≤9%	−0.39±0.12% vs placebo 0.11±0.12% p<0.01	−0.65±0.12% vs placebo 0.11±0.12% p<0.01			Significant decreases compared with an increase with placebo p<0.0001	Significant decreases compared with an increase with placebo p<0.0001
FPG	NS	−0.6±0.3 mmol/l vs placebo 0.4±0.3 mmol/l p<0.05	NS	Difference 10 μg and placebo averaged −1.4 mmol/l p=0.0001	−0.5±0.2 mmol/l, vs placebo 0.8±0.2 mmol/l p<0.0001	−0.6±0.2 mmol/l vs placebo 0.8±0.2 mmol/l p<0.0001
Postprandial glucose			Significant reductions compared with placebo p=0.03	Significant reductions compared with placebo p=0.004	Significant reductions compared with placebo p=0.0001	Significant reductions compared with placebo p=0.0001

continued

	Sulfonylurea-treated participants[159]		Metformin-treated participants[160]		Metformin- and sulfonylurea-treated participants[161]	
	5 µg	10 µg	5 µg	10 µg	5 µg	10 µg
Body weight	NS	−1.6±0.3 kg/m vs placebo −0.6±0.3 kg/m² p<0.05	−1.6±0.4 kg vs placebo −0.3±0.3 kg p≤0.05	−2.8±0.5 kg vs placebo −0.3±0.3 kg	−1.6±0.2 kg vs placebo −0.9±0.2 kg p≤0.01	−1.6±0.2 kg vs placebo −0.9±0.2 kg p≤0.01
Insulin	NS	NS	NS	NS		
Proinsulin	NS	−16 pmol/l (CI −26.1 to −6.0) vs placebo p<0.01	NS	NS		
Lipids	Small reduction vs placebo p<0.05	Small reduction vs placebo p<0.05				
Hypoglycaemia	Mild-to-moderate 14% (3% with placebo)	Mild-to-moderate 36% (3% with placebo)	Mild-to-moderate 4.5% (5.3% with placebo)	Mild-to-moderate 5.3% (the same as placebo)	19.2% – one case of severe hypoglycaemia, the remaining were mild-to-moderate (12.6% for placebo)	Mild-to-moderate 27.8% (12.6% for placebo)
AEs	Nausea 39% (7% with placebo)	Nausea 51% (7% with placebo)	Nausea 36% (23% with placebo)	Nausea 45% (23% with placebo)	Nausea 39.2% (20.6% with placebo)	Nausea 48.5% (20.6% with placebo)
Discontinuation	24.0% (7.2% with placebo)	29.5% (7.2% with placebo)	24.0% (39.8% with placebo)	29.5% (39.8% with placebo)	15.9% (23.9% with placebo)	17.8% (23.9% with placebo)

Table 10.12 Exenatide 5 µg and 10 µg compared with placebo – *continued*

▷ Open-label extension phase

The three RCTs in the table above[159–161] had a further open-label extension phase of 52 weeks, which was open to those participants who had been originally randomised to exenatide, N=668, analysis completed on N=314.[162] This study showed that at the end of 82 weeks that the reductions in HbA_{1c} and in FPG which had been identified at the end of week 30 were maintained to week 82.

The reduction in body weight was progressive to week 82, week 30 the body weight changes for the 10 µg BD dose were −1.6 to −2.8 kg, at week 82 the change from baseline was −4.4±0.3 kg (95% CI: −3.8 to −5.1 kg), or 4.4% of baseline body weight. Higher levels of weight reduction were noted in those participants who had had a higher BMI at baseline; participants with baseline BMI <25 had a mean weight reduction of 2.9% of baseline body weight, those with a baseline BMI of ≥40 had a mean reduction of 5.5% of baseline body weight.

▷ Exenatide 2.5 µg, 5 µg, 7.5 µg and 10 µg BD doses compared with placebo

This phase II study compared four doses of exenatide with placebo in participants treated either with diet modification and exercise alone or a stable dose of metformin, N=156.[163]

HbA1c

There was a decrease in HbA_{1c} compared with an increase with placebo (0.1±0.1%), for all doses: 2.5 µg (−0.3±0.1%), 5 µg (−0.4±0.1%), 7.5 µg (−0.5±0.1%), 10 µg (−0.5±0.1%), p<0.01.

Fasting blood glucose

There was a decrease in FBG compared with an increase with placebo (6.8±4.1 mg/dl), for all doses: 2.5 µg (−20.1±5.2 mg/dl), 5 µg (−21.2±3.9 mg/dl), 7.5 µg (−17.7±4.8 mg/dl), 10 µg (−17.3±4.4 mg/dl), p<0.01.

Body weight

Reductions in body weight with exenatide were significant for the 7.5 µg (−1.4±0.3kg) and 10 µg (−1.8±0.3 kg) groups, p<0.01, compared with the placebo group who were weight neutral.

Subgroup analysis

This used data from the 5 µg and 10 µg groups and considered those treated with diet/exercise compared with those treated with metformin. This found that the effects of exenatide were similar in both groups for HbA_{1c}, FPG and body weight.

Adverse events and discontinuation

40.7% of participants taking exenatide had nausea (6.5% severe nausea) compared with 12.1% of those taking the placebo (3.0% severe nausea). The nausea appeared to be dose dependent as it had a higher occurrence in the higher dose groups; 2.5 µg (23.3%), 5 µg (25.8%), 7.5 µg (61.3%) and 10 µg (51.6%). **Level 1+**

▷ Exenatide vs insulin glargine

The phase III study compared exenatide and insulin glargine in participants who had not achieved adequate glycaemic control with a combination of metformin and sulfonylurea at maximally effective doses, with N=551 participants.[164]

HbA1c

Exenatide was as effective as insulin glargine in improving glycaemic control with both groups showing a reduction of 1.11% from baseline. The percentage of participants who achieved the target HbA_{1c} of 7% or less were also similar, 46% for exenatide and 48% for insulin glargine.

Fasting plasma glucose

Those taking insulin glargine showed a greater reduction in FPG than those receiving exenatide (−2.9 vs −1.4 mmol/l), p<0.001. Significantly more of the insulin glargine group (21.6%) achieved a FPG of less than 5.6 mmol/l compared with 8.6% in the exenatide group (p<0.001).

Self-monitored blood glucose

Mean daily self-monitored glucose levels were similar between the treatments, however, those using insulin glargine had lower glucose levels at fasting (p<0.001), before meals (pre-lunch p=0.023; pre-dinner p=0.006), at 3.00 am (p<0.001) and evening (p<0.001) compared with exenatide.

Adverse events and discontinuation

There were higher incidences of the most frequent AEs of nausea and vomiting in the exenatide group (57.1% and 17.4% respectively) compared with insulin glargine (8.6% and 3.7%).

Overall rates of hypoglycaemia were similar across both treatment groups (7.4 events/patient year with exenatide and 6.3 with insulin glargine).

A higher number of participants discontinued the study with exenatide (N=54) compared with insulin glargine (N=25), for N=27 in the exenatide group the withdrawal was due to AEs. **Level 1+**

The second exenatide and insulin glargine study considered the treatments in respect to patient reported health outcome measures, N=549.[165] Both treatment groups showed baseline to endpoint improvements on several of the health outcome measures; these were not significant between the groups. Glycaemic control results were not reported. **Level 1+**

▷ Exenatide vs biphasic insulin aspart

This study reported that HbA_{1c} reduction in exenatide-treated patients (N=253) was non-inferior to that achieved with biphasic insulin aspart (N=248). In relation to body weight gain, the study showed a statistically significant difference favouring those receiving exenatide.[166]

Table 10.13 Exenatide vs biphasic insulin aspart

Nauck[166] N=501 T=52 weeks	Exenatide	Biphasic insulin aspart	Size effect
HbA_{1c}	−1.04	−0.89	NS
Fasting serum glucose	−1.8 mmol/l	−1.7 mmol/l	NS
Body weight	Exenatide-treated patients lost weight, while patients treated with biphasic insulin aspart gained weight. Between group difference −5.4kg (95% CI −5.9 to −5.0 kg)		
AEs	The incidence of GI AEs was higher with exenatide than with aspart. Nausea (33% incidence, 3.5% discontinuation) observed with exenatide. Vomiting (15% incidence). The overall hypoglycaemia rates were similar across treatment groups at endpoint		

▷   Exenatide + glitazone vs placebo + glitazone

This multicentre, double-blinded RCT compared the addition of exenatide to a glitazone with glitazone and placebo in a population of 233 suboptimally controlled people with Type 2 diabetes.[167]

Overall, the RCT showed that exenatide in combination with a glitazone improved glycaemic control in patients with Type 2 diabetes that is suboptimally controlled with a glitazone, either alone or in combination with metformin.

Table 10.14 Exenatide + glitazone vs placebo + glitazone

Zinman[167] N=233 T=16 weeks	Glitazone + placebo	Glitazone + exenatide	Size effect
HbA$_{1c}$	+0.09%	−0.89%	−0.98% (95% CI −1.21 to −0.74%, p<0.01)
Fasting serum glucose	+0.10 mmol/l	−1.59 mmol/l	−1.69 mmol/l (95% CI −2.22 to −1.17 mmol/l, p<0.001)
Body weight	−0.24 kg	−1.75 kg	−1.51 kg CI −2.15 to −0.88 kg, p<0.001)
Lipid profile	The study reported that no clinically significant changes occurred		
AEs	The most frequent AE was nausea, which was the reason for withdrawal of 9% and 1% of patients in the exenatide and placebo groups respectively The incidence of treatment-emergent oedema was similar in both groups (5.8% and 8% of patients in the exenatide and placebo groups respectively) The overall incidence of hypoglycaemia was also low and similar between groups (10.7% and 7.1% of patients in the exenatide and placebo groups respectively)		

10.4.4 Health economic evidence statements

The analysis by Ray et al. was based on a 26-week trial which found exenatide was associated with a 0.99% reduction in HbA$_{1c}$ compared to 1.07% with glargine. Exenatide was found to improve BMI, SBP, TC and LDL-C compared to glargine. No cost for exenatide in the UK was available as it had not been licensed at the time of publication so various proportions of the US price were tested from 20% to 100%. Exenatide was found to have a cost per QALY of £22,420 compared to glargine. The results were most sensitive to variation in the disutility values applied for weight change and nausea. The cost per QALY increased to £39,763 when disutility values for set levels of BMI were used rather than changes in weight.[169]

The health economic analysis of exenatide as a third-line agent in Type 2 diabetes is described in appendix C available at www.rcplondon.ac.uk/pubs/brochure.aspx?e=247. In the base-case analysis (see table 23) exenatide is shown to have an ICER of £280,495. Recognising the difficulties of factoring in the potential benefits of weight loss with exenatide, various sensitivity analyses were performed, but the ICER remained consistently high and in only one case became cost-effective, (£29,865 per QALY gained when exenatide patients were started with an initial

BMI of 27 kg/m^2 compared to a 33 kg/m^2 for all other treatments and a utility gain of 0.064 due to 3% weight loss on exenatide, no nausea, compared to weight gain for other treatments). In this model therefore, human insulin is a consistently more cost-effective option in any patient in whom it is an acceptable form of treatment.

10.5 Oral glucose control therapies (2): other oral agents and exenatide; from evidence to recommendations

10.5.1 Thiazolidinediones (glitazones)

This section updates both the previous NICE inherited guideline and the previous NICE TA guidance on the use of glitazones for the treatment of Type 2 diabetes. NICE TA guidance 63 (2003).[113]

Significant further evidence was available for pioglitazone and rosiglitazone; these studies fell into three groups.

- Comparison of glucose-lowering (and other metabolic) outcomes.
- Durability of blood glucose control.
- True health outcome studies including safety issues.

The glucose-lowering studies appeared to add little to what was already known about these drugs. The positive effects of pioglitazone on HDL-C and TGs were also noted, and were believed to have contributed to the results of the PROactive study. The effects of rosiglitazone on total and LDL-C were noted. They were difficult to interpret because of the drug effects on the changes to the nature of LDL-C particles. Other surrogate outcomes of therapy were noted to be broadly positive, including minor effects on BP.

From the PROactive study on pioglitazone (the only study with this drug with real health outcomes as a primary endpoint) appeared to be broadly positive despite statistical concerns and the selected population (secondary prevention study). However, the magnitude of the effect size on CV outcomes appeared no better than for the active treatment policy group of the UKPDS study, principally sulfonylurea therapy, the results of which were also noted to be not entirely conclusive when considered in isolation.

There are concerns over fluid retention and hospitalisation for cardiac failure with both thiazolidinediones. Recent safety data has identified a clinically significant risk of distal fracture in women using these drugs. For rosiglitazone the meta-analysis of investigator reported MI from two major studies (one not in people with diabetes) and the manufacturer's trials database raised real concerns at the time of conclusion of the draft of the current guideline. These were only partly assuaged by the report of unchanged CV death compared to sulfonylureas/ metformin in the RECORD interim analysis. The GDG therefore undertook a review of further meta-analyses published since that time up to December 2007, together with EMEA, FDA, and MHRA pronouncements, also up to December 2007. Although there was no definitive evidence of excess myocardial ischaemia from rosiglitazone, the GDG felt that there was certainly a 'signal' of increased risk of non-fatal MI for rosiglitazone. The regulators' position seemed to be of confirmation of benefit: safety ratio, and continuing to allow marketing of rosiglitazone even though an alternative was available, albeit with warnings and restrictions. The GDG was also given to understand that pricing of these drugs would become similar. On balance, despite reservations over rosiglitazone, it was not felt to be possible to unequivocally recommend a preference for pioglitazone in all circumstances, but rather to allow the choice of agent to rest with the person with diabetes and their advisor, taking account of the then current regulatory advice (which may yet change).

However, the issues over fractures and fluid retention/cardiac failure and the costs of these drugs led the GDG to conclude that thiazolidinediones could not generally replace sulfonylureas as second-line therapy, except where sulfonylureas were contraindicated by particular risk of hypoglycaemia.

The health economic modelling appeared to identify that these drugs, and in particular the then more highly priced rosiglitazone, were not cost-effective compared to human insulin therapy. However, the GDG were concerned that quality of life aspects of insulin therapy, including fear of hypoglycaemia, and the education and support costs of modern intensity of dose titration, were not adequately captured by the model. Furthermore, people of higher body weight and more insulin insensitive phenotype, as identified clinically by features of the metabolic syndrome (usually abdominal adiposity), respond better than average to thiazolidinediones, but often have barriers to insulin therapy related to weight gain, and respond less well to insulin. Accordingly they were content to allow the choice of either thiazolidinedione taking into account cost and the safety issues raised above where insulin injection therapy is likely to be poorly tolerated. This was noted to be in line with the thiazolidinedione NICE TA (guidance 63, 2003) the current guideline updates. As the initiation threshold for insulin is suggested as an $HbA_{1c} \geq 7.5$ %, it followed this should be adopted for thiazolidinediones too.

The evidence of durability of effect on blood glucose control of thiazolidinediones was noted. This was not part of the economic modelling. The GDG noted that there would be some cost offset and possible quality of life gain from any delay to initiation of insulin therapy, and perhaps from decreased requirement for uptitration of insulin doses over the years. This added to the uncertainty of the findings in regard of the cost-effectiveness of thiazolidinediones compared to insulin.

As thiazolidinediones worked in combination with metformin, fixed-dose combination products would be suitable for use where there were no cost implications or where improved drug adherence issues increase cost effectiveness. The GDG was not presented with specific evidence on this latter point.

10.5.2 Exenatide

Exenatide is a relatively new therapy, it is expensive, and has licensing restrictions within the glucose-lowering therapy pathway. The GDG did not consider it therefore for general use, but sought to determine those people in whom its use might be cost-effective as a third-line therapy.

There was little evidence comparing exenatide with other third-line therapies. Exenatide successfully lowered HbA_{1c}, though the extent of this was not impressive compared to other therapies even allowing for the rather better baseline values of modern studies. Significant weight loss compared to all other therapies was clearly found, though the extent of this was not large, and required continued therapy to be maintained. Nausea appeared to be a significant problem, and it was unclear if this was related to (causative of) the weight loss to any extent.

The studies comparing exenatide to insulin did not achieve the HbA_{1c} reduction with insulin expected from other studies, suggesting, together with the low doses used, that dose titration of the insulin comparator was inadequate. This was taken as suggesting that insulin might still be preferred for glucose lowering, even after considerations of hypoglycaemia, injection anxieties, and weight gain with insulin had been addressed.

Exenatide therapy is expensive, and the health economic modelling suggested it was not cost-effective for an unselected population as compared to commencing human insulin therapy. However, the GDG did not consider comparison with an unselected population to be applicable to some reasonably common clinical situations. They noted that all other third-line options were dominated by human insulin therapy in the economic model and that for obesity issues the costs of other aspects of obesity management (e.g. orlistat and bariatric surgery) had not been included. It was noted that previous NICE TAs had approved agents that were dominated in this economic model, including the glitazones (as second-line therapy when metformin and a sulfonylurea cannot be taken in combination) and insulin glargine. The GDG was uncertain that these agents (including exenatide) would be found to be not cost-effective if the model fully reflected the negative quality of life issues of insulin, including fear of hypoglycaemia, and the costs of support and patient education for modern intensity of insulin dose titration.

Furthermore, the more obese require much higher insulin doses, such that insulin costs alone can easily exceed those of exenatide (depending on the mix of insulin types chosen for comparator) though the benefit from insulin could be expected to be higher than in the trials (for reasons of dose titration given above). In these circumstances a confident judgment of costs and benefits to be gained from HbA_{1c} and weight change, and side effects, could not be made. However the GDG's judgment was that costs of insulin and exenatide by the end of the first year would be equivalent on average for people with a starting BMI (before these medications) of approximately >33 kg/m^2, while in this obese group the small metabolic advantage to insulin on HbA_{1c} would easily be outweighed by the metabolic advantage of 4 kg weight loss on exenatide. In this restricted circumstance, and particularly at higher BMI's, the cost-effectiveness of exenatide would then be at least as good as that of insulin.

The GDG noted an issue over the definition of obesity as it affects different ethnic groups, a problem also identified in the NICE guideline on obesity management,[12] although with no specific recommendations as to how to allow for it. Accordingly the GDG could only recommend that clinicians took ethnic group issues into account when judging the BMI above which exenatide might be indicated.

The GDG strongly felt that there was a role for third-line agents since this would allow delay of starting insulin therapy, and it was recognised that some individuals were very reluctant to switch to insulin. In circumstances where it was clinically desirable not to commence insulin, it was noted that the third-line agents were cost-effective compared to no action (continued poor blood glucose control). If human insulin was dropped from the economic model, exenatide would still be dominated by thiazolidinedione. However, it was not clear that the model adequately incorporated the divergence in body weight trend with these two types of medication, and thiazolidinediones have contraindications and safety issues of their own. Nevertheless the GDG concluded again that exenatide could only be recommended in a limited role.

As an expensive injectable the GDG therefore concluded the therapeutic positioning of exenatide should be after use of the conventional oral glucose-lowering drugs, in those people with significant body weight issues affecting health and quality of life, and should be considered only as an alternative where newer medications such as a thiazolidinedione were to be commenced, or insulin started therapy. The GDG reached a consensus on the thresholds of these criteria for this guideline in the absence of evidence to guide them.

Exenatide will be updated by NICE as part of a rapid update to this guideline which will also encompass other glucose-lowering therapies such as the gliptins.

ORAL GLUCOSE CONTROL THERAPIES (2): OTHER ORAL AGENTS AND EXENATIDE; RECOMMENDATIONS

For oral agent combination therapy with insulin please refer to chapter 11.

Thiazolidinediones (glitazones)*

R40   If glucose concentrations are not adequately controlled (to HbA_{1c} <7.5 % or other higher level agreed with the individual), consider, after discussion with the person, adding a thiazolidinedione to the combination of metformin and a sulfonylurea if human insulin is likely to be unacceptable or ineffective because of employment, social or recreational issues related to putative hypoglycaemia, injection anxieties, other personal issues, or obesity/metabolic syndrome.
Consider adding a thiazolidinedione as second-line therapy to:
- metformin as an alternative to a sulfonylurea where the person's job or other issues make the risk of hypoglycaemia with sulfonylureas particularly significant
- sulfonylurea monotherapy when blood glucose control remains or becomes inadequate ($HbA_{1c} \geq 6.5\%$) if the person does not tolerate metformin (or it is contraindicated).

R41   Warn a person prescribed a thiazolidinedione about the possibility of significant oedema and advise on the action to take if it develops.

R42   Do not commence or continue thiazolidinedione in people who have evidence of heart failure, or who are at higher risk of fracture.

R43   When selecting a thiazolidinedione for initiation and continuation of therapy, take into account up-to-date advice from the relevant regulatory bodies (the European Medicines Agency and the Medicines and Healthcare products Regulatory Agency), cost and safety issues (note that only pioglitazone can be used in combination with insulin therapy, see recommendation 49).**

Gliptins: GLP-1 enhancers

No recommendations are made on the use of gliptins as these drugs are not covered in this guideline.

Exenatide: GLP-1 mimetics

R44   Exenatide is not recommended for routine use in Type 2 diabetes.*

---

* A short clinical guideline 'Newer agents for blood glucose control in Type 2 diabetes' is in development and is expected to be published by NICE in February 2009.
** The summary of product characteristic for rosiglitazone was last updated in March 2008 – further updates regarding rosiglitazone and pioglitazone may occur in the lifetime of this guideline.

R45   Consider exenatide as an option only if all the following apply for the individual:

- a body mass index over 35.0 kg/m^2 in those of European descent, with appropriate adjustment in tailoring this advice for other ethnic groups
- specific problems of a psychological, biochemical or physical nature arising from high body weight
- inadequate blood glucose control (HbA$_{1c}$ $\geq$7.5 %) with conventional oral agents after a trial of metformin and sulfonylurea
- other high-cost medication, such as a thiazolidinedione or insulin injection therapy, would otherwise be started.

R46   Continue exenatide therapy only if a beneficial metabolic response (at least 1.0 % HbA$_{1c}$ reduction in 6 months and a weight loss of at least 5% at 1 year) occurs and is maintained.

11 Glucose control: insulin therapy

11.1 Oral agent combination therapy with insulin

11.1.1 Clinical introduction

People with Type 2 diabetes with inadequate blood glucose control on oral agents have the pathogenetic problems which caused their diabetes, and still have significantly preserved islet B-cell function. There remains the possibility that medication designed to enhance insulin secretion, reduce insulin insensitivity, or otherwise improve blood glucose control might be useful in combination with insulin therapy, in improving blood glucose control, reducing insulin dose requirement, or mitigating side effects of insulin therapy.

The clinical question is which oral agents, singly or in combination, should be continued when starting insulin therapy.

11.1.2 Methodological introduction

Studies were identified which compared insulin in combination with oral hypoglycaemic agents (OHAs) with insulin monotherapy in insulin naive Type 2 diabetic patients. A Cochrane review[170] was identified which included 20 RCTs in a search performed in March 2004. Ten additional RCTs were identified, five of which were excluded due to methodological limitations.[171–175]

Of the remaining five RCTs the treatment comparisons were:
- insulin and metformin vs insulin and placebo (most patients in each group on pre-mixed twice daily insulin regimens)[176]
- neutral protamine hagedorn (NPH) insulin (bedtime) and sulfonylurea and metformin vs NPH insulin 30/70 (twice daily)[177]
- insulin glargine (once daily) and glimepiride and metformin vs NPH insulin 30/70 (twice daily)[178]
- biphasic insulin aspart 30/70 (twice daily) and pioglitazone vs biphasic insulin aspart 30/70 (twice daily)[147]
- NPH insulin (bedtime) and glimepiride vs NPH insulin (twice daily) vs NPH insulin 30/70 (twice daily)[179]
- biphasic insulin vs biphasic insulin and metformin vs glibenclamide and metformin (although only the biphasic insulin vs biphasic insulin and metformin comparison will be considered here).[64]

It should be noted that the number of different drug combinations and comparisons, dosing and titration regimens limit direct comparison between the studies. Furthermore, all of the studies with the exception of one[176] were open-label.

Of the five trials presented above, it can be noted that only two included a biphasic insulin arm with metformin or a sulfonylurea.[64,176] Further details of the five trials in the Cochrane review, which included biphasic insulin regimens in combination with OHAs (all published between 1987 and 1998, prior to this update), are given where this data was available in the Cochrane review at the request of the GDG. These trials compared:

- mixed insulin (25% regular, 75% protamine insulin) plus glibenclamide vs mixed insulin (25% regular, 75% protamine insulin) and placebo (N=140, Cochrane methodological quality score 2/7) (Bachman 1988)
- mixed insulin (intermediate acting NPH plus regular insulin) twice daily and glibenclamide vs mixed insulin (intermediate acting NPH plus regular insulin) twice daily and placebo (N=20, Cochrane methodological quality score 2/7) (Gutniak 1987)
- insulin (combination of short and intermediate acting insulin) once or twice daily plus glibenclamide vs insulin alone (combination of short and intermediate acting insulin) once or twice daily (N=27, Cochrane methodological quality score 2/7) (Ravnik-Oblak 1995)
- mixed insulin (70% NPH, 30% soluble) at suppertime plus glibenclamide vs mixed insulin (70% NPH, 30% soluble) and placebo (N=21, Cochrane methodology score 7/7) (Riddle 1992)
- mixed insulin (70% NPH, 30% regular human insulin) at suppertime plus glimepiride vs mixed insulin (70% NPH, 30% regular human insulin) and placebo (N=145, Cochrane methodology score 6/7) (Riddle 1998).

It is notable that some of these studies had small sample sizes and/or low methodological quality scores.

11.1.3 Health economic methodological introduction

Only one economic evaluation was identified.[180] The analysis was conducted over a short time period (4 months) and intermediate outcomes were reported. For economic analysis to inform resource allocation it is important to consider the impact on final health outcomes such as mortality and morbidity.[181] The incremental costs and benefits of using insulin glargine compared to conventional insulin treatment were not reported.

An economic model was constructed based upon the UKPDS outcomes model to inform the GDG with regard to choice of glitazones or exenatide as third-line therapy in comparison to other third-line options. This is presented in appendix C available at www.rcplondon.ac.uk/pubs/brochure.aspx?e=247

11.1.4 Evidence statements

▷ Glycemic control

Overall the data seems to suggest that patients receiving a combination treatment with insulin (NPH or pre-mixes) and metformin or a sulfonylurea showed significantly lower HbA$_{1c}$ levels when compared to those treated with insulin monotherapy. FPG values were not consistently assessed by most of the studies.

Table 11.1 HbA$_{1c}$

Comparison	Study	Change in HbA$_{1c}$ %
NPH insulin + OHAs (SU or SU + metformin) vs insulin monotherapy (two or more daily injections)	Cochrane review[170] 1++	NS
NPH insulin (once daily) + SU vs NPH insulin (once daily)	Cochrane review[170] 1++	Significantly lower HbA$_{1c}$ in the combination arm. Difference 0.3% (95% CI 0.0 to 0.6, p=0.03)
NPH or mixed insulin (once daily) + OHAs vs insulin (twice daily)	Cochrane review[170] 1++	Significantly lower HbA$_{1c}$ levels in the insulin monotherapy arm (mean difference 0.4% (95% CI 0.1 to 0.8, p=0.03))
NPH insulin (bedtime) + SU vs NPH insulin (twice daily) vs NPH insulin 30 (twice daily)	1 study[179] 1+	Significantly lower HbA$_{1c}$ levels in the combination arm (p<0.001)
Insulin (pre-mix twice daily) + metformin vs insulin (pre-mix twice daily)	1 study[176] 1++	Significantly lower HbA$_{1c}$ levels in the combination arm (adjusted difference 0.5% 95% CI 0.1 to 0.9, p=0.02)
Insulin aspart (twice daily) + metformin vs insulin aspart (twice daily)	1 study[64] 1+	Significantly lower HbA$_{1c}$ levels in the combination arm (mean treatment difference 0.39±0.15% (p=0.007))
Insulin glargine (once daily) + OHA (SU or metformin) vs NPH insulin 30/70 (twice daily)	1 study[178] 1+	Significantly lower HbA$_{1c}$ levels in the combination arm (−1.64 vs −1.31%, p=0.0003)
Insulin aspart 30/70 (twice daily) + pioglitazone vs biphasic insulin aspart 30/70 (twice daily)	1 study[147] 1+	Significantly lower HbA$_{1c}$ levels in the combination arm (mean difference −0.60% SD 0.22%, p=0.008)

SD, standard deviation; SU, sulfonylurea

▷ Insulin dose

A Cochrane review[170] reported that insulin–OHA combination therapy was associated with a significantly lower insulin dose compared to insulin monotherapy. An RCT[176] reported the same trend for the combination of insulin and metformin.

▷ Well-being and quality of life

The few studies that objectively assessed well-being, quality of life or treatment satisfaction did not report significant differences between insulin–OHA combination and insulin monotherapy. However, there was a trend towards higher levels of satisfaction for patients in the combination group (especially those receiving metformin).

▷ Hypoglycaemia

Non-significant differences in the incidence of hypoglycaemic events between insulin–OHA and insulin monotherapy were reported across most of the studies identified. However, a higher number of hypoglycaemic events were observed in patients receiving monotherapy with biphasic insulin regimens (e.g. NPH 30/70).

Table 11.2 Hypoglycaemic events

Comparison	Incidence	Statistical significance
Insulin and metformin vs insulin and placebo (most patients in each group on pre-mixed twice daily insulin regimens)[176]	Insulin and metformin 82% with at least one episode vs insulin and placebo 66%	RR=1.24, 95% CI 1.02 to 1.52, p=0.027
	Severe hypoglycaemia metformin (13%) vs placebo (1%)	RR=9.48, 95%CI 1.24 to 72.2, p=0.009
NPH insulin (bedtime) and sulfonylurea and metformin vs NPH insulin 30/70 (twice daily)[177]	Insulin–OHA group mean number of hypoglycaemic events 2.7 vs insulin monotherapy 4.3	p=0.02
Insulin glargine (once daily) and glimepiride and metformin vs NPH insulin 30/70 (twice daily)[178]	Glargine plus OHA mean number of confirmed AEs 4.07 vs insulin 9.87 (all hypoglycaemic events)	p<0.0001
	Glargine plus OHA 2.62 vs insulin 5.73 (symptomatic events)	p<0.0009
	Glargine plus OHA 0.51 vs insulin 1.04 (nocturnal events)	p<0.0449
Biphasic insulin aspart 30/70 (twice daily) and pioglitazone vs biphasic insulin aspart 30/70 (twice daily)[147]	Minor hypoglycaemic episodes % of patients: BIAsp 30, 15% vs BIAsp 30+POI 12% Number of episodes: BIAsp 30, 47 and BIAsp 30+PIO, 15 Symptoms only % of patients: BIAsp 30, 40% vs BIAsp 30+PIO 34% Number of episodes: BIAsp 30, 171 and BIAsp 30+PIO, 115 Incidence (per patient-week for all episodes) BIAsp 30=0.132 vs BIAsp 30+PIO=0.083	Not reported
NPH insulin (bedtime) and glimepiride vs NPH insulin (twice daily) vs NPH insulin 30/70 (twice daily)[179]	Number of patients with at least one hypoglycaemic event: NPH insulin (bedtime) and glimepiride, 61.6% NPH insulin (twice daily), 71.6% NPH insulin 30/70 (twice daily), 72.4%	Not reported
Biphasic insulin aspart 30 (twice daily) and metformin vs biphasic insulin aspart 30 (twice daily)[64]	No major hypoglycaemic episodes during the trial, minor hypoglycaemic episodes were similar amongst treatment groups	NS

▷ Weight gain

It was observed across most of the studies that treatment with insulin and other OHA (especially metformin) was associated with significantly less weight gain when compared with insulin monotherapy.

Only one study[147] comparing the combination of BIAsp 30 plus pioglitazone with BIAsp monotherapy showed a greater weight gain in patients treated with the combination therapy.

▷ Other adverse events

Overall, no significant differences in frequency or severity of AEs were found for patients receiving insulin alone or combination therapy regimens. However, one study[147] found that more patients experienced product-related AEs in the biphasic aspart 30/70 plus pioglitazone group (28%) compared with patients receiving biphasic insulin aspart 30/70 monotherapy (20%). The combination group was also associated with a higher proportion of patients experiencing peripheral edema (6%) compared with aspart monotherapy (0%).

11.1.5 From evidence to recommendation

The new evidence continued to support the view that metformin should be continued when starting insulin therapy. The evidence was stronger than previously for sulfonylureas, for acarbose if used, and also for the thiazolidinediones. For sulfonylureas the situation was further complicated by much of the newer data coming from use with basal insulin regimens, while there was more uncertainty and concern over use with biphasic insulin (pre-mix) regimens due to risks of hypoglycaemia and the risk this might worsen achieved blood glucose control. Positive advice was tempered by concerns that the combination might cause excessive weight gain, and it was not possible to conclude whether this was clinically significant or otherwise a concern to the individual with Type 2 diabetes.

The cost and cost-effectiveness issues of continuing thiazolidinediones were considered at the time of review of the health economic modelling, although this issue was not specifically addressed by the modelling. Being high cost, it was unclear that the thiazolidinediones could give cost-effective health gains when continued at the time of starting insulin. However, it was noted that some people (often markedly obese) get a combination of reductions of insulin doses from high levels together with markedly improved blood glucose control when thiazolidinediones were added to insulin therapy.

RECOMMENDATIONS

R47 When starting basal insulin therapy:
- continue with metformin and the sulfonylurea (and acarbose, if used)
- review the use of the sulfonylurea if hypoglycaemia occurs.

R48 When starting pre-mixed insulin therapy (or mealtime plus basal insulin regimens):
- continue with metformin
- continue the sulfonylurea initially, but review and discontinue if hypoglycaemia occurs.

R49 Consider combining pioglitazone with insulin therapy for:
- a person who has previously had a marked glucose lowering response to thiazolidinedione therapy
- a person on high-dose insulin therapy whose blood glucose is inadequately controlled.

Warn the person to discontinue pioglitazone if clinically significant fluid retention develops.

11.2 Insulin therapy

11.2.1 Clinical introduction

Blood glucose control deteriorates inexorably in most people with Type 2 diabetes over a period of years, due to a waning of insulin production.[55] In these circumstances oral glucose-lowering therapies can no longer maintain blood glucose control to targets and insulin replacement therapy becomes inevitable. Insulin deficiency is however only relative, not absolute, as there is still considerable endogenous insulin secretion occurring in response to the insulin insensitivity that is also usual in people with Type 2 diabetes. This means that the insulin regimens used in Type 1 diabetes (a condition of absolute insulin deficiency) may not be those needed in people with Type 2 diabetes.

The clinical question is which of the various pharmaceutical types of insulin, and in what combinations, are optimal for the management of Type 2 diabetes, both when initiating insulin and as insulin deficiency further progresses over the years.

11.2.2 Methodological introduction

▷ Biphasic insulin preparations vs NPH

A limited number of clinical studies were identified which compare pre-mixes with NPH insulin.

There were three relevant RCTs. One study[182] compared biphasic insulin aspart 30/70 and NPH insulin in a population of 403 patients with a follow-up of 16 weeks. The other study[183] compared the combination of insulin aspart 30/70 and metformin with the combination of NPH insulin and metformin in a population of 140 patients with a follow-up of 12 weeks. The third study, a cross-over trial, compared a preprandial and basal regimen with insulin lispro and NPH, with a basal only regimen with twice daily NPH in 30 patients spending 12 weeks in each arm before cross-over.[184]

Differing populations, dosing and titration regimens may limit direct comparison between studies.

▷ Biphasic human insulin preparations vs biphasic analogue preparations

A limited number of clinical studies were identified which compare biphasic analogue preparations with biphasic human insulin preparations.

One Cochrane review and meta-analysis was identified on this question.[185] This review was excluded as 88% of the included studies were judged to be of limited methodological quality. Eight studies in Type 2 diabetics had been identified and six studies in Type 1 and Type 2 diabetics. Of the studies included in the meta-analyses on HbA_{1c} and hypoglycaemic episodes outcomes, only one study published post-2001 was included in each analysis.

Two RCTs were identified comparing once daily biphasic insulin analog formulation (insulin aspart containing 30% soluble insulin aspart and 70% insulin aspart crystallised with protamine) with human pre-mixed insulin (30% regular, 70% NPH insulin).[186,187]

The study by Boehm[187] was an extension RCT of Boehm[186] comparing the long-term efficacy of these two formulations. An additional RCT compared three times daily biphasic insulin analog formulation (insulin aspart containing 30% soluble insulin aspart and 70% insulin aspart crystallised with protamine) with once daily human pre-mixed insulin (30% regular, 70% NPH insulin).[188] One RCT compared a three times daily biphasic insulin analog formulation (50% insulin lispro and 50% neutral protamine lispro suspension) with once daily human pre-mixed insulin (30% regular insulin and 70% NPH).[189]

One RCT compared patients on metformin plus either once daily biphasic insulin analog formulation (insulin aspart containing 30% soluble insulin aspart and 70% insulin aspart crystallised with protamine), NPH insulin or human pre-mixed insulin (30% regular, 70% NPH insulin).[183] Another RCT compared a biphasic insulin analogue (insulin aspart containing 30% soluble insulin aspart and 70% insulin aspart crystallised with protamine) with a daily basal-bolus regimen with insulin aspart before meals and evening human isophane insulin (NPH).[190] All studies were on patients with Type 2 diabetes except for one that included patients with Type 1 and Type 2 diabetes.[186]

Three open-label, single dose RCTs with methodological limitations were not considered further.

Differing populations, dosing and titration regimens may limit direct comparison between studies.

▷ Multiple analogue insulin injection regimens compared to basal insulin or biphasic insulin regimens

A limited number of clinical studies were identified in this specific area.

A cohort study relevant to the question[191] conducted in India compared a multiple analogue insulin regimen with a pre-mix regimen in a cohort of 145 participants with a follow-up of 12 weeks.

The cohort study had the following limitations.
- Although described as a prospective study, it seems to be a retrospective collection of patients' data.
- It did not have a placebo-controlled arm.

Only one RCT was found that partially addressed the question.[192] This RCT did not directly compare multiple analogue insulin injection regimens with basal insulin or biphasic insulin regimens. The study was primarily designed to compare two different initiation treatment algorithms with insulin glargine (physician visit-base titration vs patient self-titration) in people with Type 2 diabetes suboptimally controlled on their previous antidiabetic treatment. A separate abstract reported the results for a subgroup of study participants who changed from once daily pre-mix insulin to once daily insulin glargine alone or with prandial insulin and/or oral antidiabetics (OADs). This reported baseline and endpoints values for HbA_{1c} along with incidence of hypoglycaemia among seven groups of patients receiving different basal-bolus regimes with or without OADs.

This subgroup analysis should be interpreted with caution because:
- there was no subgroup treatment protocol to ensure consistent management
- there was only a historical control arm to demonstrate greater clinical efficacy of a multiple insulin regimen over a biphasic insulin regimen.

▷ Long-acting insulin analogues (insulin glargine compared to NPH insulin, biphasic insulins or multiple daily injections)

A NICE technology appraisal (TA)[193] previously reviewed the evidence available until the end of 2001 and made recommendations on the use of insulin glargine in Type 2 diabetes. This guideline updates this appraisal and the GDG considered whether the appraisal recommendations should change in the light of new evidence.

Two meta-analyses[194,195] and 14 further RCTs[178,196–208] were identified which compared a regimen containing insulin glargine with another insulin containing regimen in those with Type 2 diabetes. One RCT compared morning and evening administration of insulin glargine.[209] One RCT compared insulin glargine with an optimised oral diabetic agent treatment arm.[210]

A recent meta-analysis by Horvath[195] compared the long-acting insulin analogues (insulin glargine and insulin determir) with NPH insulin. Only the results of the insulin glargine and NPH comparison are considered here. In this meta-analysis six RCTs were included in the glargine and NPH comparison.[196,199,211–214] A further RCT by Yokohama was mentioned in the study but not included in the meta-analysis.[208]

An older meta-analysis by Rosenstock[194] which contained some of the same studies as the Horvath analysis combined four RCTs[211–214] which compared insulin glargine once daily with NPH insulin once or twice daily (in three studies NPH insulin was administered once daily,[211–213] and in the other study it was administered once or twice daily).[214] Four further RCTs compared once daily insulin glargine with once daily NPH insulin.[196,199,200,206] One RCT was excluded for methodological reasons.[208]

Eight RCTs compared insulin glargine with biphasic insulins.[178,198,201–205,207] In two studies[201,202] an insulin lispro mix 75/25 (75% insulin lispro protamine suspension and 25% insulin lispro) administered twice daily was compared with bedtime insulin glargine. Two further studies compared intensive mixed preprandial regimens with insulin lispro before each meal compared to once daily insulin glargine.[203,205] Another study[178] compared insulin glargine once daily with human pre-mixed insulin (30% regular, 70% NPH insulin) twice daily, however these groups were not directly comparable as metformin and glimepiride were given with the insulin glargine and not with the pre-mixed insulin. Three studies[198,204,207] compared a once daily biphasic insulin analog formulation (insulin aspart containing 30% soluble insulin aspart and 70% insulin aspart crystallised with protamine) with once daily insulin glargine, although in one of these studies[204] glimepiride was added to the glargine arm and metformin to the biphasic arm.

The study that compared morning and evening administration of insulin glargine included glimepiride in both arms.[209]

The review commissioned by NICE,[197,215] on which previous appraisal recommendations were based, noted that in studies where insulin glargine is demonstrated to be superior in controlling nocturnal hypoglycaemia, this may only be apparent when compared with once daily NPH and not twice daily NPH. It is thus notable that no new studies were identified which compared insulin glargine with NPH insulin administered twice daily.

The range of definitions of hypoglycaemia used and differing populations may limit direct comparison between studies.

11.2.3 Meta-analysis

Meta-analyses were conducted (using the Cochrane Collaboration's RevMan software) to investigate the choice of third-line therapies where more than one study was available for a comparison. Interventions considered were:

- human insulin – NPH or a pre-mix of unmodified NPH 30/70
- biphasic analogues (either lispro or aspart) – twice daily
- insulin glargine – once daily
- glitazones (pioglitazone and rosiglitazone)
- exenatide.

Because of the high acquisition costs of these third-line therapies, the pooled point estimates and CI of efficacy were used in a health economic model comparing these treatment options (see below. Full results are shown in appendix C available at www.rcplondon.ac.uk/pubs/brochure.aspx?e=247). The economic model was an adaptation of the UKPDS risk calculations, and in order to supply the risk factors in UKPDS, the following outcomes were sought:

- HbA_{1c}
- systolic blood pressure (SBP)
- total high-density lipoprotein cholesterol (HDL-C)
- smoking status.

Of these, the only outcome where more than one study could be pooled was HbA_{1c}. Change in weight or BMI was not one of the risk factors in UKPDS, and so was addressed in the economic model by sensitivity analyses (see appendix C for more detail available at www.rcplondon.ac.uk/pubs/brochure.aspx?e=247).

Hypoglycaemia was not an outcome variable which could be varied in the UKPDS-based analysis. Accordingly a sensitivity analysis was performed by improving quality of life in insulins in evidence with less hypoglycaemia (see appendix C for more detail available at www.rcplondon.ac.uk/pubs/brochure.aspx?e=247).

The following studies were pooled:

- biphasic analogue vs human insulin: six studies, total N=1,001[182,183,186–189]
- glargine vs human insulin: two studies, total N=591[196,199]
- biphasic analogue vs glargine: three studies, total N=435.[198,201,202]

None of the comparisons had significant heterogeneity but the two studies comparing glargine to human insulin[196,199] had notably different baseline demographics and so a random effects analysis was used in this instance.

The comparison of biphasic analogues with human insulin showed no significant difference.

The comparison of glargine with human insulin showed no significant difference.

The comparison of biphasic analogue with glargine had a pooled weighted mean difference of 0.43% HbA_{1c} (95% CI 0.40 to 0.46) in favour of biphasic analogues. This analysis was dominated by one large trial[198] but all three trials showed significant differences in the same direction of effect, which supports the validity of the pooled result.

11.2.4 Health economic methodological introduction

Two studies were found that compared the cost-effectiveness of glargine insulin with other forms of insulin.[193,216] Both studies were based on meta-analysis and used the UKPDS outcomes model to predict events and costs. However, they did not take in to account the impact on quality of life of AEs such as weight gain and vomiting.

For this guideline, an economic model was constructed based upon the UKPDS outcomes model to inform the GDG with regard to the cost-effectiveness of various third-line therapy options. This is presented in appendix C available at www.rcplondon.ac.uk/pubs/brochure.aspx?e=247

11.2.5 Evidence statements

Insulin glargine was not included in the Type 2 diabetes guideline 2002 under review. However, it was the subject of a NICE TA at that time, and the current review is an update of that.

▷ Biphasic insulin preparations vs NPH

HbA$_{1c}$

The two studies[182,183] found that HbA$_{1c}$ levels decreased linearly and statistically significantly in both treatment groups (biphasic insulin aspart 30/70 and NPH insulin) compared to baseline values. There was not a significant statistical difference between the two interventions. **Level 1+**

The third study found a significantly greater reduction in HbA$_{1c}$ in the lispro and NPH arm than in the twice daily NPH arm (p<0.01).[184] **Level 1+**

▷ Fasting blood glucose/fasting plasma glucose

In patients receiving either biphasic insulin aspart 30/70 or NPH insulin, studies[182,183] showed similar reductions from baseline in FBG/FPG values. There was however no statistically significant difference between the two interventions. **Level 1+**

▷ Postprandial blood/plasma glucose

One study[182] reported that the mean prandial glucose increment over the three main meals was significantly lower in the aspart 30/70 group than in the NPH group, (0.69 mmol/l lower; p<0.0001, between groups.) **Level 1+**

The other study[183] found no significant differences between the groups regarding the mean values for the 8-point self-monitoring of blood glucose (SMBG) profile at week twelve. The study reported that SMBG values for before breakfast and before lunch values tended to be lower for the NPH insulin group, while after dinner and 10 pm, values tended to be higher for the NPH insulin group as compared to the biphasic insulin aspart. **Level 1+**

In the insulin lispro vs NPH comparison, the postprandial glucose excursion was significantly lower in the lispro arm (p<0.001).[184] **Level 1+**

▷ Body weight

Two studies[183,184] found non-significant differences in terms of body weight gain between the biphasic insulins and NPH. **Level 1+**

▷ Adverse events

Both studies comparing insulin aspart with NPH[182,183] concluded that the number and type of AEs were similar for each of the treatment groups with non-significant differences between them. **Level 1+**

One study[182] found that in terms of incidence of hypoglycaemia, the RR was not statistically significantly different between treatments (RR=1.21 (95% CI 0.77 to 1.90), p=0.40). The other study reported that there was no significant difference between regimens for either overall or nocturnal hypoglycaemia.[184] **Level 1+**

The other study[183] found that nocturnal hypoglycaemia (midnight–6 am) was less frequently reported for patients receiving biphasic insulin aspart (seven patients) as compared to patients in the NPH insulin group (11 patients). No statistical analysis was reported. **Level 1+**

▷ Lipid profile

One study[184] reported changes in lipid measures between groups and found a significantly lower fasting low-density lipoprotein cholesterol (LDL-C) and LDL-C/HDL-C ratio in the biphasic insulin (lispro) and NPH arm compared with twice daily NPH (p=0.035). After a standard meal both LDL-C (p=0.012) and HDL-C (p=0.004) were significantly higher in the biphasic insulin (lispro) and NPH arm compared with twice daily NPH arm. **Level 1+**

Table 11.3 Biphasic human insulin preparations vs biphasic analogue preparations

	RCT[188] Three times daily biphasic insulin aspart vs once daily human pre-mixed insulin N=177 Duration: 24 weeks	RCT[186] Twice daily biphasic insulin aspart vs once daily human pre-mixed insulin N=294 Duration: 12 weeks *Type 1 and 2 diabetes	RCT[187] Twice daily biphasic insulin aspart vs once daily human pre-mixed insulin N=125 Duration: 24 months	RCT[183] Metformin plus: once daily biphasic insulin aspart or NPH insulin or human pre-mixed insulin N=140 Duration: 12 weeks	RCT[189] Three times daily biphasic insulin aspart vs once daily human pre-mixed insulin N=40 Duration: 12 weeks	RCT[190] Three times daily biphasic insulin aspart vs a basal-bolus regiment using insulin aspart before meals and NPH at bedtime N=394 Duration: 16 weeks
Mean HbA$_{1c}$ at endpoint	NS	NS	NS	NS	7.6±1.1 vs 8.1±1.4%; p=0.021, mean change from baseline (favouring biphasic insulin aspart)	Mean difference in HbA$_{1c}$ at end: –0.05 (upper limit of 95% CI 0.14% (which is below the non-inferiority criterion of 0.4%) non-inferiority demonstrated)

continued

Table 11.3 Biphasic human insulin preparations vs biphasic analogue preparations – *continued*

	RCT[188] Three times daily biphasic insulin aspart vs once daily human pre-mixed insulin N=177 Duration: 24 weeks	RCT[186] Twice daily biphasic insulin aspart vs once daily human pre-mixed insulin N=294 Duration: 12 weeks *Type 1 and 2 diabetes	RCT[187] Twice daily biphasic insulin aspart vs once daily human pre-mixed insulin N=125 Duration: 24 months	RCT[183] Metformin plus: once daily biphasic insulin aspart or NPH insulin or human pre-mixed insulin N=140 Duration: 12 weeks	RCT[189] Three times daily biphasic insulin aspart vs once daily human pre-mixed insulin N=40 Duration: 12 weeks	RCT[190] Three times daily biphasic insulin aspart vs a basal-bolus regiment using insulin aspart before meals and NPH at bedtime N=394 Duration: 16 weeks
FPG	–	NS	–	NS	Pre-breakfast: 177.7±9.6 vs 147.4±6.3 mg/dl, p<0.001 (favouring human pre-mixed insulin)	–
PPG	Lunch (156 vs 176 mg/dl, p=0.0289), Before dinner (142 vs 166 mg/dl, p=0.0069) After dinner (154 vs 182 mg/dl, p=0.0022) Mean blood glucose range: 104 vs 123 mg/dl; p=0.0111 blood glucose increment (over all three meals) 25 vs 37 mg/dl; p=0.02111 (all favouring biphasic insulin aspart)	After breakfast (10.40 (0.37) vs 11.40 (0.36); p<0.05) Before lunch (6.64 (0.28) vs 7.57 (0.27); p<0.02) After dinner (9.22 (0.33) vs 10.20 (0.32); p<0.02) Bedtime (8.22 (0.31) vs 9.10 (0.30); p<0.05) blood glucose increment (over all three meals) 1.66 (0.22) vs 2.34 (0.19 mmol/l; p<0.02) (all favouring biphasic insulin aspart)	–	–	After lunch (155.6±5.8 vs 192.2±8.5 mg/dl; p<0.001) After dinner (166.3±7.2 vs 198.2±10.0 mg/dl; p<0.001) (flavouring biphasic insulin aspart)	No statistically significant difference between the treatments found in 8-point PG profiles, mean values of PG, average prandial PG increment profiles
Body weight	–	NS	NS	NS	–	NS
Hypoglycaemia Major	NS	NS	2nd year N=0 (0%) vs N=6 (10%; p=0.04) (favouring biphasic insulin aspart)	NS	NS	NS
Minor	NS	NS	NS	NS	NS	NS
Nocturnal	NS	NS (major and minor)	–	NS	–	NS
AEs	NS	NS	NS	NS	NS	NS

PPG, postprandial glucose

▷ HbA$_{1c}$

Overall, on endpoint means HbA$_{1c}$ levels biphasic analogue preparations were comparable to human pre-mixed insulin,[183,186,187,188] as well as to a basal-bolus regimen of insulin aspart and NPH.[190] **Level 1+**

One RCT found three times daily biphasic insulin lispro (50/50) gave a significantly greater reduction from baseline in mean HbA$_{1c}$ values compared with once daily pre-mixed human insulin 30/70.[189] **Level 1+**

▷ Fasting blood glucose

Two RCTs found no significant differences among the treatment groups on FBG.[186,183] **Level 1+**

One RCT found that FBG was significantly increased in patients on three times daily biphasic analogue insulin compared with once daily human pre-mixed insulin.[189] **Level 1+**

▷ Postprandial glucose

In terms of PPG, three RCTs reported significant treatment differences in favour of biphasic insulin aspart.[188,186,189] **Level 1+**

▷ Bodyweight

No studies reported any significant differences between treatment groups.[186,187,183,190] **Level 1+**

▷ Adverse events

Studies reported similar AEs profiles for biphasic analogue insulin and biphasic human insulin.[188,186,187,183,189,190] **Level 1+**

▷ Hypoglycaemia

Overall, few major hypoglycaemic episodes were associated with either biphasic analogue or human insulin.[188,186,183,189,190] **Level 1+**

A longer-term efficacy study found that during the second year of treatment significantly fewer patients in the once daily biphasic analogue insulin than the human pre-mixed insulin group experienced a major episode.[187] **Level 1++**

No study reported any significant differences between treatments on minor or nocturnal hypoglycaemic episodes.[188,186,183,190] **Level 1+**

▷ Multiple analogue insulin injection regimens compared to basal insulin or biphasic insulin regimens

HbA$_{1c}$

For HbA$_{1c}$ levels the cohort study reported that both multiple insulin regimen and pre-mix insulin regimen lowered HbA$_{1c}$ levels significantly compared to baseline values. Pre-mix insulin analogue fared better than the basal-bolus analogue therapy in lowering HbA$_{1c}$ (1.58%

vs 1.16% respectively, p<0.05). Also 41% more patients in the pre-mix group could achieve target HbA$_{1c}$ of <7% at the end of 12 weeks (45.61% vs 32.26%). **Level 2+**

▷ FPG/PPPG

Both regimes lowered FPG and postprandial plasma glucose (PPPG) levels significantly as compared to baseline. No statistical comparison was performed between groups. **Level 2+**

▷ Body weight

The body weight did not change significantly in either group at the end of the study. **Level 2+**

▷ Hypoglycaemia events

The percentage of patients experiencing minor hypoglycaemia was significantly lower in the pre-mix group than in the basal-bolus group at 12 weeks (16.7% vs 58.06%, p<0.05). **Level 2+**

Throughout the study period of 12 weeks, there were no major hypoglycaemic episodes reported in both the treatment groups. **Level 2+**

▷ Subgroup analysis

The analysis of the sub-population previously receiving pre-mix insulin suggests that optimisation of basal insulin therapy with once daily insulin glargine is safe (according to the low incidence of severe hypoglycaemic events) and results in significant improvements in glycaemia control.

The same analysis indicates that once daily insulin glargine in combination with prandial therapies (prandial insulin and/or OADs) offers additional glycaemic benefits.

▷ Long-acting insulin analogues (insulin glargine compared to NPH insulin, biphasic insulins or multiple daily injections)

NB. Glargine and its comparators are often used in these studies in combination with OAD medications. For simplicity, references to these drugs are not included in the evidence statements unless they differ between the two groups.

Table 11.4 Insulin glargine vs NPH insulin

	Meta-analysis[195] Bedtime insulin glargine vs NPH once or twice daily N=3,151 Duration: 6–12 months	Meta-analysis[194] Bedtime insulin glargine vs NPH once or twice daily N=2,304 Duration: 24–28 weeks	RCT[196] Bedtime insulin glargine vs bedtime NPH N=110 Duration: 36 weeks	RCT[200] Insulin glargine once daily vs once daily NPH N=204 Duration: 4 weeks	RCT[199] Bedtime insulin glargine vs bedtime NPH N=481 Duration: 24 weeks	RCT[206] Bedtime insulin glargine vs bedtime NPH N=443 Duration: 24 weeks
Proportion achieving 7% HbA_{1c} target	–	NS	–	–	NS (7.5% target)	NS (7.5% target)
Mean HbA_{1c} at endpoint	WMD of change of HbA_{1c} from baseline to study endpoint: NS	NS	NS	NS	NS	Change in mean HbA_{1c} at endpoint greater in glargine group (−0.99% vs −0.77%, p=0.003)
FPG	–	8±0.1 vs 9±0.0 mmol/l (p=0.02) at endpoint	5.75±0.02 vs 5.96±0.03 mmol/l (p<0.001) (mean values in last 12 weeks of the study)	NS	NS (FBG)	NS
Insulin dose	–	NS	NS	NS	–	NS
Body weight	–	–	NS	NS	–	NS
Hypoglycaemia: overall rates	Symptomatic and overall hypoglycaemia. RR 0.84 (0.75, 0.95) p=0.005 in favour of glargine	11% risk reduction with insulin glargine in documented symptomatic hypoglycaemia (p=0.0006). 46% risk reduction with insulin glargine in documented severe hypoglycaemia (p=0.04)	4.1±0.8 vs 9.0±2.3 episodes/patient year (p<0.05) of symptomatic but not confirmed hypoglycaemia during the first 12 weeks. NS thereafter	NS	27% risk reduction with insulin glargine in documented symptomatic hypoglycaemia (p=0.042)	Number of hypoglycaemic episodes lower in glargine group (682 vs 1019; p<0.004)
Nocturnal	Symptomatic nocturnal hypoglycaemia. RR 0.66 (0.55, 0.80) p<0.0001 in favour of glargine	26% risk reduction in nocturnal hypoglycaemia (p<0.0001). 59% risk reduction in severe nocturnal hypoglycaemia (p<0.02)	–	7.3% vs 19.1%; (p=0.0123) of patients experienced symptomatic nocturnal hypoglycaemia	22% risk reduction with insulin glargine compared to NPH insulin (p<0.001) and this was 19% for confirmed nocturnal events (p<0.01)	Number of hypoglycaemic episodes lower in glargine group (221 vs 620; p<0.001)
Daytime	–	NS	–	NS	–	–
AEs	NS (no meta-analysis)	NS	NS	NS	NS	NS

Table 11.5 Insulin glargine vs biphasic insulins

	RCT[201] Bedtime insulin glargine vs twice daily insulin lispro mix 75/25 N=105 Duration: 32 weeks	RCT[202] Bedtime insulin glargine vs twice daily insulin lispro mix 75/25 N=97 Duration: 32 weeks	RCT[198] Bedtime insulin glargine vs a twice daily biphasic insulin analogue 70/30 N=233 Duration: 28 weeks	RCT[207] Bedtime insulin glargine vs a twice daily biphasic insulin analogue 70/30 N=157 Duration: 28 weeks	RCT[205] Bedtime insulin glargine vs insulin lispro thrice daily vs insulin lispro mid mixture (50% lispro/50% NPL) thrice daily N=159 Duration: 24 weeks	RCT cross over[203] Bedtime insulin glargine vs insulin lispro 50/50 at breakfast and lunch and lispro 25/75 in evening N=60 Duration: 8 months	RCT[178] Morning insulin glargine plus glimepiride and metformin vs twice daily human remixed insulin 70/30 N=371 Duration: 24 weeks	RCT[204] Insulin glargine once daily plus glimepiride vs biphasic insulin analogue 70/30 twice daily plus metformin N=255 Duration: 26 weeks
Decrease in HbA$_{1c}$ from baseline	$-0.9\%\pm0.9$ vs $-3.1\%\pm1.0\%$ p=0.003	$-0.42\%\pm0.92\%$ vs $-1.0\%\pm0.85\%$ p<0.001	$-2.36\%\pm\pm0.11\%$ vs $-2.79\%\pm0.11\%$ p<0.01	$-2.46\pm1.6\%$ vs $-2.89\pm1.6\%$ p=0.035	$-0.3\pm1.1\%$ vs $-1.1\pm1.1\%$ (p=0.001) vs $-1.2\pm1.1\%$ p<0.001	$-1.76\pm0.11\%$ vs -1.98 ± 0.11 p=0.0083	-1.64 vs -1.31%, p=0.0003	Mean difference in HbA$_{1c}$ from baseline: -0.5 (-0.8, -0.2) p=0.0002 (corrected for baseline)
Mean HbA$_{1c}$ at endpoint	$7.8\%\pm1.1\%$ vs $7.4\%\pm1.1\%$ p=0.002	$8.14\%\pm1.03\%$ vs $7.54\%\pm0.87\%$ p<0.001	$7.41\pm1.24\%$ vs 6.91 ± 1.17 p<0.01	$7.4\pm1.3\%$ vs $7.0\pm1.3\%$ p=0.035	–	$7.34\pm0.11\%$ vs $7.08\pm0.11\%$ p=0.003	–	$7.9\pm1.3\%$ vs $7.5\pm1.1\%$ p=0.01
Proportion achieving 7% HbA$_{1c}$ target	18% vs 42% p=0.002	12% vs 30% p=0.002	40% vs 66%, p<0.001 (HbA$_{1c}$ <7.0%)	41% vs 65% p=0.03	24.5% vs 40.4% vs 59.3% (p not given)	31% vs 44% NS	NS	NS
Mean FBG at endpoint	123.9 mg/dl±34.9 vs 139.3±36.6 mg/dl p<0.001	7.39±1.96 vs 7.9±1.92 mmol/l p=0.007	–	Mean reduction in FPG NS	Mean reduction -2.6 ± 2.4 mmol/l vs -0.9 ± 2.2 mmol/l (p<0.001 vs $+0.9\pm1.8$ mmol/l (p<0.001)	NS	-0.9 mmol/l (95%CI -1.3 to -0.6) adjusted mean between treatment difference in favour of glargine	NS
Insulin dose	0.57±0.37 U/kg vs 0.62±0.37 U/kg p<0.001	0.36±0.18 U/kg vs 0.42±0.20 U/kg p<0.001	0.55±0.27 U/kg vs 0.82±0.40 U/kg p<0.05	0.57±0.30 IU/kg vs 0.91±0.40 IU/kg p not given	0.43±0.22 IU/(kg day) vs 0.50±0.23 IU/(kg day) 0.59±0.30 IU/(kg day) p<0.005	0.276±0.207 IU/kg vs 0.353± 0.256 IU/kg p=0.0107	28.2 IU vs 64.5 IU	0.39 IU/kg vs 0.40 IU/kg p=0.65

Mean change in body weight	1.6±4.0 kg vs 2.3±4.0 kg p=0.006	0.06±2.49 kg vs 0.82±2.56 kg p=0.001	3.5±4.5 kg. vs 5.4±4.8 kg p<0.01	3.0±4.3 kg vs 5.6±4.6 kg p=0.0004	0.7±3.8 kg vs 2.3±4.3 kg vs 1.8±3.4 kg (p not given) BMI increase significantly greater in lispro vs glargine	NS	NS	–
Hypoglycaemia: overall rates	0.39±1.24 vs 0.68±1.38 episodes/patient per 30 days p=0.041	NS	0.7±2.0 vs 3.4±6.6 episodes per patient year p<0.05	Proportion of participants reporting at least one hypoglycaemic event: 42% vs 68% p=0.0013	1.0 per 100 patient days vs 1.4 per 100 patient days vs 1.5 per 100 patient days (p not given)	2.57±3.22 vs 3.98±4.74 episodes/patient/30 days p=0.0013	4.07 vs 9.87 mean number of confirmed hypo-glycaemic events; p<0.0001	Proportion of patients experiencing minor hypoglycaemic episodes; 9% vs 20.3% p=0.0124
Nocturnal	NS	0.34±0.85 vs 0.14±0.49 episodes/patient/30 days p=0.002	–	Proportion reporting nocturnal hypoglycaemia: 10% vs 25% p=0.021	–	NS	0.51 vs 1.04 mean number of confirmed nocturnal hypoglycaemic events per patient years p<0.0449	–
Daytime	–	0.10±0.51 vs 0.46±1.28 vs episodes/patient/30 days p=0.003	–	–	–	–	–	–
AEs	NS	NS	NS	NS	NS	–	NS	NS

IU, A/Q; WMD, weighted mean differences

None of the studies[194–196,199,200,206] reported differences between the insulin glargine and NPH groups in terms of proportion of patients achieving target HbA$_{1c}$, insulin dose, body weight, daytime hypoglycaemia or AEs. One study found a significantly greater reduction in the mean HbA$_{1c}$ at endpoint in the insulin glargine arm.[206] Five studies[194–196,199,206] found significant risk reductions in overall risk of hypoglycaemia with insulin glargine compared to NPH insulin (one only in the first 12 weeks)[196] while the shorter study found no difference.[200] Five studies[194,195,199,200,206] reported significant risk reductions in terms of nocturnal hypoglycaemia with insulin glargine compared to NPH insulin. Additionally, FPG values were significantly lower at endpoint in the glargine groups in two studies[196,214] but showed no significant difference in the shorter study.[200] **Level 1+**

Seven studies[198,201–205,207] reported better HbA$_{1c}$ outcomes with the insulin mixes compared to insulin glargine. The other study found significantly higher reductions in HbA$_{1c}$ with insulin glargine from baseline, however insulin glargine was combined with OAD drugs which were not received by the insulin mix group.[178] With respect to decreases in FBG from baseline results, they were less consistent. Statistically significant decreases in FBG were reported in insulin glargine groups compared to the insulin mix groups in four studies,[178,201,202,205] although three studies did not find a significant difference.[203,204,207] Insulin doses were higher in the insulin mix groups in all studies.[178,198,201–205,207] In five studies the insulin mix groups had significantly increased body weight from baseline compared with insulin glargine.[198,201,202,205,207] Two studies found no significant difference in body weight change between the groups[178,203] and the remaining study[204] reported a greater weight increase in the insulin glargine and glimepiride group than in the biphasic insulin analogue and metformin group although they did not report if this was statistically significant. In terms of hypoglycaemia, one study found no significant difference[202] in overall hypoglycaemia rates, while the remaining studies[178,198,201,203–205,207] found overall hypoglycaemia rates were better with insulin glargine than insulin mixes. For nocturnal hypoglycaemia, two studies reported no significant difference between the groups,[201,203] another found higher rates in the glargine group[202] and two others found significantly reduced rates in that group compared to the insulin mix group.[178,207] Only one study reported daytime hypoglycaemia rates and these were found to be significantly higher in the insulin mix group.[202] No significant differences between the groups were reported in terms of AEs.[178,198,201,202,204,205,207] **Level 1+**

▷ Morning vs evening administration of insulin glargine

Standl et al.[209] compared insulin glargine delivered at different times of the day to determine the impact on glycaemic control and rates of hypoglycaemia. It was found that morning and evening administration of glargine was equivalent with respect to the incidence of nocturnal hypoglycaemia. Similar improvements in HbA$_{1c}$, FBG and the proportion of patients achieving an HbA$_{1c}$ of less than 7% was demonstrated in the two arms of the study, without any difference in the incidence of AEs. **Level 1+**

▷ Insulin glargine vs oral therapy

Gerstein et al.[210] compared the addition of insulin glargine to current treatment with the intensified oral glucose-lowering therapy. HbA$_{1c}$ outcomes were reported to be significantly better in the glargine group even after adjusting for baseline HbA$_{1c}$ and oral therapy. FPG was also significantly lower and lipid parameters were significantly improved in the glargine group.

There was no significant difference in hypoglycaemia, and the glargine group had a significantly greater weight increase. **Level 1+**

11.2.6 Health economic evidence statements

In the long-acting insulin TA[193] there was an estimated cost-effectiveness ratio of £33,000 compared to NPH insulin, using the price of a vial of glargine. Using cartridges or pens gave higher cost-effectiveness ratios, £41,000 and £43,000 respectively. The results were most sensitive to the assumption on utility gained from reducing fear of hypoglycaemia. If it was assumed that there was no utility gain from this then the cost-effectiveness ratio rose to approximately £10 million per QALY.

The second study[216] found a cost-effectiveness ratio of £13,000 per QALY gained compared to NPH insulin. But it did not take into account the disutility associated with the side effects of insulin glargine and no comparison was made with other third-line therapies.

The base-case results of the analysis of third-line therapy conducted for this guideline (see appendix C available at www.rcplondon.ac.uk/pubs/brochure.aspx?e=247) found that human insulin was as effective but less expensive than biphasic insulin, and more effective and less expensive than insulin glargine.

11.2.7 From evidence to recommendations

▷ Pre-mix insulin

There was limited evidence for comparisons of pre-mix insulin with NPH insulin in people with diabetes. Because of the use of unselected populations of people with Type 2 diabetes taking little account of factors such as degree of insulin deficiency, high or low mealtime insulin requirement, diurnal patterns of blood glucose control, and sensitivity to hypoglycaemia, the studies did not help inform clinical decision making. These insulins, compared to basal insulins, target postprandial blood glucose control. The issue of whether postprandial blood glucose control was of any specific importance, rather than being important because glucose levels are highest at that time, is not being addressed in this guideline. There was confidence that no health outcome studies on the issue had been published. The GDG felt that it was inappropriate to make strong recommendations promoting pre-mix insulin over NPH or the opposite, except to observe that as insulin deficiency progressed mealtime insulin therapy would be more likely to be indicated.

There was limited evidence on the comparisons between insulin analogue pre-mixes and human insulin pre-mixes. There was definite evidence statistically of some reduction in postprandial blood glucose control in the period after injection when using an analogue rather than human insulin, as was to be expected from other data with rapid-acting insulin analogues. Equally there was some data on the reduction of hypoglycaemia, consistent with other analogue data. These effects were clinically quite small and therefore of questionable cost-effectiveness, a view supported by the health economic modelling.

Unfortunately all comparative trials had been performed using different recommendations of timing of insulin injection before meals for human and analogue insulins (in line with licences). The advantage of injecting immediately before meals (usually twice a day) in daily life to people with diabetes was felt to be a significant quality of life issue justifying the use of the analogues. Studies asking whether human insulin pre-mixes could be given immediately before meals without deterioration of blood glucose control (hyperglycaemia early and hypoglycaemia late) compared to analogues had not been performed.

▷ Basal insulins including long-acting insulin analogues

The previous guidance for use of insulin glargine endorsed its use in people with Type 2 diabetes where the injections were given by a carer, where hypoglycaemia was a problem when using NPH insulin, and where insulin administration would otherwise require twice daily insulin injections. The studies performed since were a useful contribution not only to the understanding of insulin glargine, but more so, to the optimal use of insulin in people with Type 2 diabetes, in particular for people starting insulin therapy.

Very little useful information was found to assist in advising on the optimal insulin regimen once progression of islet B-cell failure had progressed further, for example in people 3–5 years or more after starting insulin therapy. The observational study from India was open to bias in patient and provider selection, and the subgroup analysis from A Trial comparing Lantus® Algorithms to achieve Normal blood glucose Targets in patients with Uncontrolled blood Sugar (AT.LANTUS) was similarly open to bias and in small numbers of people. The preferred view was that as islet B-cell deficiency progressed people tended to a state of insulin deficiency closer to those with Type 1 diabetes, suggesting that prior NICE guidelines advice for that group of patients could be applied.

The strongest of the new evidence for insulin starters appeared to relate to comparisons with NPH insulin, and of these the data on comparison with once daily (bedtime) human NPH insulin was the most novel. It was noted that these treat-to-target studies have the problem, given their limited duration, of driving control in the compared groups towards the same levels, and indeed pre-breakfast glucose levels and HbA_{1c} were similar for insulin glargine and NPH, at similar insulin doses. The differences in nocturnal hypoglycaemia were convincing, if small in absolute terms. Despite post hoc analyses of the relationship between HbA_{1c} and nocturnal hypoglycaemia showing convincing advantage of insulin glargine over NPH insulin, it was impossible to determine what the balance of advantage between the two measures would be in real clinical practice, where differences in hypoglycaemia tend to drive differences in insulin dosage and thus overall blood glucose control (which would be to the advantage of the long-acting analogue).

Although not the subject themselves of a randomised comparison, the approaches used in the treat-to-target studies of active dose titration in the context of appropriate education, self-monitoring and support were an important means of obtaining optimal blood glucose control whatever insulin was employed.

An issue relates to the choice of insulin preparation for starting insulin in people with Type 2 diabetes. As noted above, and provided that insulin was started reasonably early in the disease process before HbA_{1c} had deteriorated too far, there was little justification for the use of more intensive mealtime plus basal insulin regimens in this situation. The studies comparing insulin glargine with pre-mix insulin regimens gave mixed results, with improved HbA_{1c} apparently resulting from an ability to titrate twice daily insulin dosage faster (in total) than once daily injections, but at a cost of increased hypoglycaemia and weight gain. These results and the absence of longer term data on performance of the two regimens, together with complexities such as the possibility of using three injections of pre-mix, or of adding mealtime insulin to basal glargine, meant that the GDG was unable to identify overall advantage to one approach or the other.

The previous NICE guidance in relation to a single daily injection of insulin glargine not having to be given at any precise time was noted to be useful for those whose injections are given by others.

The GDG found the health economic modelling problematic in the area of insulin therapy. Major problems seem to relate to the difficulties of including fear of hypoglycaemia and its effect on everyday lifestyle, restrictions on lifestyle with insulin injections, and the present day educational costs associated with intensive insulin dose adjustment to achieve good target control. While some attempts had been made to incorporate some of these in sensitivity analyses, it was not possible to be sure of their validity, though the face value results all suggested that human insulin regimens were the only cost-effective approach.

RECOMMENDATIONS

R50   When other measures no longer achieve adequate blood glucose control to HbA_{1c} <7.5% or other higher level agreed with the individual, discuss the benefits and risks of insulin therapy. Start insulin therapy if the person agrees.

R51   When starting insulin therapy, use a structured programme employing active insulin dose titration that encompasses:
- structured education
- continuing telephone support
- frequent self-monitoring
- dose titration to target
- dietary understanding
- management of hypoglycaemia
- management of acute changes in plasma glucose control
- support from an appropriately trained and experienced healthcare professional.

R52   Insulin therapy should be initiated from a choice of a number of insulin types and regimens.
- Preferably begin with human NPH insulin, taken at bedtime or twice daily according to need.
- Consider, as an alternative, using a long-acting insulin analogue (insulin glargine) for a person who falls into one of the following categories:
  - those who require assistance from a carer or healthcare professional to administer their insulin injections
  - those whose lifestyle is significantly restricted by recurrent symptomatic hypoglycaemic episodes
  - those who would otherwise need twice daily basal insulin injections in combination with oral glucose-lowering medications.
- Consider twice-daily biphasic human insulin (pre-mix) regimens in particular where HbA_{1c} is elevated above 9.0 %. A once-daily regimen may be an option when initiating this therapy.

- Consider pre-mixed preparations of insulin analogues rather than pre-mixed human insulin preparations when:
  - immediate injection before a meal is preferred, or
  - hypoglycaemia is a problem, or
  - there are marked postprandial blood glucose excursions.

R53   Offer a trial of insulin glargine if a person who has started with NPH insulin experiences significant nocturnal hypoglycaemia.

R54   Monitor a person using a basal insulin regimen (NPH or a long-acting insulin analogue (insulin glargine) for the need for mealtime insulin (or a pre-mixed insulin preparation)). If blood glucose control remains inadequate (not to agreed target levels without problematic hypoglycaemia), move to a more intensive, mealtime plus basal insulin regimen based on the option of human or analogue insulins.

R55   Monitor a person using pre-mixed insulin once or twice daily for the need for a further preprandial injection or for an eventual change to a mealtime plus basal insulin regimen, based on human or analogue insulins, if blood glucose control remains inadequate.

11.3 Insulin detemir

The GDG considered including sitagliptin and insulin detemir in this guideline; however, they were advised by NICE not to do so. NICE is undertaking a rapid update of recommendations in this guideline on second- and third-line drugs for managing blood glucose, which will cover these drugs. The updated guideline will be published early in 2009. For more information see www.nice.org.uk and search for 'Type 2 diabetes newer agents'.

11.4 Insulin delivery devices

Insulin pumps are not considered here; they have been the subject of a recent NICE TA, and are not widely used in people with Type 2 diabetes.[217]

11.4.1 Clinical introduction

Insulin was previously normally delivered from syringes, necessitating accurate measuring of insulin doses drawn up from insulin vials under suitably hygienic conditions. Modern pen-injector devices obviate most of the problems of measuring up doses while avoiding most of the hygiene problems, and offer a convenient and safe means of carrying around injection equipment. However, several models of injector are available, including some designed for those with visual and physical impairments.

The clinical question addressed here was whether any particular pen-injector had an evidence-based advantage over any other, including groups of people with difficulty using such devices.

11.4.2 Methodological introduction

Six crossover RCTs were identified which compared insulin pens or other delivery systems with conventional syringes.[219–224] One study was excluded for methodological reasons.[224] Two crossover RCTs were also identified which compared different types of insulin pens.[220,225]

This area was not covered in detail by the previous guideline, and studies were only searched for from 1995 onwards to prevent the inclusion of obsolete devices.

None of these studies were of a particularly high methodological quality with few reporting any details of randomisation, concealment or a power analysis. Few studies took into account the insulin delivery method that patients had used previously. Most studies assessed patient preference by use of their own specifically developed for purpose questionnaires; it was notable that some of these contained 'leading' questions.

11.4.3 Health economic methodological introduction

No health economic papers were identified for this question.

11.4.4 Evidence statements: syringes vs other insulin delivery systems

▷ Glycaemic control

One study found pre-lunch blood glucose values were lower during pen treatment (p<0.01) but no other significant differences were found between pens and syringes for blood glucose profiles or in terms of HbA$_{1c}$.[219] Three other studies found no differences between syringes and other delivery devices in terms of glycaemic control.[221–223] **Level 1+**

▷ Hypoglycaemic episodes and adverse events

Two studies noted no significant difference in the incidence of hypoglycaemic episodes between pens and syringe treatments.[219,221] In other studies no AEs were considered by the investigator to be related to study treatment[223] or the safety profiles for pen and the vial/syringe appeared similar.[222] **Level 1+**

▷ Main patient acceptance outcomes

Operational use

In one study patients starting insulin using a pen found the insulin injections easy (63%) or very easy (33%) at the end of 12 weeks, whilst those who commenced insulin with conventional syringes found it more difficult with only 24% finding it very easy by the end of 12 weeks and 51% finding it easy (p=0.0005).[221] **Level 1+**

Other studies (which did not report significance) found that the operations needed for insulin administration with a pen compared to a syringe were faster (88%)[219] and that the pen device was found easier to use overall compared to the syringe (74% vs 21% respectively).[222] **Level 1+**

In a study of patients with motor dysfunction and/or visual problems, an insulin injection device with a large easy-to-read dial, large push button for injection and audible clicks for each unit injected, was found to be easier to use compared to a vial and syringe by 82% of patients with the practical aspects of the injection device (dosing and injecting) rated as very easy or easy by 86%.[223] **Level 1+**

A study of visually impaired patients found that 80% were able to set and dispense three insulin doses after written instructions when using the insulin injection device with easy-to-read dial, large button for injection and audible clicks for units injected. This was significantly more than those using a syringe (27%, p<0.001) or a pen device (61%, p<0.001).[220] **Level 1+**

Pre-selection of dose

A study comparing a pen with a conventional syringe and vial found that setting and drawing up the dose of insulin was significantly easier for patients using the pen (p=0.0490).[221] **Level 1+**

Other studies (which did not report significance) reported that 86% of participants found that pre-selection of insulin dose with a pen was easier than insulin withdrawal from a vial with a conventional syringe[219] and that 85% of patients reported that they found it easier to read the insulin dose scale with the pen than the vial/syringe (10% found reading the insulin dose scale easier using the vial/syringe).[222] **Level 1+**

Pain

A study found that injection pain was significantly lower with a pen than with syringes and vials (p=0.0018). Patients commencing on syringes reported a significantly lower level of injection pain after the switch to using the pen (p=0.0003).[221] Another study reported participants found insulin injections with the pen, compared to the conventional syringe, were 55% less painful, although 43% did not notice any difference.[219] **Level 1+**

Preference for a device

In the study of patients with motor dysfunction and/or visual problems, the insulin injection device with the easy-to-read dial, large button for injection and audible clicks for units injected, was significantly preferred to the vial and syringe (82% vs 10%, p<0.001).[223] **Level 1+**

In all studies comparing pens with conventional syringes more patients stated a preference for the pens over the conventional syringe and vial.[219–222] **Level 1+**

▷ Insulin delivery devices vs other insulin delivery devices

NovoPen® 3 vs HumaPen Ergo® vs Humalog Pen® vs InnoLet® vs FlexPen®

Auditory confirmation of dose setting was heard by 100% of study participants for NovoPen® 3, 98% for FlexPen®, 90% for InnoLet®, 75% for HumaPen Ergo® and 63% for the Humalog Pen®. This was significantly different between the NovoPen® 3 and the Humalog Pen® (p<0.001), the HumaPen Ergo® (p<0.001), and InnoLet® (p<0.01), and the FlexPen® and the Humalog Pen® (p<0.001), and HumaPen Ergo® (p<0.01).[225] **Level 1+**

For tactile feedback, (the proportion of patients physically sensing they had dialled a correct dose) this was 100% for the FlexPen®, 92% for the NovoPen® 3, 81% InnoLet®, 67% HumaPen

Ergo® and 50% for the Humalog Pen®. Significantly more patients reported that they had dialled the correct dose for the FlexPen® compared with the Humalog Pen® (p<0.001), HumaPen Ergo® (p<0.001) and InnoLet® (p<0.01). Significant differences were also noted between the NovoPen® 3 and Humalog Pen® (p<0.001) and the HumaPen Ergo® (p<0.01).[225] **Level 1+**

Patients reported most confidence in setting the correct dose when rating the NovoPen® 3 and FlexPen®. Scores for the NovoPen® 3 were significantly higher than those for the InnoLet® (p<0.001), HumaPen Ergo® (p<0.001) and Humalog Pen® (p<0.001), whereas the FlexPen® scored significantly higher than the Humalog Pen® (p<0.01).[225] **Level 1+**

InnoLet® vs Humulin Pen®

In a group of visually impaired patients, the InnoLet® insulin device (easy-to-read dial, large button for injection and audible clicks for units injected) was found to be significantly more effective than the Humulin Pen® in terms of visual accuracy when reading the dose scale (92% vs 45%, p<0.001). Additionally, significantly more patients using InnoLet® were able to intuitively set and dispense a 20U insulin dose (84% vs 41%, p<0.001) and InnoLet® was significantly preferred to the Humulin Pen® (87% vs 13%, p<0.001).[220]

11.4.5 From evidence to recommendations

There was no strong published evidence that insulin pen injectors were a preferred option for insulin injection, but in clinical practice this was not questionable. The studies comparing devices did not compare all devices, were inevitably unblinded, and were manufacturer sponsored in single centres for the most part. The issue of bias was real. It was considered that some devices preformed better than others, but also that this was generally known to regular prescribers. Prescribers should be fully familiar with the devices they were recommending; this would be difficult for all the devices available.

One injection device, the InnoLet®, was not a pen injector, but was aimed more at people with physical disabilities in manipulating injection systems. The studies were consistent with clinical experience in suggesting that this device was successful in enabling self-injection in some people who could not otherwise do it easily or reliably.

Please refer to the Diabetes UK guidance for the issue of disposal of devices/sharps.

RECOMMENDATIONS

R56   Offer education to a person who requires insulin about using an injection device (usually a pen injector and cartridge or a disposable pen) that they and/or their carer find easy to use.

R57   Appropriate local arrangements should be in place for the disposal of sharps.

R58   If a person has a manual or visual disability and requires insulin, offer a device or adaptation that:
- takes into account his or her individual needs
- he or she can use successfully.

12 Blood pressure therapy

12.1 Clinical introduction

People with Type 2 diabetes are at high cardiovascular (CV) risk, high risk of diabetes eye damage, and high risk of renal disease. These adverse outcomes are known to be reduced by improved blood pressure (BP) control, which can be used to lower the risk of stroke, MI, blindness and renal failure.[226] Some other forms of diabetes microvascular damage, including peripheral nerve damage, are known to be associated with higher BP.[227] BP lowering is likely to be highly cost-effective in people with Type 2 diabetes, more so than in the general population.

A number of clinical questions then face the person with diabetes and their advisors, these include:
- at what levels of BP to initiate therapy
- whether, and to what extent, those levels should be influenced by particular risk factors (in particular those involved in renal disease)
- what level of BP to aim for, and whether that should be modified by the presence of renal, eye, or macrovascular damage
- what lifestyle measure are effective and cost-effective in lowering BP
- what pharmacological interventions are effective and cost-effective in BP lowering
- how choice of agent might be modified by the presence of end organ damage.

Lifestyle measures (explored elsewhere) and monotherapy medication are known to have limited efficacy in lowering BP. Additional clinical questions arise over:
- the combinations of medications to be used after first-line therapy
- considerations including synergies of action, side effects of some combinations, and cost.

12.2 Blood pressure lowering – targets and intervention levels

12.2.1 Methodological introduction

There were eight papers identified as relevant to this question. These included four papers which further analysed data from large RCTs; two papers analysed data from the Irbesartan in Diabetic Nephropathy Trial (IDNT), N=1,590, median follow-up 2.6 years,[228] and median follow-up 2.9 years.[229] One study analysed data from the UKPDS study,[230] N=1,148, and a further study considered data from the Reduction of Endpoints in NIDDM with the Angiotensin II Antagonist Losartan (RENAAL) study, N=1,513, median follow-up 3.4 years.[231]

Two RCTs considered the effects of intensive compared with moderate treatment, one considered the effects of intensive treatment (valsartan) with moderate treatment (placebo) for BP control, mean follow-up <1–4 years (mean 1.9 years), N=129,[232] and the other, the Appropriate Blood Pressure Control in Diabetes (ABCD) trial, considered an intensive treatment with either enalapril or nisoldipine compared with moderate treatment (placebo), follow-up 5 years, N=480.[233]

A systematic review of several RCTs investigated the effects of different BP-lowering regimens on serious CV events in patients with and without diabetes.[234]

The final study was a 10 year observational study which considered a BP cut-off level for renal failure but not macrovascular complications, N=385.[235]

As with the papers considered for hypertension, studies which consider BP control have flexibility in their design to allow for the introduction of further antihypertensive therapy during the course of the study if required.

12.2.2 Health economic methodological introduction

No health economic papers were identified.

12.2.3 Evidence statements

Overall, an association could be established between low BP values and a lower incidence of CV events across three of the four studies looking at the relationship between BP levels and CV outcomes.[229,232,233,235] However, no clear BP threshold was identified as a potential therapeutic target.

An RCT[233] with a follow-up of 5 years concluded that intensive BP control (mean BP=28±0.8/75±0.3) in normotensive Type 2 diabetes patients was associated with a significantly lower incidence of CV events compared with those in the moderate BP control group (mean BP=137±0.7/81±0.3). **Level 1**

Another RCT conducted in normotensive Type 2 diabetes patients[232] showed non-significant differences in the incidence of CV events between the intensive blood control group (mean BP=118±10.9/75±5.7) and the moderate group (mean BP=124±10.9/80±6.5). **Level 1+**

The analysis completed on the IDNT data[229] identified a decreased risk in CV mortality and congestive heart failure (CHF) where the systolic blood pressure (SBP) decreased from >170 to 120–130 mmHg, with a 20 mmHg lower SBP being associated with a 39% reduction in both. An achieved SBP ≤20 mmHg compared with >120 mmHg showed a greater risk of CV mortality and CHF (see table 12.1). **Level 1+**

Table 12.1 Post hoc analysis of the IDNT study – Berl[229] N=1,590	
CV outcome	**Size effect**
CV mortality	A decrease in risk was observed where achieved SBP decreased from >170 to 120–130 mmHg. In this range a 20 mmHg lower SBP was associated with a 39% reduction in CV mortality, p<0.002
	An achieved SBP ≤120 showed a significantly greater risk of CV mortality compared to those with an achieved SBP >120 mmHg, RR 4.06 (2.11 to 7.80), p<0.0001
CHF	A decrease in risk was observed where achieved SBP decreased from >170 to 120–130 mmHg. In this range a 20 mmHg lower SBP was associated with a 39% reduction in CHF, p=0.001
	Those with an achieved SBP ≤120 had a significantly greater risk of CHF than those with an achieved SBP >120 mmHg, RR 1.80 (1.17 to 2.86), p=0.008
MI	A 10 mmHg lower mean achieved DBP was associated with a significantly higher risk of MI, RR 1.61 (1.28 to 2.02), p<0.0001
Stroke	A 10 mmHg lower mean achieved DBP was associated with a significantly lower risk of stroke, RR 0.65 (0.48 to 0.88), p=0.005
DBP, diastolic blood pressure	

A systematic review[234] identified 27 trials which included 33,395 individuals with diabetes and 125,314 without. Overall the analysis suggest that patients with diabetes achieved greater reductions in the risk of total major CV events and CV death with regimens targeting lower BP goals* than those without diabetes (see table 12.2). **Level 1+**

Table 12.2 Systematic review – by the Blood Pressure Lowering Treatment Trialists' Collaboration (BPLTTC)[234]

Stroke

More vs less intensive	More intensive	Less intensive	Δ BP mmHg	RR 95% CI	Diabetes vs no diabetes
Diabetes	63/1,731	86/1,868	–6.0/–4.6	0.64 (0.46 to 0.89)	NS differences
No diabetes	103/6,303	204/12,080	–3.7/–3.3	0.89 (0.70 to 1.13)	NS differences

Coronary heart disease

More vs less intensive	More intensive	Less intensive	Δ BP mmHg	RR 95% CI	Diabetes vs no diabetes
Diabetes	36/1,731	44/1,868	–6.0/–4.6	0.69 (0.38 to 1.25)	NS differences
No diabetes	27/6,303	31/12,080	–2.9/–3.0	1.10 (0.60 to 2.01)	NS differences

Heart failure

More vs less intensive	More intensive	Less intensive	Δ BP mmHg	RR 95% CI	Diabetes vs no diabetes
Diabetes	36/1,731	44/1,868	–6.0/–4.6	0.69 (0.38 to 1.25)	NS differences
No diabetes	27/6,303	31/12,080	–3.7/–3.3	1.10 (0.60 to 2.01)	NS differences

The observational study[235] identified that baseline SBP was lower (141±19 mmHg) for those with no complications compared with those who had an MI (154±20 mmHg), p<0.01. SBP was also lower during the observation period for those with no complications (145±16 mmHg) compared with those who had an MI (152±15 mmHg), p<0.05 and also those who had a stroke (153±15 mmHg), p<0.001. This study also noted that DBP was lower at baseline for those with no complications (84±9) compared with those who developed an MI (87±9 mmHg), p<0.05. **Level 2+**

---

* There were fives studies comparing more intensive and less intensive regimes. The target BP levels (mmHg) for these studies were as follows: MAP £92 vs 102–107; DBP £75 vs £90; DBP 10 mmHg below baseline vs 80–89; DBP £80 vs £85 OR £90 and DBP <85 vs <105.

▷ Renal outcomes

Five studies[228,231–233,235] were identified looking at several renal outcomes and their relation with BP control. On the whole, it could be ascertained that high BP levels (SBP and/or DBP) in patients with Type 2 diabetes were associated with a more rapid decline in renal function than in those with lower BP values.

RENAAL study

The RENAAL study[231] demonstrated that for SBP the baseline level of 160–179 mmHg or ≥180 mmHg compared with less than 130 mmHg had a significantly greater risk of reaching the primary endpoint (time to doubling of serum creatinine, end stage renal disease (ESRD) or death), risk of ESRD or death and risk of ESRD alone. Kaplan-Meier curve also showed that for those with a baseline SBP ≥140 compared with <140 mmHg there was a significantly higher risk of reaching the primary endpoint and risk of ESRD alone. For achieved SBP those who had a SBP of 140 to ≥180 mmHg compared with less than 130 mmHg had a significantly greater risk of reaching the primary endpoint; for those with an achieved SBP of 140–159 mmHg compared with less than 130 mmHg there was a significantly greater risk of ESRD or death and ESRD alone.

For achieved DBP those with a DBP from 90 to ≥100 mmHg compared with those with an achieved DBP of <70 mmHg had a significantly greater risk of reaching the primary endpoint (time to doubling of serum creatinine, ESRD or death), risk of ESRD or death and risk of ESRD alone[231] (see table 12.3.1). **Level 1+**

Table 12.3.1 RENAAL study – systolic blood pressure at baseline

SBP at baseline (mmHg)	Risk of doubling of SCr, ESRD or death (primary endpoint)	Risk of ESRD or death	Risk of ESRD alone
160–179 vs <130	HR 1.28 (0.97 to 1.69) p<0.001	HR 1.96 (1.40 to 2.74) p<0.001	HR 2.13 (1.39 to 3.27) p<0.001
≥180 vs <130	HR 1.85 (1.33 to 2.57) p<0.01*	HR 2.10 (1.44 to 3.06) p<0.01**	HR 2.02 (1.24 to 3.29) p=0.005***

* Kaplan-Meier curve for baseline SBP <140 vs ≥140 mmHg, a significantly higher risk for those ≥140 mmHg (HR 1.66, p<0.001)
** Every 10 mmHg rise in baseline SBP increased the risk for ESRD or death by 6.7%, p=0.007 (multivariate model adjusted for urinary ACR (log scale), creatinine, albumin, haemoglobin)
*** Kaplan-Meier curve for baseline SBP <140 vs ≥140 mmHg, a significantly higher risk for those ≥140 mmHg (HR 1.72, p<0.001)
SCr, serum creatinine ratio

Table 12.3.2 RENAAL study – systolic blood pressure achieved

SBP achieved (mmHg)	Risk of doubling of SCr, ESRD or death (primary endpoint)	Risk of ESRD or death	Risk of ESRD alone
140–159 vs <130	HR 1.49 (1.18 to 1.90) p<0.001	HR 1.33 (1.02 to 1.72) p=0.03	HR 1.52 (1.07 to 2.15) p=0.02

Table 12.3.3 RENAAL study – diastolic blood pressure achieved			
DBP achieved (mmHg)	Risk of doubling of SCr, ESRD or death (primary endpoint)	Risk of ESRD or death*	Risk of ESRD alone
90–99 vs <70	HR 1.72 (1.32 to 2.23) p<0.001	HR 1.55 (1.16 to 2.08) p=0.003	HR 1.67 (1.15 to 2.44) p=0.008
≥100 vs <70	HR 2.54 (1.70 to 3.80) p<0.001	HR 2.74 (1.78 to 4.24) p<0.001	HR 3.26 (1.90 to 5.58) p<0.001

* Every 10 mmHg rise in baseline DBP decreased the risk for ESRD or death by 10.9% (p=0.01) (multivariate model adjusted for urinary ACR (log scale), creatinine, albumin, haemoglobin)

Other studies reporting renal outcomes

The two studies which used intensive and moderate control groups showed significant differences between the groups only for adjusted log urinary albumin excretion rate (UAER) findings.[232,233] **Level 1+**

The further analysis from the IDNT study identified that baseline BP correlated significantly with doubling SCr or ESRD and that 36% of those with baseline SBP >170 mmHg compared with 18% for those with baseline SBP <145 mmHg reached renal endpoint. Following correction for estimated glomerular filtration rate (eGFR) and albumin:creatinine ratio (ACR) each 20 mmHg decrease in SBP was associated with a 30% reduction in the risk of a renal event. Though it should be noted that while there was an increasing risk for reaching a renal endpoint with seated SBP, those with SBP <120 mmHg were not substantially better than those between 120–130 mmHg.[228] **Level 1+**

The 10 year observational study identified that baseline SBP and DBP were significantly lower for those with no complications than those who developed renal failure, SBP was also lower for this during the observation period. A BP cut-off of >140 mmHg showed a NSx38.5 increase in the risk of renal failure.[235] **Level 2+**

▷ Retinopathy outcomes

The intensive (118±10.9/75±5.7) and moderate (124±10.9/80±6.5) groups found NS difference between the groups for progression or regression of retinopathy.[232] **Level 1+**

The other study which considered intensive (128±0.8/75±0.3) and moderate (137±0.7/81±0.3) groups identified less progression of retinopathy with the intensive group compared with the moderate group at both 2 years (13 vs 21%, p=0.046) and 5 years (34 vs 46%, p=0.019).[233] **Level 1+**

The analysis completed on the data from the UKPDS study on retinopathy is detailed in the table 12.4.[230] This considered the impact of tight blood pressure control (TBP) aiming for a BP less than 150/85 and less tight blood pressure control (LTBP) aiming for a BP of 180/105 or less. The TBP group had significantly lower microaneurysms, hard exudates and cotton wool spots than the LTBP group. This TBP group also had less retinopathy grading by the Early Treatment of Diabetic Retinopathy Study (ETDRS) grading and lower absolute risk events per 1,000 patient years for photocoagulation and blindness in one eye. **Level 1+**

Table 12.4 Retinopathy outcomes – Matthews study[230]	
Progression of retinopathy assessed by specific lesions	
MA % with ≥5 MA	• at 4.5 years; TBP vs LTBP (23.3% vs 33.5%) RR 0.7 (99% CI 0.51 to 0.95), p=0.003 • at 7.5 years; TBP vs LTBP (29.3% vs 44.8%) RR 0.66 (99% CI 0.48 to 0.90), p<0.001
Hard exudates	Overall increase 11.2% to 18.3% • at 4.5 years; TBP vs LTBP (12.5% vs 21.2%) RR 0.59 (99% CI 0.38 to 0.92), p=0.002 • at 7.5 years; TBP vs LTBP (14.1% vs 26.6%) RR 0.53 (99% CI 0.33 to 0.85), p<0.001
Cotton wool spots	Overall increase 14.0% to 22.4% • at 4.5 years; TBP vs LTBP (16.6% vs 17.4%) RR 0.69 (99% CI 0.47 to 1.02), p=0.02 • at 7.5 years; TBP vs LTBP (17.4% vs 32.5%) RR 0.53 (99% CI 0.35 to 0.81), p<0.001
Ocular endpoints	
Photocoagulation	• TBP vs LTBP had lower absolute risk events per 1,000 patient years (11.0 vs 17.0) RR 0.63 (99% CI 0.39 to 1.07), p=0.03 • due to maculopathy, 7.6 vs 13.0 (TBP vs LTBP) RR 0.58 (99% CI 0.32 to 1.04), p=0.02
Vision loss	
Blindness in one eye	• TBP group had lower absolute risk events per 1,000 patient years than the LTBP group (3.1 vs 4.1) RR 0.76 (98% CI 0.29 to 1.99), p=0.046
Retinopathy progression by ETDRS grading	• at 4.5 years two-step or more deterioration; TBP vs LTBP (27.5% vs 36.7%) RR 0.75 (99% CI 0.50 to 0.89), p=0.02 • at 7.5 years two-step or more deterioration; TBP vs LTBP (34.0% vs 51.3%) RR 0.66 (99% CI 0.50 to 0.89), p=0.001 • more than 1/3 (TBP) did not change compare with 1/5 (LTBP)
MA, microaneurysams	

▷ Nephropathy outcome

The intensive (118±10.9/75±5.7) and moderate (124±10.9/80±6.5) groups found NS difference between the groups for progression or regression of nephropathy.[232] **Level 1+**

The other study which considered intensive (128±0.8/75±0.3) and moderate (137±0.7/81±0.3) groups identified NS difference between the groups for progression of nephropathy.[233] **Level 1+**

12.2.4 From evidence to recommendations

The GDG noted the problems in assigning BP lowering targets in this area, and in particular the:

● problem setting a cut-off where the evidence suggests 'the lower the blood pressure the better (without adverse effects)'
● difficulties of achieving any reasonable target in some people

- individual targets that should logically vary with individual risk
- arbitrary dichotomy that arises immediately above and below any target level.

The results of some RCTs suggested that SBP well into the normal range (below usual target values) was both achievable and associated with benefit in people with Type 2 diabetes, consistent with epidemiological evidence from other studies. In some other studies tight BP control seemed difficult to achieve, consistent with the group's clinical experience. This led the group to take a simple risk approach centered on a target level of <140/80 mmHg for most people with Type 2 diabetes, and <130/80 mmHg for those at more particular risk. The latter group included people with raised albumin excretion rate (AER) (microalbuminuria or worse), eGFR <60 ml/min/1.73 m^2, those with retinopathy, and those with prior stroke or transient ischaemic attack (TIA). The concern that more active prevention was being targeted at those who had already developed end-organ damage was recognised, but it was noted that for both microalbuminuria (chapter 16) and early retinopathy (chapter 17) the recommendations on annual surveillance meant that markers of damage would be detected many years before ill health ensued.

12.3 Blood pressure lowering medications

12.3.1 Methodological introduction

The search identified a systematic review of several RCTs investigating the effects of different BP lowering therapies (i.e. angiotensin-converting enzyme inhibitors (ACEI), angiotensin II receptor (A2RB) anatgonists, calcium channel blockers (CCB), beta-blockers and diuretics) on serious CV events in patients with and without diabetes.[234]

▷ ACEI

There were 14 papers identified for this question, these included two Cochrane reviews, considering antihypertensive agents for preventing diabetic kidney disease[236] and ACEI and A2RB antagonists for preventing the progression of diabetic kidney disease.[237] There was also a meta-analysis which considered the effect of inhibitors of the renin-angiotensin system (RAS) and other antihypertensive drugs on renal outcomes.[238]

ACEI vs placebo

Three studies compared ramipril with a placebo, they were sub-analysis of the 5-year Heart Outcomes and Prevention Evaluation (HOPE) study, considering the diabetic subgroup, N=3,577 (total study population, N=9,297)[239,240] and an extension phase of 2.6 years, N=4,528.[241]

ACEI vs A2RB

The DETAIL (Diabetics Exposed to Telmisartan and Enalapril) study considered telmisartan compared with enalapril over 5 years, N=250.[242] An open-label study considered lisinopril compared with telmisartan and compared with a combination of the two treatments over 52 weeks, N=219.[243]

ACEI vs CCB

Three studies considered ACEI and CCB. One study considered lercanidipine compared with ramipril for 36–52 weeks, N=180.[244] An open-label study considered amlodipine compared with fosinopril and compared the combination of both drugs for 4 years, N=309.[245] A post hoc analysis of the Bergamo Nephrologic Diabetic Complications Trial (BENDICT) study was performed, this considered verapamil compared with trandopril compared with a combination of both drugs for 3.6 years, N=1,204.[246]

ACEI vs CCB vs diuretic

One study considered lisinopril compared with amlodipine and chlorthalidone* with a Type 2 diabetes group analysis, mean follow-up 4.9 years, N=12,063 (total study population N=31,512); the Antihypertensive and Lipid-Lowering to Prevent Heart Attack Trial (ALLHAT).[247]

ACEI + CCB vs ACEI + diuretic

One study considered verapamil + trandopril compared with enalapril + hydrochlorothiazide over 6 months, N=103.[248]

ACEI + CCB vs beta blocker + diuretic

Another study considered N=463 participants who were dosed with verapamil SR + ACE trandopril compared with atenolol + chlorthalidone for 20 weeks.[249]

All studies were either RCTs or subgroup analysis of RCTs, the majority of which were double-blinded (two open-label studies).[243,245] All studies involved participants with Type 2 diabetes or considered a diabetic subgroup from a larger study. Many of the studies used BP target levels, if these were not achieved with the initial dose of the drug then either dose escalation or the introduction of other antihypertensive medication was allowed to ensure that target BP was maintained accordingly.

▷ A2RB

A total of 10 studies were found relevant to the question.[237,250–258]

The studies selected were RCTs with a follow-up of at least 6 months and with a sample size of more than 100. All studies involved participants with Type 2 diabetes or considered a diabetic subgroup from a larger study. Many of the studies used BP target levels, if these were not achieved with the initial dose of the drug then either dose escalation or the introduction of other antihypertensive medication was allowed to ensure that target BP was maintained according.

These 10 RCTs reviewed the evidence on the effectiveness and safety of A2RB blockers across several comparisons.

---

* The ALLHAT study randomised patients to chlorthalidone 12.5–25.0 mg/day, amlodipine 2.5–10 mg/day or lisinopril 10–40 mg/day. The doses of these drugs were increased until a BP goal of <140/90 mmHg was achieved. In addition, other drugs could be added to the baseline treatments such as atenolol (25–100 mg/day), reserpine (0.1–0.2 mg/day) or clonidine (0.1–0.3 mg bid) at the discretion of the investigator. Also, hydralazine 25–100 mg bid could be added as a step three drug.

A2RB vs placebo

One Cochrane review[237] was identified analysing data from five studies placebo-controlled trials i.e. Brenner et al. 2001 (RENAAL), Lewis et al. 2001 (Renal data – IDNT), Parving et al. 2001 (IRMA), Tan et al. 2002 and, Berl et al. 2003 (CV data – IDNT).

Three post hoc analyses of large placebo-controlled trials were also identified: two post hoc studies of the RENAAL trial[253,254] and one post hoc study[255] of the IRMA study.

One post hoc analysis[254] analysed the impact of renal function at baseline on disease progression and response to treatment in 1,513 patients who were enrolled in the RENAAL study.

Another post hoc analysis of the 1,513 patients enrolled in the RENAAL study[253] analysed the effect of losartan versus placebo on long-term glycaemic control and serum potassium, uric acid, and lipid levels, as well as the relationship between these baseline metabolic factors and the composite endpoint (doubling of serum creatinine, ESRD, or death) or ESRD alone.

One post hoc analysis of the IRMA study[255] assessed the reversibility of kidney function changes after withdrawal of 2 years antihypertensive therapy with irbesartan on 133 Type 2 diabetes patients.

A2RB vs CCB

Four studies looked at the comparison of an A2RB with a CCB. Irbesartan vs amlodipine,[257] valsartan vs amlodipine[252,258] and telmisartan vs nifedipine.[251] It should be noted that the study by Lewis[257] was included in the Cochrane review but no data on the head comparison between A2RB and CCB was reported.

A2RB vs sympatholytic agents

One study[256] considered A2RB (losartan) compared with a beta-blocker agent (atenolol) and another study[250] compared A2RB (irbesartan) with an alpha-blocker drug (doxazosin).

Studies comparing ACEI with A2RB have been analysed under the ACEI section.

It should be noted that differing dosing and titration regimens and the differing populations included in the studies, may limit direct comparisons between studies.

▷ Beta-blockers

There were four papers identified for this question which were not covered in other antihypertensive question. These papers included comparisons of beta-blockers with other beta-blockers, or beta-blockers with CCB (studies which considered beta-blockers and ACEI or A2RB have been covered within the ACE and A2RB evidence). All of the included papers were RCTs, three were double-blind and open was open-label.[259]

Beta-blockers vs beta blockers

One paper was identified which considered carvedilol and metoprolol in N=1,235 participants for 5 months.[260]

Beta-blockers vs CCB

There were three papers identified for this. One paper was a sub-analysis of the Controlled Onset Verapamil Investigation of Cardiovascular End Points (CONVINCE) trial, which considered control-onset extended-release (COER) verapamil with atenolol or hydrochlorothiazide in N=16,476 (N=3,239 Type 2 diabetes) for 3 years.[261] A further paper considered a subgroup of the Anglo-Scandinavian Cardiac Outcomes Trial: Blood Pressure Lowering Arm (ASCOT: BPLA) trial, with N=19,257 (N=5,145 with diabetes), which was stopped prematurely at 5.5 years.[262] The third paper reported on the International Verapamil-Trandolapril Study (INVEST) trial which considered verapamil SR with atenolol for N=22,576 (N=6,400 Type 2 diabetes) participants over 24 months.[259]

12.3.2 Health economic methodological introduction

▷ ACEI

Three studies were identified, two based in the UK and one in Germany.

Beard et al. (2001)[263] and Schadlich et al. (2004)[264] used data from the HOPE and micro-HOPE studies, which compared an ACEI, ramipril, to placebo. In both analyses the treatment effects were not continued beyond the trial period of 5 years and the continued survival of patients was considered.

Gray et al. (2001)[265] was based on UKPDS data, comparing an ACEI, captopril, to a beta-blocker, atenolol. In this study a tight BP target of <150/<85 mmHg was set and other antihypertensive treatments could be added on to achieve this target. After the trial period it was assumed that beyond the trial period the two groups had identical hazard rates.

In all three studies the outcomes of interest were CV events.

▷ A2RB

The studies identified looked at the renal protection effect of angiotension II receptor antagonists (AR2B).

Three studies were based on the IDNT. Irbesartan 300 mg to amlodipine 10 mg and to a control. All participants could take standard antihypertensive therapies which exclude ACEI, AR2B, and CCBs. This study included Type 2 diabetes patients with proteinuria. No significant difference was found between irbesartan and amlodipine in reducing BP. The control had an average of 3.3 mmHg increased BP.

The combined endpoint of the study was doubling of serum creatinine concentration, ESRD or death from any cause. Irbesartan reduced this endpoint by 23% compared to amlodopine and 20% compared to control.

Palmer et al. (2004)[266] was set in the UK, Rodby et al. (2003)[267] was set in the US, and Coyle et al. (2004)[268] was set in Canada. In these studies various time horizons were used, where a 10-year time horizon was the base case, 25 years was tested in the sensitivity analysis.

Vora et al. (2005)[269] was based on the RENAAL study which compared Losartan 50–100 mg with a regimen of conventional antihypertensive treatment (CCBs, diuretics, alpha-blockers, beta-blockers, and centrally acting agents). Patients had Type 2 diabetes and nephropathy. The same combined endpoint as the IDNT was used. Losartan was found to reduce this by 25% compared with control. This analysis was set in the UK and a lifetime time horizon was used.

Smith et al. (2004)[270] was based on the Microalbuminuria Reduction with Valsartan (MARVAL) study comparing the AR2B, to the CCB amlodipine. Patients with Type 2 diabetes and microalbuminuria were included. The study found that valsartan significantly reduced urinary excretion rate compared to amlodipine. Similar reductions in BP were found. This analysis was set in the US. An 8-year time horizon was used.

12.3.3 Evidence statements

A systematic review showed that for the outcome stroke, there was no evidence of differences in the effects of the treatment regimens between patients with and without diabetes except in the comparison that included A2RB-based regimens. In this comparison, A2RB provided lesser protection to patients with diabetes compared with those without diabetes (see table 12.5.1).[234]

For the outcomes coronary heart disease (CHD) and heart failure, the review did not show differences between patients with and without diabetes for any comparison, again except for the comparison that included A2RB. Diabetic patients treated with A2RB experienced a significantly greater protection compared to those without diabetes for the outcome heart failure.[234]

According to their review, there was also some evidence of a difference between the two patient groups in protection against CV death and total mortality favouring patients with diabetes in the comparison of ACEI-based regimens vs placebo (see table 12.5.1).[234]

Table 12.5.1 Stroke – systematic review by the BPLTTC[234]

ACEI	ACE	Placebo	Δ BP mmHg	RR 95% CI	Diabetes vs no diabetes
Diabetes	125/2,378	174/2,336	−3.6/−1.9	0.69 (0.55 to 0.86)	NS differences
No diabetes	347/6,733	485/6,782	−5.8/−2.7	0.73 (0.62 to 0.85)	
CCB	**CCB**	**Placebo**	**Δ BP mmHg**	**RR 95% CI**	**Diabetes vs no diabetes**
Diabetes	21/911	45/900	−6.3/−3.0	0.47 (0.28 to 0.78)	NS differences
No diabetes	52/2,883	72/2,788	−9.2/−3.7	0.70 (0.49 to 0.99)	
AR2B	**ARB-based regimen**	**Control regimen**	**Δ BP mmHg**	**RR 95% CI**	**Diabetes vs no diabetes**
Diabetes	143/2,226	173/2,793	−2.1/−0.9	0.96 (0.77 to 1.19)	p=0.05 by X^2 test of homogeneity
No diabetes	253/6,186	342/6,153	−1.4/−0.6	0.74 (0.63 to 0.86)	

Table 12.5.2 Coronary heart disease – systematic review by the BPLTTC[234]

ACEI	ACE	Placebo	Δ BP mmHg	RR 95% CI	Diabetes vs no diabetes
Diabetes	96/2,378	105/2,336	–3.6/–1.9	0.88 (0.67 to 1.16)	NS differences
No diabetes	123/6,733	164/6,782	–5.8/–2.7	0.78 (0.62 to 0.98)	
CCB	**CCB**	**Placebo**	**Δ BP mmHg**	**RR 95% CI**	**Diabetes vs no diabetes**
Diabetes	94/868	75/858	–6.3/–3.0	1.29 (0.97 to 1.72)	NS differences
No diabetes	10/2,514	13/2,416	–9.2/–3.7	1.07 (0.43 to 2.62)	
ARB	**ARB-based regimen**	**Control regimen**	**Δ BP mmHg**	**RR 95% CI**	**Diabetes vs no diabetes**
Diabetes	150/2,226	208/2,793	–2.1/–0.9	0.92 (072 to 1.17)	NS differences
No diabetes	285/6,186	269/6,153	–1.4/–0.6	1.05 (0.89 to 1.24)	

Table 12.5.3 Heart failure – systematic review by the BPLTTC[234]

ACEI	ACE	Placebo	Δ BP mmHg	RR 95% CI	Diabetes vs no diabetes
Diabetes	96/2,378	105/2,336	–3.6/–1.9	0.88 (0.67 to 1.16)	NS differences
No diabetes	123/6,733	164/6,782	–5.8/–2.7	0.78 (0.62 to 0.98)	
CCB	**CCB**	**Placebo**	**Δ BP mmHg**	**RR 95% CI**	**Diabetes vs no diabetes**
Diabetes	94/868	75/858	–5.9/–3	1 1.29 (0.97 to 1.72)	NS differences
No diabetes	10/2,514	13/2,416	–9.3/–3.9	1.07 (0.43 to 2.62)	
ARB	**ARB-based regimen**	**Control regimen**	**Δ BP mmHg**	**RR 95% CI**	**Diabetes vs no diabetes**
Diabetes	181/1,916	346/2,507	–2.0/–0.9	0.70 (0.59 to 0.83)	p=0.002 X² test of homogeneity
No diabetes	121/4,019	106/3,979	–0.8/–0.0	1.13 (0.87 to 1.46)	

Table 12.5.4 CV DEATHS – systematic review by the BPLTTC[234]

ACEI	ACE	Placebo	Δ BP mmHg	RR 95% CI	Diabetes vs no diabetes
Diabetes	145/2,378	211/2,336	–3.6/–1.9	0.67 (0.55 to 0.82)	p=0.05 X^2 test of homogeneity
No diabetes	330/6,733	389/6,782	–5.8/–2.7	0.86 (0.75 to 0.99)	
CCB	**CCB**	**Placebo**	**Δ BP mmHg**	**RR 95% CI**	**Diabetes vs no diabetes**
Diabetes	42/868	62/858	–5.9/–3.1	0.54 (0.21 to 1.42)	NS differences
No diabetes	61/2,514	73/2,416	–9.3/–3.9	0.64 (0.24 to 1.68)	

Finally, the review did not report significant differences between different BP lowering regimens (i.e. head-to-head comparisons) in terms of stroke, CHD, heart failure in patients with diabetes. The exception being CCBs, which were associated with a higher risk of heart failure when they were compared with diuretics or beta-blockers,[234] (see tables 12.6.1–12.6.3 for outcomes). In the same way, no differences were seen in the head-to-head comparisons for total major CV events, CV deaths, and total mortality in patients with diabetes.

Table 12.6.1 Head-to-head comparisons. Stroke – systematic review by the BPLTTC[234]

ACE vs D/BB	ACE	D/BB	Δ BP mmHg	RR 95% CI
Five studies	282/4,385	405/6,614	2.2/0.3	1.02 (0.88 to 1.19)
CCB vs D/BB	**CCB**	**D/BB**	**Δ BP mmHg**	**RR 95% CI**
Eight studies	279/6,276	427/8,550	0.7/–0.8	0.94 (0.81 to 1.09)
ACE vs CCB	**ACE**	**CCB**	**Δ BP mmHg**	**RR 95% CI**
Five studies	246/4,101	227/4,222	1.6/1.2	1.09 (0.88 to 1.36)

BB, beta-blockers; D, diuretics

Table 12.6.2 Head-to-head comparisons. CHD – systematic review by the BPLTTC[234]

ACE vs D/BB	ACE	D/BB	Δ BP mmHg	RR 95% CI
Five studies	402/4,385	623/6,614	2.2/0	3 0.83 (0.62 to 1.12)
CCB vs D/BB	**CCB**	**D/BB**	**Δ BP mmHg**	**RR 95% CI**
Eight studies	431/6,276	638/8,550	0.7/–0.8	1.00 (0.89 to 1.13)
ACE vs CCB	**ACE**	**CCB**	**Δ BP mmHg**	**RR 95% CI**
Five studies	358/4,101	407/4,222	1.6/1.2	0.76 (0.51 to 1.12)

Table 12.6.3 Head-to-head comparisons. Heart failure – systematic review by the BPLTTC[234]

ACE vs D/BB	ACE	D/BB	Δ BP mmHg	RR 95% CI
Four studies	251/4,076	384/6,351	2.5/0.4	0.94 (0.55 to 1.59)
CCB vs D/BB	**CCB**	**D/BB**	**Δ BP mmHg**	**RR 95% CI**
Six studies	337/5,276	399/7,521	0.5/–0.8	1.27 (1.01 to 1.61)
ACE vs CCB	**ACE**	**CCB**	**Δ BP mmHg**	**RR 95% CI**
Five studies	263/4,101	325/4,222	1.6/1.2	0.92 (0.67 to 1.27)

ACEI

Overall, the evidence appraised showed no significant differences in terms of CV outcomes when treatment with ACEI was compared with other antihypertensive therapies or with placebo. ACEI also failed to demonstrate superiority over other agents on the basis of BP lowering power (unless combination therapy is compared with monotherapy). However, the evidence suggested that treatment with ACEI is related to greater benefits in terms of renal outcomes in patients with Type 2 diabetes as compared with other BP lowering agents.

▷ Cardiovascular outcomes

All cause mortality

The Cochrane review on antihypertensives for preventing diabetic kidney disease found NS difference for ACEI vs placebo (three trials, N=2,683) and for ACEI vs CCBs (six trials, N=1,286).[236] These findings were supported by the Cochrane review on ACEI and A2RB for preventing the progression of diabetic kidney disease for ACEI vs placebo (21 trials, N=7,295)* and ACEI vs A2RB (five studies, N=3,409).[237] **Level 1++**

---

* Though a subgroup analysis which used ACE at maximum tolerable dose did find a significant decrease vs placebo (five trials; N=2,034, RR 0.78, 0.61 to 0.98).

ACEI vs CCB vs diuretic

The diabetes ALLHAT analysis showed NS difference between the treatments for the incidence of total mortality.[247] **Level 1+**

▷ Major cardiovascular events

ACEI/placebo

The extension phase of the HOPE study showed a NS trend towards reduction in major CV events and risk of MI, with ramipril, stroke and CV death as NS. At follow-up of the study and extension there was a significant risk reduction with ramipril for the outcomes of MI, stroke and CV death.[241] **Level 1+**

ACEI vs CCB vs diuretic

The diabetes analysis of ALLHAT identified NS difference in the incidence of fatal CHD and non-fatal MI for lisinopril vs chlorthiadone in any of the three glycaemic strata that were analysed diabetes mellitus, impaired fasting glucose and normoglycaemia. This was also evident for diabetes mellitus and normoglycaemia for amlodipine vs chlorthalidone.[247] **Level 1+**

▷ Blood pressure

BP reduction with all hypertensive treatments was a consistent feature of the studies and therefore only studies where there were significant differences between the treatments will be highlighted.

ACEI/A2RB

At the 52-week follow-up point, the combination of lisinopril and telmisartan showed significantly greater reductions in both SBP and DBP than the individual monotherapies (p=0.003 for both SBP and DBP).[243] **Level 1+**

ACEI/CCB + diuretic

Similarly, the combination of amlodipine and fosinopril showed a reduction in sitting BP of 28.7/17.1 compared with 17.2/11.8 (fosinopril, p<0.01) and 19.9/12.8 (amlodipine, p<0.01).[245] **Level 1+**

ACEI + CCB/beta-blocker + diuretic

The study which compared verapamill + trandopril with atenolol + chlorthalidone identified that while both treatments significantly reduced BP that comparison between the groups showed a difference of 4.85 mmHg SBP (1.94 to 7.76, p=0.0011) and 1.79 mmHg DBP (0.26 to 3.32, p=0.0222) favouring atenolol + chlorthalidone.[249] **Level 1++**

ACEI/CCB

A post hoc analysis of the BENEDICT[246] study considered the impact on BP control and ACEI therapy on new-onset microalbumuniuria. Baseline SBP, DBP, mean arterial pressure (MAP) and pulse pressure did not predict the onset of microalbuminuria. Participants who developed micro-albuminuria had significantly lower reductions in SBP than those who did not develop micro-albuminuria (7.9 ± 11.5 vs 10.6 ± 11.9, $p<0.05$). This study also identified that those with follow-up BP below the medians or with BP reduction above the medians were more frequently on ACE therapy (particularly trandopirl + verapamil) and less frequently on concomitant treatment with diuretics, beta-blockers or CCBs.[246] **Level 1+**

▷ Renal outcomes

The Cochrane review, ACEI and A2RB antagonists for preventing the progression of diabetic kidney disease, identified ACE compared with placebo reduced the progression from micro- to macroalbuminuria, increased the regression from micro- to normoalbuminuria, and reduced the risk of ESRD.[237]

The Cochrane review, antihypertensive agents for preventing diabetic kidney disease, identified that ACEI compared with placebo/no treatment reduced the development of microalbuminuria, and ACEI compared with CCB reduced the risk of developing kidney disease.[236]

The meta-analysis identified that an ACEI or A2RB compared with other treatments only showed significant reduction in UAER.[238]

The HOPE study identified that ramipril compared with placebo reduced the risk of new microalbuminuria and that both new microalbuminuria and progression of proteinuria was higher for the diabetic group than the non-diabetic group.[240]

Combination compared with monotherapy

The combination of lisinopril and telmisartan identified higher reduction with AER compared with the monotherapies.[243]

The combination of fosinopril + amlodipine reduced UAE compared with amlodipine monotherapy (all time points) and with fosinopril monotherapy (after 18 months).[245]

Renal outcomes are detailed in the table 12.7, including study results which identified NS difference between treatments.

Table 12.7 ACEI – renal outcomes

Progression of proteinuria

HOPE study[240] Level 1+	ACEI/placebo Progression higher with non-diabetic participants than diabetic (34% vs 17%, p<0.01) Diabetes was the factor most strongly associated with the progression of proteinuria (OR 2.45, 2.148 to 2.75, p<0.05)* Ramipril vs placebo NS (adjustment for baseline reduced proteinuria by 22%, p=0.0495)

New microalbuminuria/risk of developing microalbuminuria

Cochrane review[236] Level 1++	ACEI vs placebo/no treatment, reduced development of microalbuminuria (six trials, N=3,480, RR 0.58, 0.40 to 0.84) ACEI vs CCB reduced the risk of developing kidney disease (micro- or macroalbuminuria) (four trials, N=1,210, RR 0.58, 0.40 to 0.84) ACEI vs beta-blockers NS difference
Cochrane review[237] Level 1++	ACE vs placebo/no treatment significantly reduced the progression from micro- to macroalbuminuria (17 trials, N=2,036, RR 0.49, 0.29 to 0.69) ACEI vs A2RB NS difference
HOPE study[240] Level 1+	ACEI/placebo New microalbuminuria was higher in diabetic than in non-diabetic participants (38.2% vs 18.1%) Ramipril reduced the risk of new microalbuminuria by 10% p=0.046 vs placebo, in those with diabetes

Regression from micro- to normoalbuminuria

Cochrane review[237] Level 1++	ACEI vs placebo/no treatment ACEI significantly increased regression (16 studies, N=1,910, RR 3.06, 1.76 to 5.35) ACEI vs A2RB NS difference
Dalla VM (2004)[244] Level 1+	ACEI/CCB Ramipril vs lercanidipine NS for those who reverted to normoalbuminuria
Fogari R (2002)[245] Level 1+	At 48 months 46% (fosinopril), 33% (amlodipine) and 67% (combination fosinopril + amlodipine) had moved to non-microalbuminuric status

Doubling of creatinine

Cochrane review[236] Level 1++	ACEI vs placebo NS difference
Meta-analysis[238] Level 1+	ACEI or A2RB vs other active interventions NS, those with diabetes (six trials, N=3,044) and NS those without diabetes

Serum creatinine

Meta-analysis[238] Level 1+	ACEI or A2RB vs other treatments NS, those with diabetes (18 trials, N=4,615), those without diabetes, small reduction
HOPE study[240] Level 1+	ACEI/placebo No evidence of effect on ramipril on serum creatinine levels
Barnett (2004)[242] Level 1+	ACEI/A2RB Enalapril vs telmisartan NS difference

continued

Table 12.7 ACEI – renal outcomes – *continued*

GFR

Meta-analysis[238] Level 1+	ACEI or A2RB vs other treatments NS, those with diabetes (37 studies, N=15,742), NS those without diabetes
HOPE study[240] Level 1+	ACEI/placebo Ramipril vs placebo NS difference
Barnett (2004)[242] Level 1+	ACEI/A2RB Mean change in GFR: the lower treatment boundary in favour of enalapril was −7.6, greater than the pre defined level of −10.0 indicating no difference between the treatments Enalapril vs telmisartan NS difference in annual decreases in GFR

AER

Dalla VM (2004)[244] Level 1+	ACEI/CCB Ramipril vs lercanidipine NS difference Proportion of participants with reduction >50% was 22.2% with ramipril and 34.2% lercanidipine
Sengul AM (2006)[243] Level 1	ACEI/A2RB Lisinopril vs telmisartan NS difference Combination of lisinopril + telmisartan vs monotherapies AER reduction was significantly higher (p<0.001)

ESRD

Cochrane review[237] Level 1++	ACEI vs placebo/no treatment reduction in the risk of ESRD (10 studies, N=6,819, RR 0.68, 0.39 to 0.93)
Meta-analysis[238] Level 1+	ACEI or ARB vs other treatments, NS reduction in ESRD occurrence, those with diabetes (four trials, N=14,437), those without diabetes there was a reduction with ACE or A2RB
Meta-analysis[238] Level 1+	ACEI or A2RB vs other treatments showed a reduction in UAER for those with diabetes, (34 trials, N=4,772, RR −12.21, −21.68 to −2.74), for those without diabetes (44 trials, N=5,266, RR −15.73, −24.75 to −6.74, p=0.001)
Fogari R (2002)[245] Level 1+	ACEI/CCB Combination of fosinopril + amlodipine showed significantly greater reduction vs amlodipine monotherapy at any time and vs fosinopril from 18 months onwards
Barnett (2004)[242] Level 1+	ACEI/A2RB Enalapril vs telmisartan, annual changes were small with large CI in both groups. % changes were NS difference

* The association with smoking, hypertension, male gender and peripheral vascular disease was less strong
GFR, glomerular filtration rate

▷ Metabolic outcomes

Risk of diabetes

The extended HOPE trial identified that at the end of the extension phase there was a significant further reduction in risk for diabetes for ramipril vs placebo (2.7% vs 4.0%, RR 0.66, 0.46 to 0.95).[241] **Level 1+**

HbA$_{1c}$ and glycaemic control

The study which considered fosinopril and amlodipine monotherapy, and in combination, found that HbA$_{1c}$ was NS changed by any treatments and body weight remained unchanged.[245] **Level 1+**

The study which compared verapamil SR + trandopril and atenolol + chlorthalidone found that HbA$_{1c}$ remained stable with verapamilSR + trandopril but increased with atenolol + chlorthalidone 7.8 (1.26) at baseline and 8.6 (1.77) at last visit, treatment difference, p=0.0001; fasting glucose and fructosamine treatment difference, p=0.0001.[249]

Similarly, fasting glucose and fructosamine remained stable with verapamil SR + trandopril but increased with atenolol + chlorthalidone, treatment difference p=0.0001.[249] **Level 1++**

The study which considered verapamil + trandopril vs enalapril + hydrochlorothiazide identified that HbA$_{1c}$ remained stable with verapamil + trandopril but increased with enalapril + hydrochlorothiazide (baseline 5.96±1.25% to final 6.41±1.51%), difference between groups, p=0.040.[248] Crude blood glucose changes were 23±69 mg/dl for verapamil + trandopril (16.8% reduction) and 1±32 mg/dl (0.8% reduction) with enalapril + hydrochlorothiazide. The percentage of participants with glycaemic control (<126 mg/dl) increased from 50% to 72% with verapamil + trandopril, but did not change with enalapril + hydrochlorothiazide.[248] **Level 1++**

Adverse events

Both Cochrane reviews identified an increased risk of cough with ACE vs placebo/no treatment (four trials, N=3,725, RR 1.79, 1.19 to 2.69),[236] (10 trials, N=7,087, RR 3.17, 2.29 to 4.38).[237] **Level 1++**

Throughout the other studies the incidence of discontinuation due to AEs was small and the AEs reported were mainly; progression of diabetes, unsatisfactory therapeutic response, hypotension, ankle oedema, tachycardia, headache, cough, nausea, stomach upset, respiratory infection, and dizziness. **Level 1+**

A2RB

In summary, A2RB therapy was associated with greater benefits for Type 2 diabetes patients in terms of renal outcomes (e.g. progression to ESRD, doubling of serum creatinine, proteinuria) than treatment with placebo, CCB or sympatholytic agents. In addition, treatment with A2RB was also associated with a better metabolic and BP profile than sympatholytic therapy but non-significant differences were observed over those treated with CCB.

▷ A2RB vs placebo

Cardiovascular outcomes

All-cause mortality

A Cochrane review[237] did not find a statistically significant reduction in the risk of all-cause mortality in the five studies (3,409 patients) of A2RB vs placebo/no treatment. RR 0.99, 95% CI 0.85 to 1.17. **Level 1++**

Hospitalisations for heart failure

A post hoc analysis[254] compared the incidence of hospitalisation for heart failure within three tertiles of baseline serum creatinine concentration (highest, 2.1 to 3.6 mg/dl; middle, 1.6 to 2.0 mg/dl; lowest, 0.9 to 1.6 mg/dl). The study reported that the crude incidence of first hospitalisations for heart failure was higher in the highest (16.4%) and middle (15.0%) tertiles than in the lowest (11.1%) tertile (trend test across tertiles, p=0.02).

The study concluded that losartan decreased the hospitalisations for heart failure by 50.2 and 45.1, in the highest and middle tertile, respectively but was associated with a non-significant increased risk (42.5%) of hospitalisations in the lowest tertile. **Level 1+**

Renal outcomes

Progression to ESRD

A Cochrane review[237] found a significant reduction in the risk of ESRD with A2RB compared to placebo/no treatment (three studies, N=3,251): RR 0.78, 95% CI 0.67 to 0.91. **Level 1++**

A post hoc analysis[254] compared the incidence of ESRD within three tertiles of baseline serum creatinine concentration (highest, 2.1 to 3.6 mg/dl; middle, 1.6 to 2.0 mg/dl; lowest, 0.9 to 1.6 mg/dl). The study reported that the observed crude incidence of ESRD was significantly higher in the highest (40.5%) and middle (19.3%) tertiles as compared with the lowest (7.3%) tertile (trend test across tertiles, p<0.0001).

The study concluded that losartan decreased the risk of ESRD by 24.6, 26.3, and 35.3% in highest, middle, and lowest tertiles respectively. **Level 1+**

Doubling of serum creatinine

A Cochrane review[237] found a significant reduction in the risk of doubling of serum creatinine concentration with A2RB compared to placebo/no treatment (3 studies, 3,251 patients): RR 0.79 95% CI 0.67 to 0.93. **Level 1++**

Progression from micro- to macroalbuminuria

A Cochrane review[237] showed that the use of A2RB versus placebo/no treatment was also associated with a significant reduction in the risk of progression from micro- to macroalbuminuria (three studies, 761 patients); RR 0.45, 95% CI 0.32 to 0.75. **Level 1++**

Regression from micro- to normoalbuminuria

A Cochrane review[237] found a significant increase in regression from micro- to normo-albuminuria with A2RB versus placebo/no treatment (16 studies, 1,910 patients) RR 1.42, 95% CI 1.05 to 1.93. **Level 1++**

Proteinuria

A post hoc analysis[254] compared the median proteinuria reduction (%) within three tertiles of baseline serum creatinine concentration (highest, 2.1 to 3.6 mg/dl; middle, 1.6 to 2.0 mg/dl; lowest, 0.9 to 1.6 mg/dl). The study showed a significantly (p<0.0001) greater median percentage proteinuria reduction (versus baseline) on losartan than on placebo in the highest (24 vs –8%), middle (16 vs –8%), and lowest (15 vs –10%) tertiles respectively. **Level 1+**

A post hoc analysis of the IRMA study[255] reported that after 2 years of follow-up UAER decreased by 34% (95% CI 8 to 53), and 60% (95% CI 46 to 70) in the irbesartan 150 mg and irbesartan 300 mg groups respectively (p<0.05 vs baseline). No significant reductions in UAER were found in patients receiving placebo.

One month after withdrawal of irbesartan therapy, the same post hoc analysis[255] found no significant increases in UAER in patients receiving placebo or irbesartan 150 mg when compared with baseline values. However, the study reported that UAER remained persistently reduced by 47% (95% CI 24 to 63) in the irbesartan 300 mg group (p<0.05 vs baseline). This persistent reduction in the irbesartan 300 mg group, as compared with baseline, was highly significantly different from irbesartan 150 mg (p<0.01). This difference occurred although the regain in GFR between the two irbesartan groups were nearly identical. **Level 1+**

Blood pressure

A post hoc analysis of the IRMA study[255] found that after 2 years of treatment there were no significant differences in mean arterial blood pressure between patients treated with placebo or irbesartan (150 or 300 mg). However, 1 month after withdrawal of irbesartan therapy mean arterial blood pressure was unchanged in the placebo group, but increased significantly in the irbesartan groups to 109±2 and 108±2 in the 150 mg and 300 mg groups respectively (p<0.01). **Level 1+**

Metabolic outcomes

A post hoc analysis of the RENAAL study[253] found no significant differences between patients treated with losartan or placebo in terms of glycaemic levels, lipid profile or serum uric acid after 3.4 years of follow-up. **Level 1+**

Adverse events

A Cochrane review[237] found a significant increase in the risk of hyperkalaemia with A2RB compared to placebo/no treatment (two studies, 194 patients); RR 4.93, 95% CI 1.87 to 15.65. A2RB were not found to be associated with an increased risk of cough compared to placebo/no treatment. **Level 1++**

A2RB vs CCB

Cardiovascular and renal outcomes

One RCT[257] with a follow-up of 2.6 years, found that treatment with irbesartan significantly reduced the risk of doubling serum creatinine concentration, development of ESRD, or death from any cause, by 23% compared to the amlodipine therapy (p=0.006). **Level 1++**

When individual endpoints were analyzed the RCT[257] reported:

A significantly lower risk of a doubling in the serum creatinine concentration in patients receiving irbesartan compared to amlodipine-treated patients (37% lower in the irbesartan group than in the amlodipine group, p< 0.001).

Non-significant differences in terms of progression to ESRD between irbesartan-treated patients and those receiving amlodipine (risk 23% lower in the irbesartan group p=0.07).

Non-significant difference in the rates of death from any cause between patients treated with irbesartan and those treated with amlodipine. **Level 1++**

The same study[257] did not find a significant benefit associated with irbesartan as compared with amlodipine in reducing the secondary composite endpoint of death from CV causes, non-fatal MI, heart failure resulting in hospitalisation, a permanent neurologic deficit caused by a cerebrovascular event, or lower limb amputation above the ankle. **Level 1++**

An RCT[258] comparing therapy with valsartan and amlodipine reported results for a pre-specified subgroup of Type 2 diabetes patients and found non-significant differences between the two treatment arms for the primary composite cardiac outcome which looked at cardiac mortality and morbidity.* **Level 1+**

Another RCT[252] which also compared treatment with valsartan and amlodipine, found that after 24 weeks there was a significant reduction in UAER in patients receiving valsartan as compared with those treated with amlodipine (p<0.001; 95% CI for ratio, 0.520 to 0.710). The UAER at 24 weeks with valsartan was 56% (95% CI, 49.6 to 63.0) of baseline, equivalent to a 44% reduction. The UAER for amlodipine at week 24 was 92% (95% CI, 81.7 to 103.7) of baseline, a reduction of only 8%. **Level 1++**

The same RCT[252] showed a significantly greater percentage of patients returning to normo-albuminuria status by week 24 with valsartan (29.9%) than with amlodipine (14.5%). Treatment difference 15.4% 95% CI, 5.6 to 25.8, p<0.001. **Level 1++**

Blood pressure

One RCT[257] did not find significant differences in mean arterial pressure in patients treated with irbesartan and amlodipine after 2.6 years of follow-up. **Level 1++**

Metabolic outcomes

One RCT[251] reported that at 12 months there were no significant changes from baseline in HbA_{1c}, FPG, BMI, triglycerides and high-density lipoprotein cholesterol (HDL-C) in patients treated with telmisartan or nifedipine gastrointestinal therapeutic system (nifedipine GITS) and there were no significant differences in any of these parameters between treatments. **Level 1+**

The same RCT[251] showed that reduction in total cholesterol and low-density lipoprotein with telmisartan were significantly greater than those with nifedipine GITS (p<0.05). **Level 1+**

Adverse events

One RCT[257] reported that the incidence of hyperkalaemia (necessitating discontinuation of the study medication) was significantly higher in patients receiving irbesartan as compared to those receiving amlodipine. **Level 1++**

---

* The primary endpoint was time to first cardiac event (a composite of sudden cardiac death, fatal MI, death during or after percutaneous coronary intervention or coronary artery bypass graft, death as result of heart failure, and death associated with recent MI at autopsy, heart failure requiring hospital management, non-fatal MI, or emergency procedures to prevent MI).

One RCT[252] found that ankle oedema occurred significantly less frequently in valsartan-treated patients compared to those treated with amlodipine (1.2% vs 7.4% difference –6.2% 95% CI –12.9% to –0.4%, p<0.006). **Level 1+**

A2RB vs sympatholytic agents

Cardiovascular outcomes

One RCT[256] with a follow-up of 4.7 years found that treatment with losartan significantly reduced the risk of CV death, stroke, or MI compared to atenolol therapy. RR 0.76 (95% CI 0.58 to 0.98), p=0.031. **Level 1++**

When individual endpoints were analysed the RCT[256] reported:

- a statistically significant reduction in the risk of all-cause mortality in losartan-treated patients compared to those receiving atenolol. RR 0.61 (95% CI 0.45 to 0.84), p=0.002
- a statistically significant reduction in the risk of CV death favouring the losartan group. RR 0.63 (95% CI 0.42 to 0.95), p= 0.028
- non-significant difference in the incidence of stroke or MI between patients treated with losartan and those treated with atenolol.

Blood pressure*

One RCT[250] found that after 12 months, patients treated with irbesartan had significantly lower SBP and DBP levels as compared to those receiving doxazosin, (p<0.05). **Level 1+**

Metabolic outcomes

One RCT[250] found significantly lower HbA_{1c} levels in doxazosin-treated patients as compared to patients receiving irbesartan after 12 months of follow-up. **Level 1+**

The same RCT[250] found that patients treated with doxazosin had significantly higher levels of HDL-C as compared to those treated with irbesartan (p<0.05). **Level 1+**

Adverse events

One RCT[256] showed that albuminuria was reported less frequently (p=0.002) as an AE in the losartan than in the atenolol group (losartan 7% vs atenolol 13%). **Level 1++**

The same RCT[256] found that chest pain was more frequently reported in the losartan arm (p=0.036) (losartan 2% vs atenolol 8%). **Level 1++**

Beta-blockers

The evidence appraised suggested that treatment with beta-blockers in patients with Type 2 diabetes failed to demonstrate a better CV profile when compared with CCB therapy. Furthermore a landmark RCT showed a significant reduction in the incidence of CV outcomes in patients receiving CCB as compared with those treated with beta-blockers. In terms of BP

---

* BP reduction with all hypertensive treatments was a consistent feature of the studies and therefore only studies where there were significant differences between the treatments will be highlighted.

control, the evidence did not demonstrate differences between beta-blocker therapy and other antihypertensives.

Cardiovascular outcomes

All reported CV outcomes were for beta-blockers vs CCBs.

For the study considering COER verapamil and atenolol or hydrochlorothiazide there was NS difference between the groups for both the composite of acute MI, stroke or CV related death and also for the incidence of any component of the composite in the diabetic subgroup.[261] **Level 1+**

The ASCOT-BPLA study found that for the diabetes subgroup for total CV events and procedures there was significantly lower occurrence with the amlodipine based group vs the atenolol based group (HR 0.87, 0.76 to 0.99, p=0.0283), this was also found for the non-diabetic study participants.[262] **Level 1++**

The INVEST study found NS difference in the treatments (verapamilvSR and atenolol) for death or first occurrence of non-fatal MI or non-fatal stroke in both the diabetic and non-diabetic groups.[259] **Level 1+**

Blood pressure

Within all the papers included that reported BP outcomes the treatments reduced BP and there was NS difference found between the treatment groups.[260–262]

Renal outcomes

Only the study comparing two beta-blockers reported on renal outcomes.

The study considering carvedilol and metoprolol found that carvedilol reduced the albumin:creatinine ratio vs metoprolol (relative reduction 16%, p=0.003).[260] This study also identified those with albuminuria of 30 mg or less at baseline, fewer in the carvedilol group vs the metoprolol group progressed to microalbuminuria (6.4%, 25/388 vs 10.3%, 56/542), or from carvedilol vs metoprolol, 0.60, 0.36 to 0.97, p=0.04).[260] **Level 1++**

Metabolic outcomes

Only the study comparing two beta-blockers reported on metabolic outcomes.

The study considering carvedilol and metoprolol found that carvedilol treatment had no HbA$_{1c}$ changes from baseline while metoprolol increased HbA$_{1c}$. The mean difference was 0.12%, p=0.006. More participants withdrew due to worsening glycaemic control with metoprolol (16/737, 2.2%) than with carvedilol (3/498, 0.6%), p=0.04.[260] **Level 1++**

Adverse events

The study comparing COER verapamil with atenolol or hydrochlorothiazide[261] reported that participants assigned COER verapamil withdrew more often due to adverse signs or symptoms compared with those assigned atenolol of hydrochlorothiazide (p=0.02); the most common reason was constipation (216 in the COER verapamil compared with 28 in the atenolol of hydrochlorothiazide group). However, fewer participants assigned COER verapamil (N=115) atenolol of hydrochlorothiazide withdrew because of poor BP control compared with those assigned atenolol of hydrochlorothiazide (N=207) (p<0.001 by log-rank). **Level 1+**

The INVEST study[259] showed that verapamil and atenolol were generally well tolerated in each treatment group. Patients in the verapamil group reported constipation and coughs more frequently than patients in the atenolol group, while atenolol-treated patients had more dyspnoea, lightheadedness, symptomatic bradycardia, and wheezing. **Level 1+**

The RCT comparing carvedilol with metoprolol did not report significant differences between groups in overall safety profile. However, the study stated that no participant taking carvedilol had a respiratory event in contrast with seven events in six participants taking metoprolol. **Level 1+**

The ASCOT-BPLA study concluded that the most frequent AEs found in the amlodipine based group were peripheral oedema 23%; cough 19%; joint swelling 14%; dizziness 12%; chest pain 8%; fatigue 8%. In the atenolol based group the most frequent AEs were dizziness 16%; fatigue 16%; dyspnoea 9%; cough 8%; erectile dysfunction 7%. **Level 1+**

12.3.4 Health economic evidence statements

▷ ACEI

Ramipril was found to be cost-effective compared to placebo, £2,971/LYG, Beard et al. (2001),[263] and €2,486/LYG, Schadlich et al. (2004),[264] (£1,699/LYG, exchange rate 0.68, 13 March 2007).[271]

No statistically significant difference was found between captopril and atenolol. Atenolol had significantly lower mean costs.[265]

▷ A2RB

Irbesartan was found to be both more effective and cost saving than amlodipine and standard antihypertensive treatment. Palmer et al. (2004),[266] Rodby et al. (2003),[267] and Coyle et al. (2004).[268]

Losartan was found to be both more effective and cost saving than standard antihypertensive treatment, Vora et al. (2005).[269]

Valsartan was found to be both more effective and cost saving compared to amlodipine, Smith et al. (2004).[270]

12.3.5 From evidence to recommendations

The GDG used as its starting point the 2006 update of the NICE hypertension guidelines and the NICE Type 2 diabetes hypertension guideline from 2002, available at www.nice.org.uk. The group noted that the health economic model for the former did not include renal or retinopathy outcomes, both of particular importance when considering choice of therapies for use in people with Type 2 diabetes. Thus 25% of people with Type 2 diabetes develop diabetic nephropathy within 20 years of diagnosis, while the drugs studied in the UKPDS hypertension study had strong effects on retinopathy progression. Therefore, the GDG was particularly interested in reviewing the evidence as to whether there were any differential effects in terms of different classes of antihypertensive agent on microvascular as well as cardiovascular outcomes in people with Type 2 diabetes.

The GDG noted a wealth of new evidence in this area since the previous guideline was published, and were cognisant of the recently published early revision of the NICE hypertension guidelines, albeit these applying to people without diabetes. Much of the new evidence seemed to be driven by studies in people with diabetes with increased AER (microalbuminuria or worse). The high known prevalence of renal damage in people with Type 2 diabetes and the need to prevent this and its progression were noted to emphasise the importance of BP control. Little new evidence on retinopathy prevention was available to the GDG, but it was aware of the positive data previously assessed for ACEI and a beta-adrenergic blocker. New published CV outcome data was noted to be of limited quality in some studies due to under powering in studies with other primary endpoints, even when combined for meta-analysis.

The GDG noted that the evidence did not distinguish between medications on the basis of degree of BP lowering. The issues of importance revolved around differences of evidence of effectiveness in renal related outcomes and metabolic worsening. Some classes of medications, notably A2RB and alpha-adrenergic blockers, were only available in more expensive proprietary form, and thus without added evidence of efficacy would not be cost-effective compared to older drugs.

Overall it was felt that the best evidence for prevention of renal disease and limitation of metabolic worsening related to the renin angiotensin system-blockers (RAS-blockers) (ACEI and A2RB) as a class.

With regard to non-renal outcomes, no evidence was identified that caused the GDG to reach any different conclusions from the review of the evidence carried out for the NICE hypertension guideline. The GDG recognised there was good evidence of efficacy for thiazide diuretics and CCBs, including when used in combination with RAS-blockers.

Given the benefits in terms of reno-protection and retinopathy of RAS blockade, it was felt appropriate to recommend RAS-blockers as first-line medication in the treatment of hypertension in Type 2 diabetes. This was the one change in sequencing that the GDG felt was appropriate to make to the NICE hypertension guidelines. On the grounds of cost a generic 24-hour ACEI should be used first line. A2RB (also selected on grounds of cost) should only be substituted in the event of significant ACEI intolerance, usually troublesome chronic cough (and not if hyperkalaemia or decreased renal function is the problem). An exception was highlighted in the NICE hypertension guideline where people of African-Caribbean descent are noted to respond less well to RAS-blockers, and for someone in this group either combination ACEI + diuretic therapy or CCB was thought appropriate first line. Little specific information was available for other ethnic groups.

Thiazide diuretics and CCBs are recommended as second-line medications, though it was noted that it would be usual to need at least two drugs or more, so these would be added to a RAS-blocker and each other for the most part. There was some concern about the adverse metabolic effects of thiazides (in contrast to the positive effects of RAS-blockers and neutral effects of CCB), though the standard dose of bendroflumethiazide was thought not to be a problem in this regard.

Many people with diabetes do require four or even five antihypertensive agents to approach target levels. After three classes of medication had been used the GDG felt that reasons for distinguishing between other drug classes were poor. It was felt that any alpha-blocker, beta-blocker, or potassium-sparing diuretic could be added at this stage. If an RAS-blocker is used with a potassium-sparing diuretic, the potassium levels should be carefully monitored, the clinician being alert to the possibility of hyperkalaemia.

While in general this was felt to be the appropriate positioning of the beta-blockers, particularly because of their metabolic effects when used in combination with thiazides, it was recognised that some people would have a clearer indication for these drugs through having angina, heart failure, or previous heart attack. In these circumstances the drugs would already be being prescribed. One study suggested that carvedilol was superior to metoprolol both in metabolic terms and for renal protection. The GDG found the evidence interesting but incomplete in regard of target groups and active comparisons with the RAS-blockers; accordingly no out-of-class recommendations are made.

There is a need to emphasise caution over the use of some drug classes in the increasing numbers of women with Type 2 diabetes who might become pregnant. The GDG felt comfortable that the decision to use, or not use, such drugs should be one of informed agreement between each woman and their professional advisor.

Issues of adherence and the use of fixed-dose combination therapy were considered. The evidence was not formally available to the GDG, but clinical experience over the combined burden of medications faced by many people with Type 2 diabetes led to an overall view that combination tablets could be appropriate in reducing that burden, and possibly improving outcomes through better adherence. No formal recommendations can be made.

The GDG were aware of the issues that arose from the burden of use of multiple therapies. In this area in particular it was therefore felt appropriate to further emphasise communication, discussion and agreement about medication use.

An issue considered of importance, but not covered in the evidence review was that of BP monitoring, including the role of self-monitoring and of ambulatory BP monitoring. The GDG was happy to defer to the NICE hypertension guideline on these issues.

RECOMMENDATIONS

R59   Measure blood pressure at least annually in a person without previously diagnosed hypertension or renal disease. Offer and reinforce preventive lifestyle advice.

R60   For a person on antihypertensive therapy at diagnosis of diabetes, review control of blood pressure and medications used, and make changes only where there is poor control or where current medications are not appropriate because of microvascular complications or metabolic problems.

R61   Repeat blood pressure measurements within:
- One month if blood pressure is higher than 150/90 mmHg
- Two months if blood pressure is higher than 140/80 mmHg
- Two months if blood pressure is higher than 130/80 mmHg and there is kidney, eye or cerebrovascular damage.

Offer lifestyle advice (diet and exercise) at the same time.

R62   Offer lifestyle advice (see dietary recommendations in section 6.1 of this guideline and the lifestyle recommendations in section 1.2 of 'Hypertension: management of hypertension in adults in primary care')[272] if blood pressure is confirmed as being consistently above 140/80 mmHg (or above 130/80 mmHg if there is kidney, eye or cerebrovascular damage).

R63   Add medications if lifestyle advice does not reduce blood pressure to below 140/80 mmHg (below 130/80 mmHg if there is kidney, eye or cerebrovascular damage).

R64   Monitor blood pressure 1–2 monthly, and intensify therapy if on medications, until blood pressure is consistently below 140/80 mmHg (below 130/80 mmHg if there is kidney, eye or cerebrovascular disease).

R65   First-line blood pressure-lowering therapy should be a once daily, generic angiotensin-converting enzyme (ACE) inhibitor. Exceptions to this are people of African-Caribbean descent or women for whom there is a possibility of becoming pregnant (see recommendation 66 and 67).

R66   The first-line blood pressure-lowering therapy for a person of African-Caribbean descent should be an ACE inhibitor plus either a diuretic or a generic calcium channel blocker.

R67   A calcium channel blocker should be the first-line blood pressure-lowering therapy for a woman for whom, after an informed discussion, it is agreed there is a possibility of her becoming pregnant.

R68   For a person with continuing intolerance to an ACE inhibitor (other than renal deterioration or hyperkalaemia), substitute an angiotensin II-receptor antagonist for the ACE inhibitor.

R69   If the person's blood pressure is not reduced to the individually agreed target with first-line therapy, add a calcium channel blocker or a diuretic (usually bendroflumethiazide, 2.5 mg daily). Add the other drug (that is, the calcium channel blocker or diuretic) if the target is not reached with dual therapy.

R70   If the person's blood pressure is not reduced to the individually agreed target with triple therapy (see recommendation 69), add an alpha-blocker, a beta-blocker or a potassium-sparing diuretic (the last with caution if the individual is already taking an ACE inhibitor or an angiotensin II-receptor antagonist).

R71   Monitor the blood pressure of a person who has attained and consistently remained at his or her blood pressure target every 4–6 months, and check for possible adverse effects of antihypertensive therapy – including the risks from unnecessarily low blood pressure.

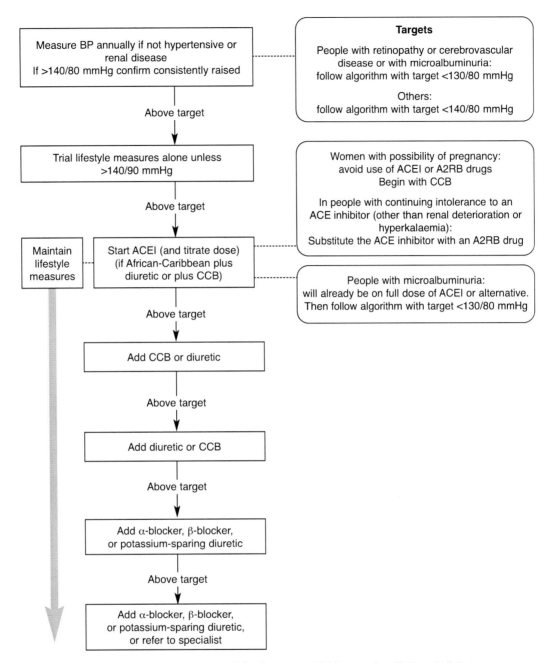

Figure 12.1 Scheme for the management of blood pressure (BP) for people with Type 2 diabetes
ACEI, angiotensin-converting enzyme inhibitor; A2RB, angiotensin 2 receptor blocker (sartan); CCB, calcium channel blocker

13 | Cardiovascular risk estimation

13.1.1 Clinical introduction

Nearly all people with Type 2 diabetes are at high cardiovascular (CV) risk – high enough to justify statin therapy without further assessment.[273] Others are at more extreme risk.[273] Other therapies in addition to cholesterol-modifying drugs used to ameliorate CV risk include blood glucose lowering, blood pressure (BP) lowering, and anti-platelet therapies (see recommendations in these areas), together with lifestyle measures. Logically the intensity with which these therapies are used should be determined in part by the level of risk. To a limited extent this can be assessed clinically by summation of presence of risk factors (high waist circumference, low-density lipoprotein cholesterol (LDL-C) level, HbA_{1c}, BP, smoking, family history of premature vascular disease, ethnic group, abnormal serum high-density lipoprotein cholesterol (HDL-C) and triglyceride (TG)) or the presence of particular risk factors (microalbuminuria, previous CV event). However, many of these variables are continuous distributions so it makes sense to ask whether tools are available that make full use of the data which could be made available from their measurement. As diabetes itself is a risk factor, any such approach would have to be diabetes specific.

The clinical questions addressed were whether any risk calculator (risk engine) or risk chart, specifically designed for people with diabetes, gave valid and useful assessments of CV risk in people with diabetes, and in what circumstances they might be used.

13.1.2 Methodological introduction

A total of five studies were identified as relevant to the question.[274–278] It should be noted that studies reporting internal validations of their models (i.e. a first level of validation in which the model is required to reproduce the data originally used in its calibration) were excluded.

The five studies included compared the prognostic value of several methods of risk prediction (either computerised tools or chart/table-based tools). These tools aim at identifying high-risk patients and determine whether a patient will receive a therapy that modifies cardiovascular disease/coronary heart disease (CVD/CHD) morbidity and mortality.

One observational study[277] assessed differences between absolute CHD risks calculated by the Joint British Societies' (JBS) risk calculator chart and UKPDS risk engine. The study had a median follow-up of 4.2 years and compared the two methods on a cohort of diabetic populations from guideline 26 NHS-general practices.

One study[275] assessed differences between absolute CHD risks calculated by the Framingham study risk equation and UKPDS risk engine. The study compared the two methods by using clinical records from UK diabetic patients.

One study[276] compared the prognostic value of four methods to predict CVD and CHD risk (JBS risk calculator, the CardioRisk Manager, the Prospective Cardiovascular Münster (PROCAM) calculation and the UKPDS risk engine) using data from a UK clinical-based population database of diabetic patients.

One study[278] assessed the prognostic value of three risk calculators for CVD and CHD (Framingham study risk equation, Systematic Coronary Risk Evaluation (SCORE) project risk score and Diabetes Epidemiology Collaborative Analysis of Diagnostic criteria in Europe (DECODE) risk equation) using UKPDS data.

One study[274] reported 74 validation exercises involving 18 clinical trials for the Archimedes diabetes model. (No studies were found comparing the Archimedes diabetes model with other risk calculators.)

It should be noted that the likelihood of variation in terms of risk prediction is greatest between the tools in the format of either a chart or a table. This is because patient characteristics are either dichotomised or approximated resulting in broad categories of risk. The computer-based tools have similar patient characteristics as inputs and should therefore give similar answers. However, important differences exist in the number and type of equations used and assumptions made about missing patient data.*

▷ Methods of risk prediction analysed

Framingham-based risk assessments

The Framingham CV risk function, which is widely employed to estimate CVD and CHD risk, is a survival model based on the Weibull distribution and derived from the risk profiles of 5,573 CHD-free members of the Framingham cohort, aged 30–74 years and followed for 12 years, 6% of whom had diabetes (N=337). The JBS charts and the CardioRisk Manager program make use of modified versions of the Framingham model.

JBS risk calculator chart utilises eight risk factors (age, sex, systolic or diastolic BP, smoking status, presence or absence of diabetes mellitus, left ventricular hypertrophy (LVH) and total and HDL-C) to calculate absolute CHD risk in those patients aged between 30 and 74 years.

The CardioRisk manager program (computer-based) calculates and displays an individual's absolute and relative 10-year risks of CHD, stroke, or various other endpoints of CVD and can be used to estimate the expected benefit of modifying risk factors. The model uses the full Framingham risk score (rather than an approximation of it). The eleven variables included are: age, sex, systolic or diastolic BP, smoking status, presence or absence of diabetes mellitus and LVH and total and HDL-C, atrial fibrillation, history of CVD, antihypertensive therapy.

The UKPDS risk engine

The UKPDS risk engine (computer-based) for determining CHD risk is based on data from 4,540 participants in the UKPDS study and includes diabetes specific covariates. The UKPDS risk engine model utilises nine risk factors, these are: age at diagnosis, duration of diabetes, sex, ethnicity, smoking status, SBP, HbA_{1c}, total and HDL-C to calculate CHD risk.

The differences between the JBS risk calculator and the UKPDS risk engine are that the UKPDS model recognises glycaemic control as a continuous risk factor, rather than a dichotomous variable such as absence or presence of diabetes. Furthermore, age is replaced by two diabetes specific variables; age at diagnosis and duration of diabetes. Ethnicity is also included as a risk factor in the UKPDS equation but not in the Framingham equation.

---

* Charts and tables are easy to use and an estimate of risk can be obtained without knowledge of all the patients' characteristics. The advantage of the computer-based tools is the ability to allow fine graduations instead of broad categories of risk. The disadvantage is that patient characteristics either have to be available or be measured by the clinician.

The UKPDS modified risk engine (stroke)

There is a modified UKPDS engine used to calculate the risk of a first stroke. The equation is based on data from 4,549 patients enrolled in the UKPDS. Variables included in the final model were duration of diabetes, age, sex, smoking, systolic blood pressure (SBP), total cholesterol (TC) to HDL ratio and presence of atrial fibrillation. Not included in the model were BMI, HbA$_{1c}$, ethnicity, and ex-smoking status.

PROCAM score system

It constitutes a relatively simple point-scoring scheme for calculating the risk of CHD (fatal or non-fatal MI or acute coronary death). These scores were derived from a Cox proportional hazards model calculated from 10 years of follow-up of the cohort of middle-aged men in the PROCAM study. The model is based on 325 acute coronary events occurring within 10 years of follow-up among 5,389 men, 35 to 65 years of age at recruitment into the PROCAM study. The model uses eight independent risk variables (ranked in order of importance): age, low-density lipoprotein (LDL), HDL-C, SBP, family history of premature MI, diabetes, smoking, and TGs.

SCORE risk charts

The SCORE risk charts were intended for risk stratification in the primary prevention of CVD and CHD. The equation is based on a pooled dataset from 12 European cohort studies, mainly carried out in general population settings (N=205,178). Ten-year risk of fatal CVD was calculated using a Weibull model in which age was used as a measure of exposure time to risk rather than as a risk factor. Variables included were TC and TC/high-density lipoprotein (HDL) ratio. However, due to non-uniformity* in the ascertainment of diabetes, the SCORE study did not include a dichotomous diabetes variable into the risk function and neither produce a separate risk score system for people with diabetes.

DECODE risk score

The model used the large European DECODE cohort (25,413 patients from 14 European studies) to develop risk scores for CVD mortality over 5 year and 10-year follow-up periods. The risk factors used by the model were: age, fasting and 2-h glucose (including cases of known diabetes), fasting glucose alone (including cases of known diabetes), cholesterol, smoking status, systolic BP and BMI. The model developed a score for absolute risk (AR) based on country-specific CVD death rates for 1995. An important limitation of the model is that the lack of knowledge of whether the participants included in the DECODE cohort already had CVD at baseline.

The Archimedes model

It is a mathematical model that attempts to replicate the pathophysiology of diabetes with a high level of biological and clinical detail. The model includes the pertinent organ systems, more than 50 continuously interacting biological variables, and the major symptoms, tests, treatments, and outcomes. The several equations on which this model is built can simulate a variety of clinical trials and reproduce their results with good accuracy.

---

* Data on diabetes had not been collected uniformly in SCORE study cohorts. In a majority of the cohorts the diagnosis of diabetes was based only on a self-report (sometimes with corroborative evidence from a family doctor) and in some study cohorts information on diabetes was not available.

The Archimedes model is written at a fairly deep level of biology. It is continuous in time, and it preserves the continuous nature and simultaneous interactions of biological variables.* Structurally, it is written with differential equations and is programmed in an object-oriented language called Smalltalk.

13.1.3 Health economic methodological introduction

No health economic papers were identified.

13.1.4 Evidence statements

▷ UKPDS risk engine vs Framingham equation

One observational study was identified assessing the prognostic value of these two methods in a cohort of patients newly diagnosed with Type 2 diabetes.[277] In addition the sensitivity and specificity of both models at a 15%, 10-year CHD risk threshold (NICE guidelines) was compared with that of the ADA lipid threshold (LDL ≥2.6 mmol/l or TG ≥4.5 mmol/l). **Level 2++**

Overall

At the level of the entire cohort, the number of events predicted by the Framingham equation underestimated both true CVD and CHD events by 33% and 32% respectively, as opposed to the statistically non-significant 13% of CHD events in the case of the UKPDS risk engine. (See tables 13.1–13.3.)

Gender/hypertension treatment

The Framingham results suggested a tendency towards a greater degree of underestimation of CHD events in men than women (41% vs 26%) and for pre-treated rather than untreated BP (42 vs 31%). (See tables 13.1–13.3.)

Risk stratification

When using both risk calculation methods similar proportions were assigned, 10-year scores less than 15% (Framingham 27.3% and UKPDS 25.7%). However, the UKPDS risk engine assigned a 10-year score over 30% to 187 (43.7%) of the study participants as compared with only 88 (20.5%) when derived from Framingham.

---

* For example, in the Archimedes model the equations are not calculating the risk of an outcome such as a MI, but are rather modelling the occlusion of specific coronary arteries in specific locations. The model also includes FPG as a continuous variable, and they incorporate not only the degree of elevation in FPG but also the duration of time that the FPG has been elevated to different degrees.

Table 13.1 Proportion of actual and predicted CVD events using the Framingham equations

	N	Actual events	Predicted	Ratio P/A	Discrimination	Calibration
All cohort members	428	98	66	0.67	0.673	32.8 (p<0.001)
Males	241	63	41	0.65	0.669	*
Females	187	35	25	0.71	0.678	*
Pre-treated BP	136	40	24	0.60	0.634	*
Untreated BP	292	58	42	0.66	0.690	*

Table 13.2 Proportion of actual and predicted CHD events using the Framingham equations

	N	Actual events	Predicted	Ratio P/A	Discrimination	Calibration
All cohort members	428	60	41	0.68	0.657	19.8 (p=0.011)
Males	241	41	24	0.59	0.726	*
Females	187	19	14	0.74	0.697	*
Pre-treated BP	136	24	14	0.58	0.666	*
Untreated BP	292	36	25	0.69	0.663	*

Table 13.3 Proportion of actual and predicted CHD events using the UKPDS risk engine

	N	Actual events	Predicted	Ratio P/A	Discrimination	Calibration
All cohort members	428	60	52	0.87	0.670	17.1 (p=0.029)
Males	241	41	37	0.90	0.673	*
Females	187	19	16	0.84	0.618	*
Pre-treated BP	136	24	19	0.79	0.696	*
Untreated BP	292	36	33	0.92	0.648	*

▷ Framingham and UKPDS risk engine vs ADA lipid threshold

The 15%, 10-year CHD risk threshold with both the Framingham and UKPDS risk engines had similar sensitivity for primary CVD as the lipid level threshold 85.7 and 89.8% vs 93.9% (p=0.21 and 0.34) and both had greater specificity 33.0 and 30.3% vs 12.1% (p<0.001 and p<0.001).

▷ UKPDS risk engine vs JBS risk chart

One study[275] compared the prognostic value between these two risk calculators by using data from NHS clinical databases. **Level 3**

Overall

Overall, the UKPDS risk engine was found to calculate a significantly higher mean 10-year risk (UKPDS vs JBS, 21.5 vs 18.3%, p<0.0001) with the mean difference of 3.2% (95% CI 2.7–3.8). However, both methods identified approximately 65% of patients with Type 2 diabetes who would require primary prevention intervention and therefore have comparable accuracy in identifying these high-risk patients.

Gender differences

A bias towards men to have a much higher CHD risk with the UKPDS risk engine was reported. The mean difference in risk score between men and woman was approximately 8.4% with the UKPDS risk engine in comparison with 1.7% with the JBS calculator. For men, the UKPDS risk engine calculated CHD risk approximately 6% higher than the JBS calculator.

Risk stratification

Both methods identified similar proportions of patients with CHD risk of at least 15% over 10 years. However, the main differential feature found between the two methods was the tendency of the UKPDS risk engine to identify significantly more patients in the high-risk category (>30%) in comparison with JBS (p<0.001). (See table 13.4.)

Table 13.4 CHD 10-year risk stratification (UKPDS risk engine vs JBS risk chart)			
	<15%	**15–30%**	**>30%**
UKPDS	34.4%	43.0%	22.6%
JBS	34.4%	58.3%	7.3%

▷ JBS risk calculator, the CardioRisk Manager, the PROCAM calculation and the UKPDS risk engine

One study[276] assessed the prognostic value across four risk calculators. Analysis was conducted by accessing medical records from a cohort of diabetic patients who had attended a NHS clinic for a period of 10 years. **Level 3**

Overall, the study showed that all tests (except PROCAM) demonstrated acceptable discrimination with respect to CHD/CVD, however all underestimated the risk of future events.

Table 13.5 Discrimintation of the four methods of risk prediction		
Discrimination C-index (95% CI)		
	CVD	**CHD**
JBS	0.80 (0.75–0.85)	0.77 (0.74–0.80)
CRM	0.76 (0.72–0.79)	0.73 (0.70–0.77)
PROCAM	0.67 (0.62–0.73)	0.65 (0.59–0.71)
UKPDS	0.74 (0.70–0.78)	0.76 (0.72–0.80)
CRM, Cardio Risk Manager		

▷ Framingham study risk equation, SCORE project risk score and DECODE risk equation

One study[278] evaluated these three risk equations in patients with Type 2 diabetes using UKPDS data. **Level 3**

The 10-year fatal CVD event rate

The 10-year fatal CVD event rate (95% CI) observed in UKPDS was 7.4% (6.5–8.3). Framingham underestimated this by 32% with an AR of 5.0%, SCORE overestimated risk by 18% (AR 8.7%) whereas DECODE (AR 6.6%) yielded an acceptable estimate.

For males, only SCORE provided a reasonable estimate. In females, only Framingham performed well.

For Caucasians (N=3,207), the 7.9% (6.7–9.0) observed event rate was underestimated by 34% using Framingham (AR 5.2%), overestimated by 19% using SCORE (AR 9.4%), and estimated appropriately by DECODE (AR 7.1%).

The 10-year fatal CHD event rate

The 10-year fatal CHD event rate (95% CI) observed in UKPDS was 6.3% (5.5–7.1). Framingham underestimated this (AR 4.3%) while SCORE provided a reasonable estimate (AR 5.7%). Both equations provided reliable estimates for females but not males. For Caucasians, the observed rate of 7.2% (6.3–8.1) was underestimated by both Framingham (4.6%) and SCORE (6.2%).

Table 13.6 Discrimination of the three methods of risk prediction (aROC analysis)

Discrimination C-index (95% CI)

	CVD mortality
Framingham	0.76
SCORE	0.77
DECODE	0.67

aROC, areas under the receiver operating characteristics

▷ External validation of the Archimedes diabetes model

A study[274] reported results from a total of 74 validation exercises which were conducted involving different treatments and outcomes in 18 clinical trials (10 of which were not used to build the model).* **Level 3**

For 71 of the 74 exercises there were no statistically significant differences between the results calculated by the model and the results observed in the trial. Overall, the correlation coefficient for all 74 exercises is r=0.99.

---

* Ten of the trials (DPP, HPS, MICROHOPE, LIPID, HHS, SHEP, LRC-CPPT, MRC, VA-HIT, and WOSCOPS) were not used at all to build the physiology model; they provided external or independent validations of the model. The remaining eight trials (UKPDS, HOPE, CARE, Lewis, IRMA-2, DCCT, IDNT, and 4-S) provided internal or dependent validations.

If the outcomes in the control group and the absolute differences between the control and treated groups are compared for model and trial, the correlation coefficient is r=0.99. Focusing specifically on the absolute differences in the outcomes, which determines the number needed to treat, the correlation coefficient is r=0.97. For the 10 trials that were not used to build the model, the correlation coefficient is also r=0.99.

13.1.5 From evidence to recommendations

The UKPDS risk engine and to a lesser extent the older JBS-2 charts had some evidence of validity in people with Type 2 diabetes, at least once over the age of 40 years. However, in their latest revision JBS-2 charts for people with Type 2 diabetes are not available. Other estimations based on the Framingham population were not reliable, and the reasons for this were understood. No system included all the desirable variables, with the exception of Archimedes, but this was not intended as a clinical tool.

It was noted that a wide range of epidemiological studies suggested that people with diabetes were over twice as likely as the background population (age and sex matched) to develop CVD, and that many had confounding factors (such as use of antihypertensive or glucose-lowering medications) which prevented use of calculators. Studies such as the UK validation analysis reported above were clearly not consistent epidemiologically with UK populations at diagnosis, and furthermore excluded people already on therapy, and are therefore not reliable as a means of estimating the size of the population justifying therapy except for comparing tools. The group concluded that the normal approach, once age was considered, of managing nearly all people with Type 2 diabetes as having risk >20%/10-years was appropriate, particularly as outcome from MI is known to be worse for those with diabetes, and preventative therapy therefore more cost effective.

Particular concerns were also expressed by the GDG over people with microalbuminuria, those with more extreme family histories of CVD, and those with previous and recurrent CV events. This and the age problem meant that it was recognised that any risk estimation had a limited role. However, the GDG were also concerned that some people with Type 2 diabetes do not have the classical phenotype of the disease with abdominal adiposity (or obesity) and low HDL-C. It was concerned that such people should be recognised at diagnosis and managed more conservatively.

RECOMMENDATIONS

R72   Consider a person to be at high premature cardiovascular risk for his or her age unless he or she:
- is not overweight, tailoring this with an assessment of body weight associated risk according to ethnic group*
- is normotensive (<140/80 mmHg in the absence of antihypertensive therapy)
- does not have macroalbuminuria
- does not smoke
- does not have a high-risk lipid profile
- has no history of cardiovascular disease, and
- has no family history of cardiovascular disease.

---

* Please see the NICE Obesity guideline (CG43), www.nice.org.uk/guidance/index.jsp?action=byID&o=11000

R73   If the person is considered not to be at high cardiovascular risk, estimate cardiovascular risk annually using the UK Prospective Diabetes Study (UKPDS) risk engine.[279]

R74   Consider using cardiovascular risk estimates from the UKPDS risk engine for educational purposes when discussing cardiovascular complications with the individual.[279]

R75   Perform full lipid profile (including high-density lipoprotein cholesterol and triglyceride estimations) when assessing cardiovascular risk annually, and before starting lipid-modifying therapy.

14 | Management of blood lipid levels

14.1 Overall clinical introduction

Nearly all people with Type 2 diabetes are at high cardiovascular (CV) risk. Epidemiologically that excess risk is independently associated with their hyperglycaemia together with high blood pressure (BP) and dyslipidaemia, the last typically the low high-density lipoprotein cholesterol (HDL-C) and raised triglyceride (TG) levels found as components of the metabolic syndrome.[280] Studies have suggested that people with Type 2 diabetes without declared cardiovascular disease (CVD) are at as high a risk of a CVD event as someone without diabetes with declared CVD.[273] While this is disputed by other studies, it still leaves individuals with Type 2 diabetes as nearly always in the high CVD risk category, and accordingly it has been usual to manage them actively as if for secondary rather than primary prevention of CVD. Nevertheless, in a few people with Type 2 diabetes the clinical phenotype is not that associated with high CV risk, albeit these people being generally remarkable for not being overweight nor having features of the metabolic syndrome, and being insulin sensitive. More importantly people with Type 2 diabetes who have declared CVD are at much higher risk (>1.5–2.6) of further events or CV death as people with CVD without diabetes.[273] Such extreme risk would appear to justify more intensive management than usually offered to someone who has, for example, had a heart attack.

The management of CV risk through glucose lowering, BP lowering, and anti-platelet therapy is dealt with elsewhere in this guideline. This chapter deals with lipid-lowering therapy; dietary modification also being dealt with in a separate chapter. Paradoxically, although low-density lipoprotein cholesterol (LDL-C) levels are not particularly raised in people with Type 2 diabetes compared to the background population, the opportunity to lower risk through lipid management is currently greatest through drugs which lower LDL-C, principally the statins. Nevertheless, a variety of other lipid modifying drugs are available and will be considered in turn.

14.2 Targets and intervention levels

14.2.1 Clinical introduction

The principal aspects of the blood lipid profile recognised as risk factors for CVD include LDL-C, HDL-C, and TGs. As the means of management of these is widely available (lifestyle and drugs) it might seem logical to treat them as safe targets. Unfortunately there is no 'safe' level, nor a level at which they do not contribute to vascular risk, a situation analogous with blood glucose control and BP control. This leads to the question of the level of blood lipids that should be acceptable without intensive therapy in people with diabetes, or whether instead it is risk and not lipid levels that should be managed.

The clinical question is to what levels if any should LDL-C, HDL-C and serum TG be managed in clinical practice.

14.2.2 Methodological introduction

There were three studies which were specifically relevant to target levels for lipid levels and two meta-analysis studies.

The Cholesterol Treatment Trialists' (CTT) Collaborators completed a prospective meta-analysis in 14 randomised trials of statins, published in 2005.[281] This analysis included data from 90,056 (N=45,054 allocated a statin, N=45,002 controls) participants with diabetes. The studies included were published over 10 years from 1994–2004.

A meta-analysis was completed which considered pharmacological lipid-lowering therapy in Type 2 diabetes. This analysis included 14 studies (total N=17,749), six primary prevention studies (N=11,025) and eight secondary prevention studies (N=6,724). The studies included were published from 1987–2003.[282]

14.2.3 Health economic methodological introduction

No health economic papers were identified.

The health economic analysis performed for statin therapy (appendix D, available at www.rcplondon.ac.uk/pubs/brochure.aspx?e=247) addressed the question of target levels in part. This is considered further in the section on statin therapy.

14.2.4 Evidence statements

▷ Outcomes

CTT collaborators

The CTT collaborators meta-analysis identified that there is an approximately linear relationship between the absolute reductions in LDL-C found in the 14 studies and the proportional reductions in the incidence of coronary and other major vascular events.[281]

The proportional reductions in major vascular event rates per mmol/l LDL-C reduction were very similar in all subgroups examined (i.e. including the diabetic subgroup), including not just individuals presenting with LDL-C below 2.6 mmol/l (100 mg/dl). **Level 1++**

Table 14.1 Risk reductions in LDL-C	
	Percentage proportional reduction per mmol/l LDL-C reduction
Overall death rate	12% reduction in all-cause mortality; RR 0.88 (0.84 to 0.91, p<0.0001)
CHD death	19% reduction in CHD death; 14/1,000 fewer deaths among those with pre-existing CHD and 4/1,000 among those without pre-existing CHD
Major coronary events	23% reduction in the incidence of first major coronary events; RR 0.77 (p<0.001) Diabetic subgroup, without pre-existing vascular disease; RR 0.74 (0.62 to 0.88, p<0.001)
Coronary revascularisation	24% reduction in the incidence of first coronary revascularisation (proportional reductions in coronary artery grafting and angioplasty were similar); RR 0.76 (0.73 to 0.80, p<0.0001)
Stroke	17% reduction in the incidence of first stroke; RR 0.83 (0.78 to 0.88, p<0.0001)
Major vascular events	21% reduction in the incidence of major vascular events; RR 0.79 (0.77 to 0.81, p<0.0001) Diabetic subgroup, without pre-existing vascular disease; RR 0.75 (0.66 to 0.86)
CHD, coronary heart disease	

Meta-analysis – lipid-lowering therapy

The lipid-lowering therapy meta-analysis showed that the RR reductions were similar for both primary and secondary prevention.[282] However, the average absolute risk reduction was more than twice as high for those with coronary artery disease (secondary prevention) than for those without it (primary prevention).

Primary prevention trials – fixed effects analysis due to level of heterogeneity (p=0.18). The pooled RR for CV events with lipid-lowering therapy was 0.78 (0.67 to 0.89), with number needed to be treated (NNT) for benefit of 34.5 (for 4.3 years).

Secondary prevention analysis – random effects analysis as there was substantial between study heterogeneity (p=0.03). The pooled RR for CV events with lipid-lowering therapy was similar to that for primary prevention 0.76 (0.59 to 0.93), with NNT for benefit for of 13.8 (for 4.9 years).

The authors concluded that target cholesterol levels and the effectiveness of dose titration (or the use of multiple agents) have not been rigorously examined. Most studies compared a lipid-lowering drug with placebo but did not evaluate the effect of reaching specific cholesterol levels. Level 1++

14.2.5 From evidence to recommendations

The GDG reviewed the evidence, and their clinical experience of trying to manage the complexities of CV risk in clinical practice. They recognised the primacy of trying to control risk cost effectively against treating-to-target, but also noted the practical utility of measurements in assessing response to therapies and providing motivation to people with diabetes. Ultimately the issue of cost effectiveness could only be resolved in the context of the interventions being used to modify the lipid profile, and the evidence in this area was therefore subsumed into the recommendations on the use of CV risk estimation, statins and fibrates.

14.3 Statins and ezetimibe

14.3.1 Clinical introduction

Cholesterol lowering remained difficult, and indeed controversial, until the late 1980s when statins became available. Subsequently these drugs became the mainstay of lipid-lowering therapy, supported eventually by CV outcome studies. As discussed above, people with Type 2 diabetes are at high CV risk, and most of their morbidity and increased mortality comes from coronary, cerebral, and peripheral arterial disease. In earlier NICE technology appraisals (TAs) and the prior Type 2 diabetes guideline, statins were recommended for all people with extant CVD or at high risk thereof, states which include most people with Type 2 diabetes.[283]

Clinical questions which arise include whether more potent and more expensive statins should ever be used (and if so when), the use of statins in younger people with Type 2 diabetes, whether any people should not be routinely given statins, and the use of alternatives such as fibrates (addressed in the following fibrate section) and ezetimibe addressed by a 2007 NICE TA.[284]

14.3.2 Methodological introduction

The issues around statins initiation therapy for the prevention of CV events have been covered in a recently published NICE TA, 'Statins for the prevention of cardiovascular events',[283] which included RCTs conducted in people with Type 2 diabetes.

In addition, an ezetimibe TA[284] was in development at the time of this review (ezetimibe for the treatment of primary (heterozygous-familial and non-familial) hypercholesterolaemia). According to the scope, this TA is looking at the following clinical scenarios/comparisons.

- Patients (including Type 2 diabetes population) whose condition is not adequately controlled with a statin alone.
  - Ezetimibe + statin vs statins monotherapy.
  - Ezetimibe + statin vs statins + other lipid-lowering agent.
- Patients (including Type 2 diabetes population) in whom a statin is considered inappropriate, or is not tolerated.
  - Ezetimibe monotherapy vs placebo.
  - Ezetimibe vs other lipid-lowering agent.
- On these grounds, this review has excluded:
  - all the studies that were included by the NICE TA 94 on statins
  - any study that should be picked out by the ezetimibe TA.

Studies comparing statins with fibrates, (head-to-head comparisons or combination therapy) since these are being analysed by the fibrate question. The purpose of this review is not to repeat the statins or ezetimibe TAs, but to provide supplementary information about dose escalation, sequencing of statins, and use of alternative agents (fibrates and nicotinic acid).

Seven RCTs were identified which reviewed the effectiveness and safety of statins.[285–291] One study was excluded due to major methodological limitations.[285]

Among the remaining six studies, three RCTs were conducted specifically on patients with Type 2 diabetes, (see table 14.2).

Table 14.2 Study interventions			
Study	**N=**	**T=**	**Interventions**
Shepard J (2006)[291]	1,501	4.9 years	Atorvastatin (10 vs 80 mg)
Miller M (2004)[287]	151	6 weeks	Simvastatin (40 vs 80 mg vs placebo)
Berne C (2005)[288]	465	16 weeks	Rosuvastatin (10 mg vs atorvastatin 10 mg)

The other three studies were post hoc analyses of large trials:* Collaborative Atorvastatin Diabetes Study (CARDS) (atorvastatin 10 mg vs placebo),[289] Anglo-Scandinavian Cardiac Outcomes Trial: Lipid lowering arm (ASCOT-LLA) (atorvastatin 10 mg vs placebo),[290] and Diabetes Atorvastatin Lipid Intervention (DALI) (atorvastatin 10 vs 80 mg).[286]

It should be noted that differing dosing and titration regimens, follow-up periods and the differing populations included, may limit direct comparison between studies.

---

* These large trials were included in the statins NICE TA.

14.3.3 Health economic methodological introduction

No health economic papers were identified.

A health economic evaluation was developed by a health economist for the lipid modification group which looked at different doses of statins. This was presented to the GDG for this guideline as it was thought to be useful evidence.

The model was later further developed to consider specifically aspects of titration target and titration strategy in people with diabetes, and is described in appendix D.

In summary this considered two uptitration levels (total or LDL-C: 5.0/3.0 and 4.0/2.0 mmol/l) for people already started on simvastatin 40 mg/day, and either a one-step uptitration to 80 mg/day, or two-step to atorvastatin 80 mg/day.

14.3.4 Evidence statements

▷ Cardiovascular outcomes

Studies conducted on Type 2 diabetes population

One RCT[291] found that over the 5 years of double-blind treatment, the incidence of a major CV event* was significantly lower in patients receiving atorvastatin 80 mg than in those receiving atorvastatin 10 mg. This represented a 25% reduction in the risk of major CV events in favour of the high-dose group (p>0.026). This trend was observed across all quintiles of patient age and duration of diabetes and in patients with $HbA_{1c} \leq 7\%$ and $A_{1C} > 7\%$. **Level 1++**

The same RCT[291] reported significant differences between the groups, in favour of atorvastatin 80 mg, for the secondary outcomes of time to cerebrovascular event (p<0.037) and time to CV event (p<0.044). **Level 1++**

Post hoc sub-analysis

A post hoc analysis of the ASCOT-LLA study[290] found a significantly lower incidence of CV events in the subpopulation of people with Type 2 diabetes treated with atorvastatin –10 mg when compared with those receiving placebo. (Hazard ratio 0.77, 95% CI 0.61 to 0.98, p<0.036.) **Level 1+**

A post hoc analysis of the DALI trial[286] showed that both standard and aggressive therapy with atorvastatin (10–80 mg) did not reverse endothelial dysfunction (as measure by the surrogate marker of flow mediated vasodilatation). **Level 1+**

A post hoc analysis of the CARDS trial[289] analysed the time between initiation of atorvastatin 10 mg and the appearance of significant differences in the incidence of CV events when compared to placebo. The study demonstrated that by 1 year of follow-up the estimate of the treatment effect of atorvastatin 10 mg on the primary endpoint of major CV events was already at its final values of 37% reduction, and by 18 months the CI did not include unity. **Level 1++**

---

* Death from CHD, non-fatal, non-procedure related MI, resuscitated cardiac arrest, or fatal or non-fatal stroke.

▷ Lipid levels

Studies conducted on Type 2 diabetes population

An RCT[291] reported that end-of-treatment LDL-C levels increased by 3% to a mean of 98.6 mg/dl (2.5 mmol/l) in patients who continued atorvastatin 10 mg, while a further reduction of 19% to a mean of 77.0 mg/dl (2.0 mmol/l) was observed in those assigned to atorvastatin 80 mg (p <0.0001). **Level 1++**

The same study[291] reported significant differences between the groups, in favour of atorvastatin 80 mg, for total cholesterol (TC) levels and TG. **Level 1++**

One RCT[287] reported that simvastatin 80 mg treatment resulted in significantly lower low-density lipoprotein (LDL) levels compared with simvastatin 40 mg (p<0.001). **Level 1+**

The same study[287] showed that after a 6-week treatment, approximately 87% of patients treated with simvastatin 80 mg, and 82% of patients treated with simvastatin 40 mg, had LDL values that met or exceeded the National Cholesterol Education Program Adult Treatment Panel III (NCEP ATP III) treatment goal of <100 mg/dl (2.6 mmol/l), compared with only 14.3 of patients treated with placebo. No statistical significance was reported. **Level 1+**

An RCT[288] comparing treatment with rosuvastatin 10 mg vs atorvastatin 10 mg, reported that at the end of the study rosuvastatin-treated patients had significantly lower LDL levels compared with the atorvastatin group (p<0.0001). The study also reported that at 16 weeks, significantly more patients achieved their LDL goal with rosuvastatin compared with atorvastatin (94% vs 88%, p<0.05). **Level 1+**

Post hoc sub-analysis

The ASCOT-LLA post hoc study[290] found that among diabetic participants in the atorvastatin group, TC and LDL levels at year one of follow-up were lower than in the placebo group by ~1.3 and 1.2 mmol/l respectively. By the end of the study, these differences were 0.9 and 0.9 mmol/l respectively. However, no statistical analysis was performed. **Level 1+**

In relation to lipid levels, the DALI post hoc analysis found that after 30 weeks, patients receiving atorvastatin 80 mg had significantly lower LDL levels than those treated with only 10 mg of atorvastatin (p<0.01).

▷ Safety issues

Studies conducted on Type 2 diabetes population

An RCT[291] found no significant differences between the treatment groups (atorvastatin 10 mg and 80 mg) in the rate of treatment related adverse events (AEs), including myalgia, or persistent elevations in liver enzymes. No incidents of rhabdomyolysis were reported in either treatment group. **Level 1++**

One RCT[287] comparing different doses of simvastatin (simvastatin 40 and 80 mg) concluded that no drug related serious clinical AEs were observed in the treatment groups. However, the study reported that two patients on simvastatin 80 mg treatment had an Alanine Transaminase (ALT) and Asparte Transaminase (AST) level >3 times the upper limit of normal; one of these patients was discontinued because of these elevations (the liver function tests returned to normal after discontinuation of the therapy). **Level 1+**

An RCT[288] comparing treatment with rosuvastatin 10 mg vs atorvastatin 10 mg, reported that both treatments were well tolerated, with overall incidences of AEs being similar between the groups. According to the study ten patients discontinued because of AEs, three in the rosuvastatin group and seven in the atorvastatin group. There were no cases of myopathy. **Level 1+**

Post hoc sub-analysis

The ASCOT-LLA post hoc study[290] found that the use of atorvastatin in the diabetic population was not associated with any excess risk of adverse reactions, and there were no significant differences in liver enzyme abnormalities between those allocated statin and placebo. No cases of rhabdomyolysis were reported. **Level 1+**

14.3.5 Health economic evidence statements

The model developed for this guideline suggested that one-step titration from simvastatin 40 mg to 80 mg daily was very cost-effective in those with no previous CV event or extant CVD where TC still exceeded 4.0 mmol/l or LDL-C exceeded 2.0 mmol/l.

For those with already diagnosed CVD (or developing CVD) two-step titration (firstly to 80 mg simvastatin and then if indicated to atorvastatin 80 mg daily) was found to be cost-effective in those with already diagnosed CVD and whose TC still exceeded 4.0 mmol/l or LDL-C exceeded 2.0 mmol/l.

14.3.6 From evidence to recommendations

The GDG were cognisant of the previous NICE statin appraisal, the prior Type 2 diabetes guidelines, the ezetimibe appraisal, the deliberations of the NICE guidelines group on management of CVD, and the health economic analysis. The evidence of effectiveness and safety of generic statins, and in particular simvastatin seemed clear, and at current prices probably cost-saving in the population with Type 2 diabetes over the age of 40 years (irrespective of experience of CVD). There may be individuals in this group at lower CV risk (discussed in section 13), but these people would be uncommon and easily identified by the absence of CV risk factors (see 13.1.6). In others statin therapy should usually be with generic simvastatin at standard dosage (40 mg) in line with the prior TA[283] and the Heart Protection Study.

The group recognised that some people below the age of 40 years were also at high risk (10 year risk >20%, or 20 year risk >40%). It was considered that they would have to be identified by conventional risk factors; presence of features of the metabolic syndrome, strong family history, ethnic group, and evidence of microvascular damage such as nephropathy. Such people would then be treated with a statin, particularly as their 10-year risk horizon came to include 40 years of age or greater. However, the contraindication of the use of statins in pregnancy was felt to be great enough to deserve special mention, for any woman of childbearing potential.

The health economic analysis suggested titration to simvastatin 80 mg was highly cost-effective in those whose lipid levels were not controlled to target levels of 4.0/2.0 mmol/l (T-/LDL-C) irrespective of presence or absence of diagnosed CVD.

In those with CVD the health economic analysis suggested that uptitration from simvastatin 80 mg to a more efficacious statin (modelled as atorvastatin 80 mg daily) was cost-effective if the titration targets were not met on the simvastatin.

The GDG noted the stronger evidence base for atorvastatin than other higher efficacy statins. In regard of the use of ezetimibe (addition to simvastatin), they noted that guidance was provided by the NICE ezetimibe TA.

Unfortunately there is no easy way of calculating CV risk in people already under preventative management (which would be likely to include recent lifestyle change, aspirin, renin-angiotensin blockers and perhaps other drugs, as well as statins themselves). The alternative approach of using lipid levels was less attractive, but had the advantage of being pragmatic, and allowing monitoring of response.

14.4 Fibrates

14.4.1 Clinical introduction

Fibrates have a long and controversial history as lipid-lowering agents, beginning with clofibrate over 30 years ago and being implicated in the problems which led to withdrawal of cerivastatin in the 1990s. However, bezafibrate, fenofibrate and ciprofibrate have shown considerable staying power in the market. Statins have, however, eclipsed fibrates as primary cholesterol-lowering agents, so the issues surrounding fibrates relate to specific lipid abnormalities. In clinical practice these mostly concern hypertriglyceridaemia, itself strongly associated with low HDL-C levels, this problem being particularly common in people with Type 2 diabetes (more so than raised LDL-C levels).

The clinical question then relates to whether and when a fibrate should be initiated before statin therapy, and the circumstances under which a fibrate should be added to, or substituted for, statin therapy.

14.4.2 Methodological introduction

There were eleven studies identified which included fibrates and involved participants with Type 2 diabetes. Nine studies were reviewed, two studies comparing fenofibrate and placebo were excluded,[292,293] as the Effects of long-term fenofibrate therapy on cardiovascular events in 9,795 people with Type 2 diabetes mellitus (FIELD) study,[294] which had N=9,795 participants across 63 centres, was included.

One study considered fluvastatin and fenofibrate with fenofibrate monotherapy.[295]

There were three studies which considered fenofibrate in comparison with statin monotherapy and the combination of fenofibrate and a statin; atorvastatin,[296] rosuvastatin,[297] and simvastatin.[298]

The remaining four studies included gemfibrozil in comparison with placebo,[299] in comparison with statin monotherapy; simvastatin[300] and statin monotherapy and the combination of gemfibrozil and a statin; pravastatin,[301] and atorvastatin.[302]

14.4.3 Health economic methodological introduction

Two evaluations were identified one conducted in the UK and in one the US. In both studies no clinical evidence was found for fenofibrate and so it was assumed to be equally effective as gemfibrozil. Both studies used a 5-year time horizon. The US study was excluded as it was not generalisable to the UK setting.

14.4.4 Evidence statements

▷ Outcomes – fenofibrate

Fenofibrate vs placebo

The double-blind, multicentre FIELD study with N=9,795 participants compared fenofibrate 200 mg/day with a placebo in a Type 2 diabetes population, over a 5-year duration.[294]

Lipids

At 4 months, 1 year, 2 years and at completion of the study there were significant decreases in TC, LDL-C and TG levels and increases in HDL-C levels with fenofibrate compared with placebo.

Table 14.3 Fenofibrate outcomes			
	TC	**LDL-C**	**HDL-C**	**TG**
Absolute (mmol/l) and RR (%) differences between the treatment groups, p<0.05 for all time points				
4 months	−0.58 (−11.4%)	−0.39 (−12.0%)	0.05 (5.1%)	−0.56 (−28.6%)
1 year	−0.58 (−11.6%)	−0.38 (−11.9%)	0.05 (4.5%)	−0.58 (−30.2%)
2 years	−0.56 (−11.1%)	−0.36 (−11.7%)	0.04 (3.5%)	−0.52 (−27.4%)
Study close	−0.33 (−6.9%)	−0.17 (−5.8%)	0.01 (1.2%)	−0.41 (−21.9%)

For study participants who started other lipid-lowering therapy during the study (total N=2,720, N=944 placebo group and N=1,776 fenofibrate group) they showed smaller changes in lipid levels, but the significance between the groups remained p<0.05 at 2 years. At study close the changes remained significant for TC and TGs between the groups; however, the changes in LDL-C and HDL-C were NS.

Adverse events

There were small percentages (0.5 with placebo and 0.8% with fenofibrate) of possible serious adverse drug reactions. Four participants had rhabdomyolysis which fully resolved (N=3 with fenofibrate and N=1 with placebo). Rates of new cancer diagnosis were similar between groups.

GI events were the most frequently reported event, these were noted with N=975 (20%) of the fenofibrate and N=927 (19%) of the placebo group. **Level 1++**

Fenofibrate vs simvastatin

This single centre, double-blind study compared fenofibrate 160 mg/day with simvastatin 20 mg/day and both monotherapies with the combination of fenofibrate and simvastatin, with N=300 participants.[298]

Fenofibrate was found to have significantly greater reductions in TC and for LDL-C than simvastatin and than the combination of the drugs, differences between simvastatin and the combined group were NS.

The fenofibrate and combined groups had significantly higher decreases in TGs than simvastatin (NS between fenofibrate and combined treatments).

Adverse events

There were no serious drug related AEs. **Level 1++**

Fenofibrate vs atorvastatin

This study compared fenofibrate 200 mg/day and atorvastatin 20 mg/day monotherapies compared with the combination of fenofibrate and atorvastatin, with N=120 participants.[296]

Treatment goals

The treatment goals for LDL-C (2.4 mmol/l), TGs (2.6 mmol/l) and HDL-C (1.2 mmol/l) were reached in significantly more (reached by 97.5%, 100% and 60% respectively, $p<0.05$) participants for the combination of fenofibrate and atorvastatin than the monotherapies. The fenofibrate group compared with the atorvastatin group reached the treatment goals in a significantly higher percentage for HDL-C (30% vs 17.5%) and TGs (92.5% vs 75%), while the reverse was true for LDL-C with 80% of the atorvatstatin reaching the treatment goal compared with 5% of the fenofibrate group.

Lipids

The combination treatment reduced the TC, TGs and LDL-C significantly more than the atorvastatin or the fenofibrate as monotherapies. This combination also significantly increased HDL-C compared with atorvastatin monotherapy but not compared with fenofibrate.

Adverse events

There were no significant AEs reported in this study. **Level 1+**

Fenofibrate vs fluvastatin

This double-blind study over 12 months compared the combination of extended-release fluvastatin 80 mg and fenofibrate 200 mg and the monotherapy of fenofibrate 20 mg, N=48 participants.[295]

At 6 months the combination showed a significantly higher reduction in LDL-C compared with fenofibrate monotherapy. For the 12-month point significantly there were greater reductions in LDL-C and TG levels and increases in HDL-C with the combination group compared with the monotherapy.

Adverse events

No serious AEs were reported, N=3 discontinued in the study due to myalgia. **Level 1++**

Fenofibrate vs rosuvastatin

This multicentre study incorporated both a double-blind, fixed-dose phase and an open-label titrating dose phase, N=216.[297]

Fixed dose: the 6-week fixed-dose phase had placebo, rosuvastatin 5 mg and rosuvastatin 10 mg groups.

There were significant decreases for both rosuvastatin 5 mg and 10 mg groups compared with increases with placebo in TC (−36.6%, −31.4% vs 1.1%, p<0.001) and TGs (−24.5%, −29.5% vs 4.7%, p<0.001) and compared with decreases in LDL-C levels with placebo (−40.7%, −45.8% vs −0.6%, p<0.001). At week 6, 77.4% of those in the rosuvastatin 10 mg group had reached the LDL-C goal of <100 mg/dl, compared with 8.3% of those receiving placebo.

Titrating dose

This 18-week phase used sequential dose increases at 6-week intervals provided the LDL-C level remained >50 mg/dl (>1.3 mmol/l).

The groups were:

- placebo in fixed dose – rosuvastatin 10 mg (with possible increases to 20 and 40 mg)
- placebo in fixed dose – fenofibrate 67 mg once daily (with possible increases to BD and TID fenofibrate)
- rosuvastatin 5 mg in fixed dose – rosuvastatin 5 mg and fenofibrate 67 mg once daily (with possible increases to BD and TID fenofibrate)
- rosuvastatin 10 mg in fixed dose – rosuvastatin 10 mg and fenofibrate 67 mg once daily (with possible increases to BD and TID fenofibrate).

By the final stage of the dose-titration phase a smaller proportion of those on the groups which received rosuvastatin 10 mg required dose titration than in the other two groups.

Lipids

There was a significant decrease in LDL-C with placebo/rosuvastatin compared with a slight increase with placebo/fenofibrate. This reduction in LDL-C was also significantly greater than that found with rosuvastatin 5 mg/fenofibrate, but was NS compared with rosuvastatin 10 mg/fenofibrate.

The reductions in TG levels between the groups which had placebo in the fixed-dose phase were NS. The decrease in TG levels with rosuvastatin 10 mg/fenofibrate were significantly greater than those with placebo/rosuvastatin.

For each group those who reached the goal of LDL-C <100 mg/dl at the end of both the fixed-dose and the titrating-dose phase were; rosuvastatin 40 mg (86.0%, N=50), rosuvastatin 10 mg and fenofibrate 67 mg TID (75.5%, N=53), rosuvastatin 5 mg and fenofibrate 67 mg TID (75.0%, N=60), and fenofibrate 67 mg TID (4.1%, N=49).

Adverse events

The most frequently reported AEs in a small number of participants were GI related, myalgia and increases in ALT and creatine kinase (CK) levels. **Level 1+**

Table 14.4 Fenofibrate comparison studies

		TC	LDL-C	HDL-C	TG
Muhlestein JB (2006)[298]	Fenofibrate	−1.2% (p<0.0001 vs simvastatin and combination)	−5.6% (p<0.0001 vs simvastatin and combination)	NS vs comparisons	−38.2% (NS vs combination)
	Simvastatin	−26.2% (NS vs combination)	−34.1% (NS vs combination)	NS	−24.8% (p<0.0001 vs fenofibrate and combination)
	Combination	−27.1%	−29.1%	NS	−49.4%
Athyros VG (2002)[296]	Fenofibrate	253±17 to 213±14 (−16)	163±15 to 140±15 (−15)	NS with combination	281±24 to 167±15 (−41)
	Atorvastatin	252±17 to 174±10 (−31)	161±15 to 97±7 (−31)	34.6±3.2 to 37.7±4.5 (9)	278±24 to 195±22 (−30)
	Combination	255±19 to 159±7 (−37) (p<0.05 vs fenofibrate and atorvastatin)	163±16 to 89±6 (−46) (p<0.05 vs fenofibrate and atorvastatin)	35±3.5 to 43±4.3 (22) (p<0.05 vs atorvastatin)	278±23 to 139±12 (−50) (p<0.05 vs fenofibrate and atorvastatin)
Derosa G (2004)[295]	Fluvastatin/ fenofibrate	NS vs fenofibrate	−35% (p<0.05)	34% (p<0.05)	−35% (p<0.05)
	Fenofibrate	NS	−25%	14%	−17%
Durrington PN (2004)[297]	Placebo/ fenofibrate		0.7% (p<0.001 vs placebo/rosuvastatin)	NS between groups	NS vs placebo/rosuvastatin
	Placebo/ rosuvastatin		−46.7%	NS	−30.3%
	Rosuvastatin 5 mg/ fenofibrate		−34.1% (p<0.001 vs placebo/rosuvastatin)	NS	−47.1% (p=0.001 vs placebo/rosuvastatin)
	Rosuvastatin 10 mg/ fenofibrate		−42.4%	NS	NS vs placebo/rosuvastatin

▷ Outcomes – gemfibrozil

Gemfibrozil vs placebo

This study compared gemfibrozil 1,200 mg and a matched placebo in the Veterans Affairs High Density Lipoprotein Intervention Trial (VA-HIT) and included a subgroup diabetic, N=627.[299]

This study considered major CV events and identified in the diabetes group a significant reduction in the risk of major CV events of 32%, of CHD death 41%, and of stroke 40%, compared with placebo.

The lipid level analysis was not analysed by diabetic subgroup. **Level 1+**

Gemfibrozil vs simvastatin

This study compared gemfibrozil 1,200 mg compared with simvastatin 20 mg, N=70.[300]

This study did not complete comparisons between the groups, both treatments significantly decreased TC and TG levels, and increased HDL-C compared with the baseline. There were significant decreases in LDL-C with simvastatin compared with baseline but not with gemfibrozil.

There were small numbers of incidents of GI events with gemfibrozil and generalised weakness and muscle pain with simvastatin. **Level 1+**

Gemfibrozil vs pravastatin

This double-blind, multicentre study with N=268 participants compared gemfibrozil 1,200 mg and pravastatin matched placebo with pravastatin 40 mg and gemfibrozil matched placebo.[301]

Lipids

There were significantly greater reductions in TC and LDL-C with pravastatin than with gemfibrozil. Conversely there was a significantly greater reduction in TG levels with gemfibrozil than with pravastatin p<0.001. Changes in HDL-C were NS between the groups.

Adverse events

The AEs reported were considered not severe and the most frequent were GI related (N=28 gemfibrozil and N=24 pravastatin). **Level 1++**

Gemfibrozil vs atorvastatin

This open-label, crossover study compared gemfibrozil and atorvastatin and a combination of both drugs, in a titrating dose study, N=44.[302]

Lipids

The atorvastatin and combination groups had significantly greater reductions in LDL-C than the gemfibrozil group (reductions NS for atorvastatin vs combination). For TG levels the gemfibrozil and combination groups had significantly greater reductions than the atorvastatin group (reductions NS for gemfibrozil vs combination). There were NS differences between the monotherapies and the combination treatment for HDL-C levels.

Adverse events

GI related (abdominal discomfort, constipation, loose stools, nausea) were reported by N=6 (atorvastatin), N=11 (gemfibrozil) and N=8 (combination). **Level 1+**

Table 14.5 Gemfibrozil comparison studies		TC	LDL-C	HDL-C	TG
Schweitzer M (2002)[301]	Gemfibrozil	−0.42±0.77	−0.22±0.76	NS	−0.77±1.01, (p<0.001 vs pravastatin)
	Pravastatin	−1.35±0.67, (p<0.001 vs gemfibrozil)	−1.3±0.59, (p<0.001 vs gemfibrozil)	NS	−0.27±0.82
Wagner AM (2003)[302]	Gemfibrozil		147±2.7 to 142±2.7	NS	167±9.7 to 113±9.7
	Atorvastatin		152±2.7 to 99±2.7 (p<0.0001 vs gemfibrozil)	NS	162±9.7 to 143±9.7 (0.01 vs gemfibrozil)
	Combination		148±2.7 to 106±2.7 (p<0.0001 vs gemfibrozil)	NS	190±10.6 to 117±10.6 (p<0.05 vs atorvastatin)

14.4.5 Health economic evidence statements

Feher et al.[303] was a very simple analysis although it was unclear how the costs in the treated groups were calculated. Only costs of the drugs and a cost per CHD event were included. The costs used are now out of date and assuming the same risk reduction for statins and fenofibrate would result in statins being cost saving.

14.4.6 From evidence to recommendations

While the evidence was not as strong as for the statins, there was convincing evidence of the effectiveness of fibrates in CV protection in people with Type 2 diabetes. Some of the trials (e.g. FIELD) in which this evidence was found included people with TG levels down to the upper end of the normal range (~1.8 mmol/l). However, while the price of fibrates was considerably above that of generic statins, the more effective fibrates as judged by TG lowering were about half the price of proprietary statins when both are used at standard doses.

Hypertriglyceridaemia is a complex condition with both a genetic basis and often being secondary to other medical conditions, including poor blood glucose control. The GDG recognised it was not writing a guideline on management of hypertriglyceridaemia in people with Type 2 diabetes, but because of the interaction with blood glucose control and other medical conditions often associated with Type 2 diabetes (including renal impairment and liver disease), it could not avoid some general guidance in the area.

In drawing up the recommendations the GDG was also cognisant of the need to be aware of:

- the likely combination with statin therapy (given its recommendations on statins) and the higher rate of side effects of combined usage
- the more immediate risks of pancreatitis with higher levels of TGs
- the difficulty of assessing LDL-C levels when TG levels were above 4.5 mmol/l. A useful pragmatic compromise was felt to be to base recommendations around cut-off levels of 2.3 and 4.5 mmol/l.

There is evidence of differences between fibrates: gemfibrozil had greater interactions with other drugs commonly used in diabetes care; bezafibrate was cheaper and less effective in TG lowering and with a poorer CV evidence base than fenofibrate; and ciprofibrate was more poorly investigated. Therefore recommendations were based around fenofibrate, though with a role for bezafibrate where CV risk was less pronounced, and ciprofibrate as an alternative.

Further information on fibrate statin combinations might become available when the ACCORD trial reports.[35]

14.5 Nicotinic acid and derivatives

14.5.1 Clinical introduction

Abnormalities of blood lipid profiles, including serum HDL-C and TGs, are recognised CV risk factors, and are particularly likely to be abnormal in people with Type 2 diabetes. Nicotinic acid preparations are one approach to improving lipid profiles. Nicotinic acid administration is associated with side effects due to vasodilatation, and derivatives (acipimox) and modified-release preparations have been made available to try and reduce the problem. The clinical question is then what role nicotinic acid derivatives might have in the management of Type 2 diabetes.

14.5.2 Methodological introduction

There were four studies identified in this area. Two of the studies were multicentre, double-blind RCTs, one of which considered immediate-release nicotinic acid against placebo, N=125;[304] the other study compared different doses of an extended-release nicotinic acid with placebo, N=148.[305]

There were also two single centre studies identified, one crossover, non-blinded study which considered nicotinic acid compared with no therapy, N=13.[306] There was only one study which considered nicotinic acid with any other drug and this was, nicotinic acid compared with pravastatin, N=44.[307]

It should be noted that two of these studies used samples which were combinations of diabetic and non-diabetic participants, one study represented the outcomes entirely separately[304] and therefore the N=543 non-diabetic participants are not reported here, solely the N=125 diabetic participants. The other study gave combined results for the drug efficacy results but separate results for the glycaemic effects, with a total sample of N=44 but a Type 2 diabetic sample of N=11, therefore the results are reported pooled with the other participants for the efficacy section.[307]

14.5.3 Health economic methodological introduction

Two papers were identified. Armstrong et al.[308] was given a negative rating because the time horizon was very short and would not capture all the benefits of treatment.

Olson et al.[309] was excluded as it was not a diabetic population and did not present results according to risk.

An additional paper was suggested in the consultation comments, Roze et al.[310] The base-case analysis excluded people with diabetes, but a sensitivity analysis was conducted for a diabetic population. All patients received the same statin treatment with additional prolonged-release nicotinic acid compared to no additional treatment. This paper was excluded as this was not considered a suitable comparison for people with diabetes who have failed on statin monotherapy.[310]

14.5.4 Evidence statements

▷ Nicotinic acid vs placebo/no therapy

Table 14.6 Lipid profiles (shaded areas not measured or reported in that study)

	Nicotinic acid 3,000 mg/d vs placebo[304]	Nicotinic acid ER 1,000 mg/d and 1,500 mg/d vs placebo[305]	Nicotinic acid 1,500 mg/d vs no therapy (crossover)[306]
HDL	HDL increased by 29% vs 0% with placebo, p<0.001	1,000 mg increases in HDL of +19% vs placebo, p<0.05 1,500 mg increases of +24% vs placebo, p<0.05	Significant increase compared with placebo, p=0.0001
LDL	LDL decreased by 8% compared with 1% for placebo; p<0.001	1,000 mg NS 1,500 mg LDL decreases compared with placebo at weeks 12 and 16 (p<0.05)	NS
VLDL			Significant decrease compared with placebo, p=0.0009
TC		Statistical analysis not reported	Significant decrease compared with placebo, p=0.0001
TC/HDL ratio		1,000 mg decrease in TC/HDL ratio −12%(2.8%), p<0.01 1,500 mg decrease in TC/HDL ratio −22%(2.7%), p<0.01	Significant decrease compared with placebo, p=0.0001
TGs	TGs decreased by 23% compared with 7% with placebo, p<0.001	1,000 mg NS 1,500 mg reductions in TG of −13% to −28% vs placebo, p<0.05	Significant decrease compared with placebo, p=0.0006

Overall nicotinic acid was found to show reduction in LDL, TGs and the TC/HDL ratio and increases in HDL, compared with placebo in all three studies with more significant changes for doses of 1,500 mg/day and greater. **Level 1+**

Table 14.7 Glycaemic effects			
	Nicotinic acid 3,000 mg/d vs placebo[304]	**Nicotinic acid ER 1,000 mg/d and 1,500 mg/d vs placebo[305]**	**Nicotinic acid 1,500 mg/d vs no therapy (crossover)[306]**
HbA$_{1c}$	Nicotinic acid – no change Placebo HbA$_{1c}$ decreased by 0.3% compared with nicotinic acid, p=0.04	1,000 mg – NS 1,500 mg – HbA$_{1c}$ increased of 0.29%, p=0.48 compared with placebo	HbA$_{1c}$ increased compared with placebo, p=0.002
Fasting glucose	Nicotinic acid showed an increase in average levels; 8.1 mg/dl vs a decrease of 8.7 mg/dl with placebo, p=0.04		NS
24-hour plasma glucose profile			Increased compared with placebo, p=0.047
24-hour urinary glucose			Increased compared with placebo, p=0.016

Nicotinic acid showed some glycaemic effects compared with placebo, one study identified that HbA$_{1c}$ remained stable with nicotinic acid but had a significant decrease with placebo, this study included a downtitration of nicotinic acid if HbA$_{1c}$ exceeded 10%, this occurred in N=10 of the nicotinic acid group and N=8 of the placebo group.[304]

Two studies identified an increase in HbA$_{1c}$ with doses of 1,500 mg/d, compared with placebo for both immediate-release and extended-release formulations.[305,306] **Level 1+**

▷ Adverse events

Increases in uric acid were identified in two of the studies, for one this was from 339 to 386 μmol/l and was significant compared with placebo, p<0.001.[304] The second study noted that N=2 participants had very high uric acid levels of 684 and 761 μmol/l.[306] The third (extended-release) study found no significant differences in uric acid levels.[305]

Flushing was considered a minor complaint in one study, numbers not reported.[306] Two thirds of those taking the extended-release nicotinic acid formulation reported flushing at some point during the trial, approximately 10% of those taking placebo reported it.[305] **Level 1+**

▷ Nicotinic acid vs pravastatin

One study considered nicotinic acid 1,500 mg/day compared with pravastatin 40 mg/day, followed by a combination therapy phase of nicotinic acid 1,000 mg/day with pravastatin 20 mg/day. This study included both diabetic and non-diabetic participants (N=11, Type 2 diabetes).[307] This study considered the results for lipid profiles for the combined diabetic and non-diabetic participants. The glycaemic effect results were considered separately for diabetic and non-diabetic participants.

▷ Lipid profiles

Nicotinic acid was not found to be more effective than pravastatin as the later showed significant reductions in LDL and TC levels compared with nicotinic acid. Combination therapy showed significant decreases in LDL, TC and TG levels compared with nicotinic acid and significant increases in HDL and decreases in TG levels compared with pravastatin.

Table 14.8 Lipid profiles			
	Nicotinic acid 3,000 mg/d vs pravastatin 40 mg/d	**Nicotinic acid 1,000 mg/d with pravastatin 20 mg/d vs nicotinic acid 3,000 mg/d**	**Nicotinic acid 1,500 mg/d with pravastatin 20 mg/d vs pravastatin 40 mg/d**
HDL	NS	NS	Increased with combination compared with pravastatin (35.6±4.1 vs 16.4±5.8, p<0.001)
LDL	Pravastatin showed reductions in LDL compared with nicotinic acid (−32.1±3.0 vs −16.9±3.3, p<0.01)	Decreased with combination compared with nicotinic acid (−35.7±3.3 vs −16.9±3.3, p<0.01)	NS
TC	Pravastatin showed reductions in TC compared with nicotinic acid (−24.9±2.0 vs −9.8±2.9, p<0.001)	Decreased with combination compared with nicotinic acid (−23.8±2.9 vs −9.8±2.9, p<0.001)	NS
TG	NS	Decreased with combination compared with nicotinic acid (−39.4±6.7 vs −31.8±6.8, p=0.03)	Decreased with combination compared with pravastatin (−39.3±5.4 vs −28.0±5.1, p=0.01)
Lipoprotein-(a)	NS	NS	NS

Level 1+

▷ Glycaemic effects

Diabetic participants: nicotinic acid monotherapy showed an increase in HbA_{1c} by approximately 8% (p=0.03), pravastatin showed no change in HbA_{1c} level and the increase seen with combination therapy was non-significant. Nicotinic acid monotherapy increased FPG by approximately 26% (p=0.02), there were no changes with pravastatin or combination therapy.

Non-diabetic participants: nicotinic acid monotherapy showed an increase in HbA_{1c} by approximately 4% (p=0.02), combination therapy showed an increase of approximately 6% (p<0.01), pravastatin showed no change. None of the treatments showed changes in FPG. **Level 1+**

▷ Adverse events

All of the participants in the nicotinic acid group complained of flushing, this generally lasted from 10 to 15 minutes and was ameliorated with aspirin. Nine participants (21%) withdrew from this study with significant flushing or nausea with nicotinic acid, one participant withdrew with nausea from the pravastatin group. **Level 1+**

14.5.5 From evidence to recommendations

This group of drugs was not considered in the previous guideline (2002).[414] The limited number of studies presented suggested that nicotinic acid can have some advantageous effect on serum HDL-C and lipids, but also that it has some negative effects on blood glucose control. In the absence of outcome trials in people with Type 2 diabetes, and given also the problems of using the current preparations (notably flushing despite prophylactic aspirin, dose titration and use of modified-release preparations), no general recommendation could be given for use of nicotinic acid. The group were aware of some possible special indications in people with extreme hypertriglyceridaemia, but felt this to be outside the remit of the current guideline.

14.6 Omega 3 fish oils

14.6.1 Clinical introduction

The concept of beneficial and harmful dietary fats has come to the fore in recent years. Some evidence does exist for the use of omega 3 fish oils in certain circumstances such as post-MI. The clinical question then was what role these oils might have in the management of people with Type 2 diabetes.

14.6.2 Methodological introduction

There were seven studies identified for participants with Type 2 diabetes. A Cochrane systematic review, for which the last search had been completed in September 2000,[311] included studies that were 2–24 weeks in duration.

A second systematic review and meta-analysis[312] investigated the haematological and thrombogenic effects of omega 3 fatty acids and did not report on glycaemic and lipid control outcomes. Included studies were of 4–24 weeks duration.

There were five RCTs identified. Four of the studies compared; fish oil, eicosapentaenoic acid (EPA), docosahexaenoic acid (DHA), and placebo,[313] fish oil (one group taking EPA and one taking DHA) compared with olive oil[314] and fish oil (EPA and DHA) compared with corn oil,[315,316] all of these studies used capsules of the oils. Two of the studies were conducted in the same centre using a virtually identical patient group and research method.[315,316]

The final study compared the effects of a daily fish meal and light or moderate exercise, with no fish and light or moderate exercise.[317] These studies were of 6–8 weeks duration.

It should be noted that a systematic review including studies conducted in the general population (search performed up to February 2002) was also identified.[318] This review concluded that there was no evidence of a clear benefit of omega 3 fats on health.

Participants in these studies were often requested to follow dietary guidelines and their compliance with these may have affected the findings.

14.6.3 Health economic methodological introduction

No health economic papers were identified.

14.6.4 Evidence statements

Table 14.9 Study comparisons

	Cochrane review[311]	Jain S (2002)[313]	Petersen M (2002)[316]	Pederson H (2003)[315]	Woodman RJ (2002)[314]
Type and dose of omega 3	Any type of dietary supplement with omega 3 fatty acids included	Maxigard capsule (180 mg EPA acid and 120 mg DHA acid) BD	4 g/capsules of fish oil/day containing 2.6 g EPA and DHA/day	4 g/capsules of fish oil/day containing 2.6 g EPA and DHA – equivalent to a daily intake of 50–60g of fatty fish	4 g EPA or 4 g DHA once a day with evening meal
TGs	14 studies: decrease compared with placebo: −0.56 mmol/l (−0.71 to −0.40), p<0.00001	Decrease compared with placebo: (p<0.001) Baseline TGs mg %: Maxigard: 209.6±59.1 Placebo: 189.6±52.0	Decrease compared with corn oil: (−0.54±0.13) to (−0.04±0.17), p=0.025 Baseline TGs: Fish oil: 2.35±0.27 Corn oil: 2.76±0.46	Decrease compared with corn oil: (−0.53±0.11) to (−0.08±0.16), p=0.025. Baseline TGs: Fish oil: 2.3±0.3 Corn oil: 2.6±0.5	Decrease compared with olive oil: 19% (p=0.022) EPA and 15% (p=0.022) DHA Baseline TGs: EPA: 1.3±0.7 DHA: 1.6±0.6 Olive oil: 1.7±0.6
TC	NS	Decrease compared with placebo: (p=0.05)	NS	NS	
LDL-C	11 studies: increase compared with placebo: 0.24mmol/l (0.005 to 0.43), p=0.01	Decrease compared with placebo: (p=0.014)	NS		
HDL-C	NS	Decrease compared with placebo: (p<0.001)	NS	Increase compared with corn oil: (0.07±0.01 vs. −0.01±0.01) p=0.045	NS
HDL-C subgroups			HDL2a decreased compared with corn oil: (p=0.07). HDL2b increased compared with corn oil: (p=0.012)		Increase in HDL2 compared with olive oil: 16% (p=0.026) EPA and 22% (p=0.05) DHA. Increase in HDL3: 11% (p=0.026) EPA and NS with DHA
HbA1c	NS	Decrease compared with placebo: (p=0.009)	NS	NS	NS
FBG	NS	Decrease compared with placebo: (p=0.004)	NS	NS	Increased compared with olive oil; EPA (p=0.002) and DHA (p=0.002)
Weight	NS			NS	
BP		Decrease compared with placebo: systolic (p=0.0003), diastolic (p=0.0003)	NS		NS

Cochrane review and RCTs

The table above details the evidence from the RCTs comparing omega 3 and placebo, or corn oil or fish oil.

All studies (Cochrane review and the five RCTs) found that treatment with omega 3 significantly reduced TGs compared to placebo. **Level 1+**

The only other area where the Cochrane review identified significant changes was in LDL-C where omega 3 were associated with a significant increase compared with placebo. **Level 1++**

Subgroup analysis – Cochrane review

A subgroup analysis was undertaken with the hypertriglyceridaemic participants, doses of fish oil and trial duration.

Hypertriglyceridaemic participants (control TGs >4 mmol/l)

An increased reduction in TGs was identified in trials (N=3) with only hypertriglyceridaemic participants; −1.45 mmol/l (−2.89 to −0.01, p=0.05), compared with studies with non-hypertriglyceridaemic participants (N=11) −0.40 mmol/l (−0.61 to −0.19, p=0.0002).

Increases in LDL-C levels were significant in the hypertriglyceridaemic groups (N=2 trials), 0.6 mmol/l (0.16 to 1.04, p=0.008), but they were NS in the non-hypertriglyceridaemic groups (N=9 trials).

Dose of fish oil

Trials with high doses of fish oil (>2 g EPA, N=4) showed a significant increase in LDL-C 0.51 mmol/l (0.18 to 0.84, p=0.003), this was NS for lower doses (<2 g EPA, N=7).

Levels of TGs in the high-dose groups decreased by 1.11 mmol/l (−2.21 to −0.10, p=0.03), but in the low-dose group this was less at 0.54 mmol/l (−0.69 to −0.38, p<0.00001).

Trial duration

In trials of longer than 2 months LDL-C levels increased by 0.33 mmol/l (0.00 to 0.65, p=0.05), the increases were NS in trials shorter than 2 months.

TG levels were reduced by 0.81 mmol/l (−1.21 to −0.41, p=0.00008) in the longer trials and by less than 0.36 (−0.58 to −0.13, p=0.002) in the shorter ones. **Level 1++**

▷ Daily fish meal and exercise comparison study

Triglycerides

The study which included fish meals found that compared with the control (no fish meals, light exercise) the inclusion of a daily fish meal significantly reduced TGs, −0.9±1.3 mmol/l, p=0.0001, with fish/moderate exercise reducing by 1.21±0.3 mmol/l and fish/light exercise by 1.22±0.3 mmol/l p=0.0001. The addition of exercise without the fish also showed a significant decrease in TGs −0.7±0.3 mmol/l, p=0.03, compared with the control.[317]

HDL-C (subgroups)

The study which included fish meals found that high-density lipoprotein 2 cholesterol (HDL2-C) was significantly increased, 0.06 mmol/l, p=0.01 and high-density lipoprotein 3 cholesterol (HDL3-C) significantly reduced by the inclusion of fish compared with the low-fat control group, –0.05 mmol/l, p=0.01.[317] **Level 1+**

Cardiovascular effects

A meta-analysis found that participants who took omega 3 fatty acids had a significant reduction in diastolic BP of 1.79 mmHg (95% CI, –3.56, –0.02; p=0.05) and a non-significant reduction in systolic BP (p=0.32). There was also a non-significant reduction in heart rate (p=0.52).[312] **Level 1++**

Thrombogenic factors

The pooled analysis of the data of two studies, showed a significant increase in factor VII of 24.86% (95% CI, 7.17, 42.56; p=0.006).[312] **Level 1++**

14.6.5 From evidence to recommendations

From the evidence available fish oils as a homogeneous therapeutic concept is problematic, as the evidence included showed a variation in the fish oil dosage used. Clinical experience confirmed that large total doses of oils used to get an adequate dose of omega 3 fish oils in some preparations can cause adverse effects. From the evidence available omega 3 fish oil preparations could help lower TG levels, but overall showed minimal improvement in lipid profiles in people who had not had a MI. The GDG agreed there were financial consequences in prescribing omega 3 supplements when the evidence showed no clear benefit.

It was recognised that the recommendations made must be understood as only applying for omega 3 fish oil supplementation, and not to recommendations on sources of dietary fats.

RECOMMENDATIONS

R76   Review cardiovascular risk status annually by assessment of cardiovascular risk factors, including features of the metabolic syndrome and waist circumference, and change in personal or family cardiovascular history.

Statins and ezetimibe

R77   For a person who is 40 years old or over:
- initiate therapy with generic simvastatin (to 40 mg) or a statin of similar efficacy and cost unless the cardiovascular risk from non-hyperglycaemia-related factors is low (see recommendation 72).
- if the cardiovascular risk from non-hyperglycaemia-related factors is low, assess cardiovascular risk using the UKPDS risk engine (see recommendation 73) and initiate simvastatin therapy (to 40 mg), or a statin of similar efficacy and cost, if the cardiovascular risk exceeds 20% over 10 years.

R78   For a person who is under 40 years old, consider initiating generic simvastatin therapy (to 40 mg), or a statin of similar efficacy and cost, where the cardiovascular risk factor profile appears particularly poor (multiple features of the metabolic syndrome, presence of conventional risk factors, microalbuminuria, at-risk ethnic group, or strong family history of premature cardiovascular disease).

R79   Once a person has been started on cholesterol-lowering therapy, assess his or her lipid profile (together with other modifiable risk factors and any new diagnosis of cardiovascular disease) 1–3 months after starting treatment, and annually thereafter. In those not on cholesterol-lowering therapy, reassess cardiovascular risk annually, and consider initiating a statin (see recommendations 77 and 78).

R80   Increase the dose of simvastatin, in anyone initiated on simvastatin in line with the above recommendations, to 80 mg daily unless total cholesterol level is below 4.0 mmol/l or low-density lipoprotein cholesterol level is below 2.0 mmol/l.

R81   Consider intensifying cholesterol-lowering therapy (with a more effective statin[283] or ezetimibe,[284] in line with NICE guidance), if there is existing or newly diagnosed cardiovascular disease, or if there is an increased albumin excretion rate, to achieve a total cholesterol level below 4.0 mmol/litre (and high-density lipoprotein cholesterol not exceeding 1.4 mmol/litre) or a low-density lipoprotein cholesterol level below 2.0 mmol/litre.*

R82   If there is a possibility of a woman becoming pregnant, do not use statins unless the issues have been discussed with the woman and agreement has been reached.

Fibrates

R83   If there is a history of elevated serum triglycerides, perform a full fasting lipid profile (including high-density lipoprotein cholesterol and triglyceride estimations) when assessing cardiovascular risk annually.

R84   Assess possible secondary causes of high serum triglyceride levels, including poor blood glucose control (others include hypothyroidism, renal impairment and liver inflammation, particularly from alcohol). If a secondary cause is identified, manage according to need.

R85   Prescribe a fibrate (fenofibrate as first-line) if triglyceride levels remain above 4.5 mmol/litre despite attention to other causes. In some circumstances, this will be before a statin has been started because of acute need (that is, risk of pancreatitis) and because of the undesirability of initiating two drugs at the same time.

R86   If cardiovascular risk is high (as is usual in people with Type 2 diabetes), consider adding a fibrate to statin therapy if triglyceride levels remain in the range 2.3–4.5 mmol/litre despite statin therapy.

---

* This wording should not be read as implying that treatment might be aimed at achieving a low HDL cholesterol level. The intention here is to set limits for the validity of total cholesterol level measurement, not to set any kind of target for HDL cholesterol, which is usually regarded as protective against cardiovascular disease. Total cholesterol measurement is problematic as it includes HDL cholesterol, and so can be elevated by higher levels of HDL cholesterol. In these circumstances, treatments aimed at lowering total cholesterol further are not indicated and LDL cholesterol levels should be used to assess the results of lipid-lowering treatments.

Nicotinic acid

R87   Do not use nicotinic acid preparations and derivatives routinely for people with Type 2 diabetes. They may have a role in a few people who are intolerant of other therapies and have more extreme disorders of blood lipid metabolism, when managed by those with specialist expertise in this area.

Omega 3 fish oils

R88   Do not prescribe fish oil preparations for the primary prevention of cardiovascular disease in people with Type 2 diabetes. This recommendation does not apply to people with hypertriglyceridaemia receiving advice from a healthcare professional with special expertise in blood lipid management.

R89   Consider a trial of highly concentrated licensed omega 3 fish oils for refractory hypertriglyceridaemia if lifestyle measures and fibrate therapy have failed.

15 | Antithrombotic therapy

15.1 Antiplatelet therapy

15.1.1 Clinical introduction

Antiplatelet therapy now has an established role in the management of people at high risk of cardiovascular (CV) events. People with Type 2 diabetes are known to have CV risk higher than matched populations after allowance for other CV risk factors, and in some studies as high as those without diabetes who have declared cardiovascular disease (CVD).[273] National guidelines and the previous NICE (inherited) Type 2 diabetes guideline recommend use of aspirin in people at high CV risk.[319,320] Other antiplatelet agents (clopidogrel and dipyridamole modified release (MR)) have been the subject of a NICE technology appraisal (TA) but without specific calculation for the higher CV event rate or the specific risk reduction in people with Type 2 diabetes.[321] The increasing occurrence of Type 2 diabetes in younger people raises the additional question of the use of antiplatelet therapy in those who CV risk may be not be very high.

The guidelines are not concerned with the use of antiplatelet therapy after acute cardiological events or cardiac interventions, or after acute cerebrovascular events.

The clinical question then is whether antiplatelet medications should be used in people with Type 2 diabetes, or in which subgroups of such people, and if so which agents and in what doses.

15.1.2 Methodological introduction

▷ Aspirin

There were only two studies which were reviewed that considered aspirin and CVD in people with Type 2 diabetes from 2001 onwards. There were a number of large trials completed which evaluated aspirin in populations which had a diabetic subgroup included. A review which included the Early Treatment of Diabetic Retinopathy Study 1992 (ETDRS), Thrombosis Prevention Trial 1998 (TPT), Hypertension Optimal Treatment trial 1998 (HOT), and Primary Prevention Project 2001 (PPP), the efficacy of low- and high-dose aspirin has been evaluated and reductions on CV endpoints in high-risk patients demonstrated. However, this review also noted that these trials had small numbers of participants with diabetes and that no head-to-head comparison of low- versus high-dose therapy has been conducted in diabetics.

The two studies reviewed comprised one RCT involving participants with Type 2 diabetic nephropathy and compared aspirin with dipyridamole, a combination of aspirin and dipyridamole with placebo. The authors stated that they believed this study to be the first clinical trial of aspirin in Type 2 diabetic nephropathy.[322]

The second study was an open-label RCT which compared aspirin with vitamin E with 4,495 participants of whom 1,031 were diabetic. This study had been planned with a 5-year follow-up but was terminated early (at 3.7 years) on the advice of the independent Data Safety and Monitoring Board (DSMB) when newly available evidence on the benefit of aspirin in primary prevention was available.[323]

215

There was also a multicentre RCT with a Type 2 diabetic sample (N=1,209),[324] however, this study compared aspirin with picotamide, which is unlicensed and therefore the study was excluded.

▷ Clopidogrel vs aspirin

Six large RCTs were identified, all of which had long follow-up periods, allowing assessment of the long-term CV event risk.[325–330] The studies were conducted in the general population but included subgroup analysis of those with diabetes, none of the studies discriminated between those with Type 1 or with Type 2 diabetes.

One RCT, a post hoc sub-analysis from the Clopidogrel vs Aspirin in Patients at Risk of Ischemic Events (CAPRIE)* study (N=3,866 with diabetes) compared aspirin monotherapy with clopidogrel monotherapy.[326]

Four RCTs compared the combination of aspirin plus clopidogrel with aspirin plus placebo.

- The Clopidogrel for High Atherothrombotic Risk and Ischemic Stabilization, Management and Avoidance study (CHARISMA)[328] with a median follow-up of 28 months compared the combination of clopidogrel 75 mg/day plus a low dose of aspirin with a low dose of aspirin alone, in those with either clinically evident CVD (secondary prevention) or multiple vascular risk factors (primary prevention) (N=6,556 for those with diabetes, 42% of the total sample).

- The Clopidogrel in Unstable Angina to Prevent Recurrent Events (CURE) trial[327] included those with unstable angina or non-Q wave MI within 24 hours of an acute event, mean follow-up of 9 months. The principal objectives of this study were to compare the early and long-term efficacy and safety of the use of clopidogrel vs placebo on top of standard therapy with aspirin. 12,562 patients were given clopidogrel 300 mg bolus and then 75 mg daily plus aspirin (75–325 mg daily) or placebo plus aspirin (N=2,840 for those with diabetes, 22.6% of the total sample). The patients were followed for a maximum of 12 months (mean 9 months).

- The PCI-CURE[330] which was a sub-analysis of 2,658 CURE study patients requiring percutaneous coronary intervention (PCI). Diabetic patients represented 18.9% (N=504) of the total sample.

- The Clopidogrel Reduction of Events During Extended Observation (CREDO)[329] trial evaluated the efficacy of continuing clopidogrel on top of standard therapy with aspirin for 1 year following PCI. Participants received either a clopidogrel loading dose (300 mg) or placebo 3–24 hours before intervention. Patients in both treatments arms then received clopidogrel 75 mg/day for 28 days. Between 4 weeks and 12 months, patients in the loading-dose group received prolonged clopidogrel therapy, and those in the control group received placebo. Both treatment groups received aspirin throughout the study. Diabetic patients represented 26.4% (N=560) of the total sample.

---

* CAPRIE was a large randomised trial of the efficacy of clopidogrel and acetylsalicylic acid (ASA) in reducing the risk of a composite endpoint of ischaemic stroke, MI, or vascular death in patients with recent ischaemic stroke, recent MI, or established peripheral arterial disease (PAD) (secondary prevention). The study reported a significant benefit of clopidogrel over aspirin in relation to the primary outcome (non-fatal MI, non-fatal stroke, or vascular death) with a RR reduction of 8.7% (95% CI 0.3 to 16.5, p=0.043) compared with ASA in this broad population with a history of atherothrombosis (112 patients would need to be treated with clopidogrel rather than aspirin over this time to prevent one vascular event).

Only one RCT, Management of ATherothrombosis with Clopidogrel in High-risk patients with recent transient ischaemic stroke (MATCH), was identified comparing the combination of clopidogrel plus aspirin with clopidogrel plus placebo.[325] Patients with recent ischaemic stroke or transient ischaemic attack and at least one additional vascular risk factor were randomised to aspirin 75 mg plus clopidogrel 75 mg or clopidogrel 75 mg plus placebo for 18 months. (N=7,599 for those with diabetes, 68% of the sample.)

It should be noted that differing dosing and titration regimens and the differing populations included in the studies, such as patients with no clinical evidence of CVD,[328] to patients with recent ischaemic stroke[325] or patients undergoing a coronary surgery[330] may limit direct comparison between studies.

15.1.3 Health economic methodological introduction

One study was identified looking at aspirin compared to standard care, but the main outcomes for the trial were blood pressure (BP) targets and results of the addition of aspirin were not given for the diabetes subgroup.[331]

In the HTA clopidogrel used in combination with aspirin compared to aspirin alone in the treatment of non-ST segment elevation acute coronary syndromes (ACS), diabetes was considered as one of the risk factors contributing to high risk.[332]

In the study by Weintraub et al.[333] clopidogrel was compared to aspirin in patients hospitalised within 24 hours of onset of symptoms indicative of ACS who did not have significant ST segment elevation. A subgroup analysis was performed for diabetics.[333]

In the studies by Ringborg et al.[334] and Cowper et al.[335] the cost-effectiveness of clopidogrel plus aspirin for 12 months was compared to only 1 month of therapy. In the Ringborg study diabetes was not found to be a significant risk factor and the results for the whole population are reported here.[334] In the Cowper study diabetes was considered a high-risk factor.[335]

15.1.4 Evidence statements

▷ Aspirin and dipyridamole

This study found that there was a significant decrease in proteinuria with aspirin (−15.9%), with dipyridamole (−14.8%) and with the combination of aspirin and dipyridamole (−37.3%) compared with an increase in proteinuria found with placebo (1.9%), p=0.0007. Significant decreases were also identified in the urinary protein/creatinine ratio with the three treatment groups compared with the placebo.

There were no changes identified in BP, renal function tests and blood sugar. No adverse events (AEs) were noted during this study. **Level 1+**

▷ Aspirin and vitamin E

This study was terminated early (3.7 years) and in the diabetic subgroup there were no significant changes identified with aspirin in incidence of major CV and cerebrovascular events. **Level 1+**

▷ Clopidogrel vs aspirin

CAPRIE: Post hoc sub-analysis

This sub-analysis found a significantly lower incidence of CV events in diabetic patients receiving clopidogrel compared to those treated with aspirin. Furthermore, the incidence of rehospitalisation for any bleeding event was significantly lower with clopidogrel than with the aspirin group (see table 15.1). **Level 1+**

Table 15.1 CAPRIE: Post hoc sub-analysis			
CAPRIE (Diabetic subpopulation N=3,866)	**Aspirin**	**Clopidogrel**	**Size effect**
Primary endpoint stroke, MI, vascular death or rehospitalisation for ischaemia or bleeding	17.7%	15.6%	RRR 12.4% ARR 2.1% p=0.042 NNT 48
Incidence of rehospitalisation for any bleeding event	2.8%	1.8%	RRR 37% (95% CI 3.8–58.7) p=0.031
Subset of patients treated with insulin at baseline (N=1,134) Primary endpoint stroke, MI, vascular death or rehospitalisation for ischaemia or bleeding	21.5%	17.7%	RRR 16.7% ARR 3.8% p=0.106 NNT 26.3

ARR, absolute relative risk; NNT, number needed to treat; RRR, relative risk reduction

The authors acknowledged several limitations of this sub-analysis:

- compared with the original CAPRIE primary cluster endpoints this was a different endpoint ('softer' according to the authors)
- the study was not sufficiently powered to allow identification of specific individual endpoints
- the duration and severity of diabetes were unknown
- specific details regarding control of diabetes, such as glycosylated haemoglobin levels or glycaemic control were not collected. **Level 1+**

▷ Aspirin + clopidogrel vs aspirin + placebo

CHARISMA study

The CHARISMA study did not find a significant benefit associated with clopidogrel plus aspirin as compared with placebo plus aspirin in reducing the incidence of the primary endpoint of MI, stroke, or death from CV causes in patients with clinically evident CVD or at high risk for such disease. **Level 1++**

The same study found a moderate, though significant, benefit associated with clopidogrel plus aspirin as compared with placebo plus aspirin in reducing the secondary composite endpoint of MI, stroke, or death from CV causes, or hospitalisation for unstable angina, transient ischemic attack or revascularisation (see table 15.2). **Level 1++**

The CHARISMA study found no significant differences in the rate of severe bleeding between the two groups. However, the combination of clopidogrel and aspirin was associated with a significantly higher rate of moderate bleeding in comparison with treatment with aspirin plus placebo (see table 15.2). **Level 1++**

Table 15.2 CHARISMA study

CHARISMA	Aspirin + clopidogrel	Aspirin + placebo	Size effect
Primary endpoint MI, stroke, or CV death	NS		
Secondary endpoint MI, stroke, CV death, or hospitalisation for unstable angina, TIA, or revascularisation	16.7%	17.9%	RR 0.92 95% CI 0.86 to 0.995 p=0.04
Severe bleeding	NS		
Moderate bleeding	2.1%	1.3%	RR 1.62 95% CI 1.27 to 2.08 p<0.001

TIA, transient ischaemic attack

▷ Subgroup analysis

A subgroup analysis suggested that in the population of patients with clinically evident CVD (symptomatic) the combination of clopidogrel plus aspirin was significantly beneficial in comparison with placebo plus aspirin with respect to the primary efficacy endpoint. (Among the 12,153 symptomatic patients, there was a marginally significant reduction in the primary endpoint with aspiring plus clopidogrel. See table 15.3.) **Level 1++**

The analysis suggested that there was a risk associated with dual antiplatelet therapy in the asymptomatic group since among the 3,284 asymptomatic patients there was a 6.6% relative increase in the rate of primary events with clopidogrel plus aspirin, compared to 5.5% with placebo (see table 15.3). **Level 1++**

Furthermore, in the subgroup of asymptomatic patients, there was a significant increase in the rate of death from all causes among the patients assigned to clopidogrel plus aspirin as compared with those assigned to placebo plus aspirin, as well as a significant increase in the rate of death from CV causes among those assigned to the combination therapy (see table 15.3). **Level 1++**

The rates of severe bleeding were higher, but not significant, among both the asymptomatic and symptomatic patients receiving the combination therapy compared to those receiving aspirin plus placebo (see table 15.3). **Level 1++**

Among asymptomatic patients, there was no significant difference in the rates of moderate bleeding between the two groups. In contrast, the rates of moderate bleeding among symptomatic patients were significantly higher in those treated with aspirin plus clopidogrel than in patients receiving aspirin plus placebo (see table 15.3). **Level 1++**

Table 15.3 CHARISMA study: subgroup analysis

CHARISMA: Subgroup analysis		Aspirin + clopidogrel	Aspirin + placebo	Size effect
Patients with clinically evident CV disease (symptomatic) N=12,153	Primary endpoint MI, stroke, or CV death	6.9%	7.9%	RR 0.88 95% CI 0.77–0.998 p=0.046
	Severe bleeding	NS		
	Moderate bleeding	2.1%	1.3%	p<0.001
Patients with risk factors for CVD (asymptomatic) N=3,284	Primary endpoint MI, stroke, or CV death	6.6%	5.5%	p=0.20
	Death from all causes	5.4%	3.8%	p=0.04
	Death from CV causes	3.9%	2.2%	p=0.01
	Severe bleeding	NS		
	Moderate bleeding	NS		

▷ CREDO study

The CREDO study found that at 12 months long-term clopidogrel and aspirin treatment significantly reduced the risk of death, MI or stroke in comparison with those treated with clopidogrel and aspirin for 4 weeks and then aspirin plus placebo for 11 months. RR reduction of 27%, 95% CI (3.9%–44.4%), p=0.02. Absolute reduction 3% (p=0.02). **Level 1++**

The study also showed that the clopidogrel pre-treatment loading dose did not significantly reduce the combined risk of death, MI, or urgent target vessel revascularisation at 28 days. **Level 1++**

There was no significant difference in the risk of major bleeding between the groups, though there was a higher risk of major bleeding identified for those treated with long-term clopidogrel and aspirin compared with those taking aspirin plus placebo. **Level 1++**

▷ Clopidogrel + aspirin vs clopidogrel + placebo

MATCH study

The study found that combination treatment with aspirin plus clopidogrel did not significantly reduce the primary composite CV morbidity or mortality endpoint* compared with clopidogrel plus placebo. **Level 1++**

The secondary endpoint analysis (ischaemic stroke and/or vascular death, all-cause stroke, non-fatal events and rehospitalisation) showed no significant difference between the addition of

---

* Primary composite endpoint: first occurrence of an event in the composite of ischaemic stroke, MI, vascular death (including haemorrhagic death of any origin), or rehospitalisation for an acute ischaemic event (including unstable angina pectoris, worsening of peripheral arterial disease requiring therapeutic intervention or urgent revascularisation, or TIA).

aspirin to clopidogrel versus clopidogrel plus placebo, though rates were lower with aspirin than with placebo, added to clopidogrel. **Level 1++**

In terms of AEs, the study concluded that adding aspirin to clopidogrel resulted in significantly more bleeding complications than in the placebo and clopidogrel arm, doubling the number of events (see table 15.4). **Level 1++**

MATCH	Clopidogrel + aspirin	Clopidogrel + placebo	Size effect
Table 15.4 MATCH			
Life-threatening bleedings*	2.6%	1.3%	RR 1.26 95% CI (0.64–1.88) p<0.0001
Major bleedings	2%	1%	RR 1.36 95% CI (0.86–1.86) p<0.0001
Minor bleedings	3%	1%	p<0.0001

* Life-threatening events were more frequent in the aspirin plus clopidogrel versus clopidogrel monotherapy, irrespective of whether they were GI (1.4 vs 0.6%) or intracranial (1.1 vs 0.7%)

There was no significant difference in overall mortality between the two treatment groups. The most common type of haemorrhagic complication was GI bleeding. **Level 1++**

▷ Subgroup analysis

Post hoc analysis found no significant difference among the 5,197 diabetic patients included in the MATCH trial in terms of the incidence of primary endpoint. **Level 1++**

15.1.5 Health economic evidence statements

In the treatment of non-ST segment elevation ACS in high-risk patients the cost-effectiveness of clopidogrel used in combination with aspirin compared to aspirin alone £4,939 per QALY.[332]

A US study compared clopidogrel to aspirin in diabetic patients hospitalised within 24 hours of onset of symptoms indicative of ACS, the cost-effectiveness was $8,457–9,857 per life-year gained.[333] (In this analysis a cost-effectiveness ratio less than $50,000 was considered cost-effective.)

15.1.6 From evidence to recommendations

Little extra evidence of note on use of aspirin was available since the last review. However, there is now better understanding of the extent of the CV risk faced by people with Type 2 diabetes. The rather poor direct evidence for people with Type 2 diabetes led to difficulties in assessing the level of risk above which aspirin therapy should be advised. The GDG accepts that its view that all people at, or over, the age of 50 years should treated is somewhat arbitrary. Primary prevention below that age would be by assessment of higher CV risk (family history of premature vascular disease, abnormal lipid profile, marked abdominal adiposity). While the group were aware of some discussions over the dose of aspirin to be used in people with diabetes, they were not presented with any evidence that could lead to a variation from the usual national recommendations of 75 mg.

NICE guidance for dipyridamole MR related only to people with cerebrovascular events.

The evidence for the use of clopidogrel was noted to relate to acute and non-acute situations. The current guideline review was not concerned with acute vascular events or interventions. The CHARISMA and MATCH trials suggested that the combination of aspirin and clopidogrel carried a significant side-effect risk of a serious nature not balanced by secure health gain, and therefore could not be generally recommended. NICE guidance for secondary prevention of vascular events in people without diabetes was that clopidogrel should not be used instead of aspirin except where intolerance or hypersensitivity to the latter was present. The specific evidence for people with diabetes, mostly sub-analyses, did not suggest that advice should be varied for people with Type 2 diabetes.

RECOMMENDATIONS

R90   Offer low-dose aspirin, 75 mg daily, to a person who is 50 years old or over if blood pressure is below 145/90 mmHg.

R91   Offer low-dose aspirin, 75 mg daily, to a person who is under 50 years old and has significant other cardiovascular risk factors (features of the metabolic syndrome, strong early family history of cardiovascular disease, smoking, hypertension, extant cardiovascular disease, microalbuminuria).

R92   Clopidogrel should be used instead of aspirin only in those with clear aspirin intolerance (except in the context of acute cardiovascular events and procedures). Follow the recommendations in the NICE TA 'Clopidogrel and modified-release dipyridamole in the prevention of occlusive vascular events'.[321]

16 | Kidney damage

16.1 Diabetes kidney disease management

16.1.1 Clinical introduction

Kidney disease in people with Type 2 diabetes is becoming an ever larger health burden.[336] This reflects a number of trends including the increasing prevalence of people with diabetes, the better cardiovascular (CV) survival with modern management, and the better management of progression of kidney damage itself. The trend to younger onset of Type 2 diabetes is also likely to see more kidney damage as these people are at lower CV risk, while in the elderly the condition is ever more complicated by comorbidities disease.

Primary prevention of kidney damage from diabetes centres around the prevention of microvascular (classical diabetic nephropathy) and arterial (and thus renovascular) damage discussed in other chapters of this guideline – the current section is concerned with detection and secondary prevention of kidney damage. For reasons of coherence some recommendations overlap with, or are reproduced from, other sections of the guideline.

The clinical questions addressed here include how often and by what means to detect and confirm the possibility of diabetic renal disease, and the means of monitoring its progression. In those with detected renal disease issues arise as to the means to reduce or stop such progression, and the point at which to engage specialist renal management.

16.1.2 Methodological introduction

Both methodologically and clinically this question attempts to cover a broad research area which encompasses different key issues relevant to the diagnosis and management of renal disease (e.g. monitoring of renal function (GFR, measurement of serum creatinine, renal ultrasound) and qualitative and quantitative measurements for albuminuria (screening tests).

A total of nine studies were identified as relevant to the question.[337–345]

Given the diversity of studies the evidence has been divided into the following categories:
- studies comparing the accuracy of different equations used to estimated GFR
- studies looking at qualitative methods to detect microalbuminuria
- studies comparing several quantitative methods to assess renal disease such as renal ultrasound, serum creatinine, estimated glomerular filtration rate (eGFR) and tests for albuminuria (i.e. UAER, urinary albumin concentration (UAC), albumin:creatinine ratio (ACR).

▷ Equations estimating GFR in Type 2 diabetes population

General background

- Although GFR can be measured directly using inulin, the classic method for measuring inulin clearance requires an intravenous infusion and timed urine collections over a period of several hours. Therefore, GFR is costly and cumbersome. Several other alternative measures have been devised; however, predictive equations have proven simpler.

- In adults the equations used are the Modification of Diet in Renal Disease (MDRD) study and the Cockcroft-Gault (CG) equations.
- Both the CG and the MDRD equations were developed in predominantly non-diabetic individuals.
- The CG equation has the advantage of being more widely known, easier to remember and more extensively validated than the MDRD formula. However, the MDRD formula does not require knowledge of the patient's weight (making it far more suitable for automated laboratory reporting), and does not need correction for body surface (and therefore does not require knowledge of the patient's height).
- The MDRD study equation has not been validated in children (aged under 18 years), pregnant women, the elderly (aged over 70), racial or ethnic subgroups other than Caucasians and African-Americans, in individuals with normal kidney function who are at increased risk for CKD or in normal individuals.

Studies included

No RCTs were identified comparing the performance of different equations estimating GFR in a Type 2 diabetes population.

Two cross-sectional studies[344,345] were identified as looking at the performance of the estimating equations in patients with diabetes and CKD.

One study[344] compared the abbreviated MDRD equation with the CG in 249 CKD patients with diabetes. The study used data from the renal function laboratory at the Cleveland Clinic Foundation which performed approximately 9,000 measurements of GFR by 125 I-iothalamate renal clearance from 1982 to 2002 and maintained a database with demographic and laboratory variables.

The other study[345] compared the performance of three equations (CG, MDRD and a simplified CG).* Data for the study was taken from 200 adult diabetic patients with CKD attending a hospital in Pessac, France. GFR was evaluated by clearance of the radionuclide marker was measured after intravenous injection of 51Cr-EDTA.

Studies in which serum creatinine assays were not adjusted (calibrated) to mimic that of the MDRD study laboratory were excluded** (it should be noted that the same exclusion criteria has been adopted by the NICE CKD guideline – due to be published in September 2008). In addition, studies were excluded if gold standards test were not used as the reference test or if they had a small sample size (N<100).

---

* To protect the CG from the influence of body weight it was replaced by its mean value (76 kg) to calculate a new formula: modified CG (MCG).

** The majority of the between laboratory difference is due to calibration differences. Bias between different creatinine assays produces predictable and significant differences in estimates of GFR. Currently, there is no universally accepted standardisation for creatinine assays. A potential solution is for laboratories to align their creatinine assay to that used by the MDRD laboratory. Isotope dilution mass spectrometry (IDMS) is another alternative.

▷ Qualitative methods to assess microalbuminuria

General background

To be useful as screening tests, qualitative (or semiquantitative) tests must have high detection rates for microalbuminuria (not only increased albumin concentrations in urine). According to the US Laboratory Medicine Practice Guidelines the sensitivity of a clinically useful qualitative test should be higher than 95%.

Dipstick tests are subject to false positives because of patient dehydration, hematuria, exercise, infection, and extremely alkaline urine. Conversely, dipstick tests also are subject to false negatives as a result of excessive hydration and urine proteins other that albumin.

Studies included

No RCTs were identified addressing this issue.

Three cross-sectional studies[339,340,343] were found evaluating the performance of a qualitative method (Micral-Test II) with other methods to assess microalbuminuria in Type 2 diabetes populations.

One study[339] compared the Micral-Test II with nephelometry in 166 patients with Type 2 diabetes and essential hypertension.

Another study[340] assesses the accuracy of the Micral-Test II, UAC, and ACR in a random urine specimen in 278 diabetic patients.

One study[343] compared the Micral-Test II with UAC by immunoturbidimetric.

Studies with a small sample (N<100) were excluded.

▷ Studies comparing several quantitative methods to assess renal disease

General background

- The most commonly used measure of overall kidney function in clinical practice is serum creatinine concentration. Unfortunately, this measurement is affected by many factors other than the level of kidney function and varies markedly with age, gender and muscle mass. Moreover, as it was stated above, there is significant calibration issues associated with the measurement of serum creatinine that lead to inter-laboratory variation.
- Consequently, many guidelines, including the Kidney Disease Outcomes Quality Initiative (K/DOQI), British Renal Association and Kidney Disease Improving Global Outcomes (KDIGO) guidelines have recommended that serum creatinine concentration alone should not be used to assess the level of kidney function.
- UAC and ACR are alternative ways of estimating loss of glomerular permselectivity when using single urine samples instead of timed urine collections (i.e. UAER in a 24-hour sample).The amount of albumin lost in the urine will primarily depend on the degree of damage to the glomerular membrane, whereas UAC, in addition, will depend on the extent to which the urine has been concentrated in the tubular system.

- By dividing UAC by urinary creatinine concentrations (i.e. ACR), an attempt is made to correct for inter- and intraindividual differences in daily urine volume.

Studies included

No RCTs were identified addressing this issue.

Four cross-sectional studies[337,338,341,342] were found comparing different quantitative methods to assess renal disease.

One study[337] analysed the status of eGFR (by diethylene triamine pentaacetic acid (DTPA) renal scan) vis-à-vis other non-invasive modes of assessment of renal involvement (UAER, serum creatinine and ultrasound) in 100 diabetic patients.

One study[338] determined the diagnostic performance of albuminuria (ACR) and a serum creatinine >120 µmol to detect an eGFR <60 ml/min/1.73m^2 in a population of 4,303 diabetics.

Similarly, one study[342] examined the ability of ACR to detect clinically meaningful CKD (GFR <60 ml/min 1.73 m^2) compared with estimated GFR (by using the MDRD equation) in a population of 7,596 diabetics.

Another study[341] analysed the association between GFR (by DTPA renal scan) and UAER (timed urine collection) in 301 Type 2 diabetes patients. In particular, the study determined the prevalence and characteristics of patients with impaired renal function (GFR <60 ml/min 1.73 m^2) and an AER within the normoalbuminuric range.

16.1.3 Health economic methodological introduction

No health economic papers were identified.

16.1.4 Evidence Statements

▷ Equations estimating GFR in Type 2 diabetes population

Bias

One study[344] reported that in the whole CKD group (diabetics and non-diabetics N=828), the MDRD equation was superior to the CG equation in terms of bias. The MDRD equation slightly underestimated the measured eGFR while the CG equation significantly overestimated the eGFR (−0.5 vs 3.5 ml/min per 1.73 m^2 p<0.001). **Level 2+**

The study[344] showed that the MDRD equation was also significantly less biased than the CG in the diabetic subgroup (N=249) and in people with a measured GFR <30 ml/min per 1.73m^2 (N=546) p<0.001 in each group. **Level 2+**

The study[344] concluded that the MDRD and CG equations were significantly more biased in people with GFR >60 ml/min per 1.73 m^2 (N=117). The MDRD equation underestimated the measured eGFR, while the CG equation significantly overestimated the GFR (−3.5 vs 7.9 ml/min per 1.73 m^2, p<0.001). The equations were also biased, but to a lesser extent in patients with GFR 30–60 ml/min per 1.73 m^2. **Level 2+**

One study[345] revealed a bias for the MDRD and MCG – the differences between the predicted and the measured GFR were correlated with their means (MDRD: r=0.054, p<0.0001; MCG: r=0.27, p<0.001). There was no such bias for CG.

Test correlation

In terms of test correlation, the study[344] demonstrated that in the CKD population, both the MDRD (r=0.90) and CG equations (r=0.89) correlated highly with measured[125] I-iothalamate GFR. **Level 2+**

One study[345] showed that over the whole population the mean isotopic GFR was 56.5±34.9 ml/min/1.73 m^2, the mean CG 61.2±35.6 (p<0.01 vs isotopic), the mean MCG. 60.0±29.9 (p<0.05 vs isotopic) and the mean MDRD, 51.0±24.3 (p<0.001 vs isotopic). The MCG was better correlated with isotopic GFR than was the CG (CG: r=0.75, MCG: r=0.83; p<0.05 vs CG, MDRD: r=0.82; p=0.068 vs CG). **Level 2+**

Accuracy

In relation to accuracy, the study[344] showed that in the diabetic group, the MDRD equation was significantly more accurate (63%) than the CG equation (53%) p<0.05. **Level 2+**

One study[345] stated that the receiver operating characteristic (ROC) curves showed that the MDRD and the MCG had a better maximal accuracy for the diagnosis of moderate (N=119; area under curve (AUC): 0.866 for CG, 0.920 for MDRD, 0.921 for MCG; both 0.891 vs CG) and severe (N=52; AUC: 0.891 for CG, 0.930 for MDRD, 0.942 for MCG; both p<0.05 vs CG) renal failure. **Level 2+**

The same study[345] concluded that as the MCG was more accurate for high GFR, and the MDRD was more accurate for low GFR, the MCG could be used at low serum creatine values and the MDRD at high values.

▷   Studies looking at qualitative methods to assess microalbuminuria

One study[339] comparing the Micral-Test II with nephelometry demonstrated that the dipstick had a sensitivity of 83% and a specificity of 96%. The correlation between nephelometry and Micral Test II results was 0.81 (p<0.0001). **Level 2+**

The same study[339] showed that when the ROC curve for the Micral-Test II as a diagnostic test for microalbuminuria was analysed, the calculated mean area under the ROC curve (±SEM) was 0.91±0.03 (CI 95% 0.85–0.96) and the corresponding best cut-off value was 30.5 mg/l. **Level 2+**

One study[343] comparing the Micral-Test II with UAER (in a 24-hour timed urine collection) reported a sensitivity 88% and a specificity 80%.

When performance was assessed by different concentrations readings the study found that Micral-Test II strips performed reasonably well at 0.50 and 100 mg/l with a high percentage of true negatives (93%, 0 mg/l), true positives (81%, 50 mg/l and 91%, 100 mg/l), low percentages of false negatives (7%, 0 mg/l) and false positives (19%, 50 mg/l and 9%, 100 mg/l). However, at 20 mg/l Micral strips did not perform well (51% false positive). **Level 2+**

One study[340] assessing the accuracy of the Micral-Test II, the UAC and the ACR in a random urine specimen found the following test correlations:

- UAER vs UAC: 0.76 p<0.0001
- UAER vs ACR: 0.74 p<0.0001
- ACR vs UAC: 0.86 p<0.0001

The study[340] also reported that age and 24-hour creatinuria presented a negative correlation (278 patients, r=–0.19, p=0.002). No correlation was observed between age and UAER (r=0.02, p=0.74), age and UAC (r=0.07, p=0.22) and age and UACR (r=0.11, p=0.08). **Level 2+**

The same study[340] showed that the specificity of UAC and UACR was similar when considering the 100% sensitivity cut-off points. The sensitivity and specificity of the Micral-Test II strip for a 20 mg/l cut-off point (as indicated by manufacturer) on fresh urine samples based on ROC curve analysis (N=130) were 90 and 46% respectively. **Level 2+**

In terms of accuracy, the study[340] stated that the comparison among the areas under the ROC curves for UAC, UACR and the Micral-Test II took into account the individual results, for each single patient (N=130), of the three screening methods being tested and of the reference test method (UAER).The study concluded that a similar area was observed under the UAC (0.934±0.032) and UACR (0.920±0.035) curves (p=0.626).

The area under the curve was smaller for the Micral-Test II (0.846±0.047) than for UAC (p=0.014). **Level 2+**

▷ Studies comparing several quantitative methods to assess renal disease

Ultrasound – serum creatinine – albuminuria – GFR

One study[337] analysed the status of GFR (by DTPA renal scan) vis-à-vis other non-invasive modes of assessment of renal involvement (UAER, serum creatinine and ultrasound) in 100 Type 2 diabetes patients. Patients were divided into three subgroups depending on the duration of initial detection of Type 2 diabetes. Group A constituted patients with less than 5 years duration, group B 5–15 years and group C more than 15 years duration.

Ultrasound

The study[337] reported that most of the patients in group A and B had a large kidney with preserved corticomedullary (CM) differentiation (83.9% and 80%); only group C had a significantly higher prevalence of large kidney with loss of CM differentiation (75.9%). **Level 2+**

Serum creatinine

The study[337] concluded that there was no difference between group A and B as far as the serum creatinine was concerned. High level of serum creatinine was only significantly associated with group C (44.8%). **Level 2+**

Albuminuria

The study[337] found that normoalbuminuria and microalbuminuria were significantly higher in group A (25.8% and 74.2%). Macroalbuminuria was higher in both group B and C (80% and 69%).

For UAER group A had a significantly lower level compared to both B and C (p<0.01), however, there was no significant difference between group B and C with respect to the amount of both micro- and macroalbuminuria. **Level 2+**

Glomerular filtration rate

The study[337] showed that group A presented a significantly higher prevalence of normal and raised GFR (25.8% and 61.3%). Group B had a significantly higher prevalence of low GFR, while prevalence of very low GFR was highest in group C (37.9%).

The GFR had a progressively significant decrement from group A through group B to C (p<0.01). **Level 2+**

The study[337] concluded that GFR estimation was the only renal parameter which could singly provide a picture of the actual renal status of Type 2 diabetes patients at any duration irrespective of the status of albuminuria, azotaemia or renal size and morphology as their variability or progression is non-linear.

▷ Diagnostic performance of ACR >120 μmol to detect an eGFR <60 ml/min/1.73 m^2 (MDRD)

After ranking 4,303 diabetics based on their eGFR (>90, 90–60, 60–30 and <30 ml/min per 1.73 m^2) one study[338] showed that the proportion of individuals with abnormal serum creatinine rose with progressive fall in eGFR (0%, 1%, 37% and 100% with creatinine >120 μmol/l in eGFR >90, 90–60, 60–30 and <30 ml/min per 1.73 m^2 respectively), as did the proportion with abnormal albuminuria (33%, 27%, 42% and 77% with ACR >3.5 mg/mmol). **Level 2+**

The study[338] found that of the 1,296 individuals with an eGFR <60, 539 (42%) had abnormal serum creatinine, 579 (45%) had abnormal albuminuria and 798 (62%) had either abnormal serum creatinine or urine ACR. Thus, a creatinine and ACR based strategy would have missed the renal risk of 498 (38%) individuals since they had normal values of both despite having a significantly impaired eGFR <60 ml/min per 1.73 m^2. **Level 2+**

The same study[338] also demonstrated that the proportion missed by current markers was more marked in women (N=757) where the prevalence of those with abnormal serum creatinine, urine ACR and either were 20%, 38% and 47% respectively, compared with 72%, 54% and 83% observed in men (N=539). **Level 2+**

When the study analysed the data by ethnic origin, it was found that white people appeared to benefit the most from eGFR, with a greater prevalence of normocreatinaemic and normoalbuminuric renal insufficiency, whereas the majority of the African-Caribbean group with low eGFR had either an abnormal creatinine or ACR 39%, 42% and 59% respectively, with abnormal creatinine, ACR and either in white people (N=997); 62%, 69% and 80% respectively, in African-Caribbeans (N=84); and 44%, 54% and 69% respectively in Indo-Asians (N=210). **Level 2+**

The study did not find difference in performance when data was analysed by the type of diabetes. **Level 2+**

The study[338] concluded that GFR estimates may have a place in routine diabetes clinical care, being a more sensitive marker of risk than serum creatinine or albuminuria. eGFR also appears to eliminate the gender and ethnic bias observed with current markers and also provides an opportunity to monitor longitudinal changes.

Another study[342] using data from 7,596 diabetics found that 27.5% (N=1,715) of the population had an eGFR <60 ml/min/1.73 m^2; of these 19.4% had normoalbuminuria; 20.4% had albuminuria, the remainder not having had albuminuria determined.* The study also reported that serum creatinine was normal (£120 mmol/l) in 54.7% of those with eGFR <60 ml/min/1.73 m^2 and £150 mmol/l in 82.2%. **Level 2+**

This study[342] found that the sensitivity of abnormal serum creatinine levels in identifying eGFR <60 ml/min/1.73 m^2 is 45.3%, albuminuria is 51.2% and either an abnormal serum creatinine or albuminuria is 82.4%. **Level 2+**

The same study also reported that unidentified CKD, defined as the presence of a GFR <60 ml/min/1.73 m^2 but without any evidence of an abnormal creatinine (i.e. serum creatinine £120 mmol/l) was significantly greater in females compared with males adjusting for age, type of diabetes and secondary care setting (OR 8.22, CI 6.56 to 10.29). Using albuminuria as a screening test also failed to identify CKD in females (OR 2.22, CI 1.63 to 3.03). The presence of abnormal serum creatinine and albuminuria to identify CKD continued to display a significant bias against females (OR 7.58, CI 5.44 to 10.57). **Level 2+**

The study[342] concluded that current screening techniques based upon albuminuria and/or abnormal serum creatinine would fail to detect a significant number of participants with an eGFR <60 ml/min/1.73 m^2. Therefore, without eGFR reporting the clinician may not be alerted to the presence of CKD and be falsely reassured that renal function is normal.

▷ Association between GFR (by DTPA renal scan) and UAER (timed urine collection)

One study[341] divided 301 Type 2 diabetes patients on the basis of their GFR (i.e., < or ≥60 ml/min 1.73 m^2) and albuminuria status (i.e., normo <20 μg/min, micro 20–200 μg/min, macro >200 μg/min). The study found a significant correlation between a decreasing GFR with increasing levels of AER (r=-0.29, p<0.0001). **Level 2+**

Glomerular filtration rate status

The study[341] reported that for the 109 patients with a GFR <60 l/min 1.73 m^2 the prevalence of normo-, micro- and macroalbuminuria was 39%, 35% and 26% respectively. For the 192 patients with a GFR ≥60 ml/min 1.73 m^2 the prevalence of normo-, micro- and macroalbuminuria was 60%, 33% and 7% respectively. **Level 2+**

---

* Albuminuria was determined in only 39.8% of participants with an eGFR <60 ml/min/1.73m^2 over the 2-year period of our study despite current recommendations in the UK for annual screening. A greater proportion of participants (70%) receiving diabetes management in a secondary care setting had albuminuria quantified.

UAER status

When the study[341] stratified the 301 patients according to their AER status regardless of their GFR, 52% had normo-, 34% had micro-, and 14% had macroalbuminuria. For the 158 normoalbuminuric patients, 27% had a corresponding GFR <60 ml/min 1.73 m^2 and 73% had a GFR ≥60 ml/min 1.73 m^2. **Level 2+**

The study also demonstrated that normoalbuminuric patients were significantly older (p<0.01) and more commonly female (p<0.01) in comparison to those with macroalbuminuria. There were no differences in the duration of diabetes, BMI, prevalence of retinopathy, history of CVD, smoking history, HbA$_{1c}$ levels, systolic blood pressure, diastolic blood pressure (DBP), total cholesterol, low-density lipoprotein, high-density lipoprotein and triglyceride levels among patients with a GFR <60 ml/min 1.73 m^2 associated with normo-, micro-, or macroalbuminuria.

Overall, the study did not find significant differences in the use of any antihypertensive agent (specifically renin-angiotensin system inhibitors (RAS-inhibitors)) for patients with a GFR <60 ml/min 1.73 m^2 and normo-, micro- or macroalbuminuria. **Level 2+**

The study[341] calculated the prevalence of a GFR <60 ml/min 1.73 m^2 and normoalbuminuria after excluding 23 of 43 patients whose normoalbuminuric status was possibly altered by the use of RAS inhibitors. After this adjustment the prevalence of a <60 ml/min 1.73 m^2 and normoalbuminuria was 20 of 86 (23%). **Level 2+**

16.1.5 From evidence to recommendations

The GDG noted the importance to health in delaying or preventing the progression of diabetes renal damage, and the certainty of evidence that this could be done. Detection of early diabetes kidney damage at a stage when therapy could be usefully intensified was now nearly universally through urinary ACR – review of the evidence showed no reason to doubt this was appropriate. This measure is also a CV risk factor, and accordingly features elsewhere in chapter 13.

Some discussion of the logistics of collection of first-pass morning urine samples revealed there was no single right answer to establishing a sound process for ensuring samples were obtained annually. No changes in the process for confirming presence of microalbuminuria were felt necessary.

It was noted that laboratory estimation of serum creatinine was now reported with an eGFR result using the method abbreviated MDRD (4-variable) equation. The group recognised some problems with these calculations (worse overall in people with diabetes than in the general population) but could see no better alternative.

The management of diabetic nephropathy when confirmed was felt not to have changed from that of the previous NICE guideline and that for Type 1 diabetes, centring around renin-angiotensin system blockade, tight blood pressure control, and specialist referral. Non-diabetic renal disease will also occur in people with diabetes and needs not to be confused with diabetic nephropathy. The group noted that there were a series of markers which suggested when renal disease in people with diabetes was not diabetic nephropathy.

The group noted that there is a NICE CKD clinical guideline which also considers people with diabetes. This guideline is due to be published in September 2008.

RECOMMENDATIONS

R93   Ask all people with or without detected nephropathy to bring in a first-pass morning urine specimen once a year. In the absence of proteinuria/urinary tract infection (UTI), send this for laboratory estimation of albumin:creatinine ratio. Request a specimen on a subsequent visit if UTI prevents analysis.

R94   Make the measurement on a spot sample if a first-pass sample is not provided (and repeat on a first-pass specimen if abnormal) or make a formal arrangement for a first-pass specimen to be provided.

R95   Measure serum creatinine and estimate the glomerular filtration rate (using the method-abbreviated modification of diet in renal disease (MDRD) four-variable equation) annually at the time of albumin:creatinine ratio estimation.

R96   Repeat the test if an abnormal albumin:creatinine ratio is obtained (in the absence of proteinuria/UTI) at each of the next two clinic visits but within a maximum of 3–4 months. Take the result to be confirming microalbuminuria if a further specimen (out of two more) is also abnormal (>2.5 mg/mmol for men, >3.5 mg/mmol for women).

R97   Suspect renal disease, other than diabetic nephropathy and consider further investigation or referral when the albumin:creatinine ratio (ACR) is raised and any of the following apply:
- there is no significant or progressive retinopathy
- blood pressure is particularly high or resistant to treatment
- had a documented normal ACR and develops heavy proteinuria (ACR >100 mg/mmol)
- significant haematuria is present
- the glomerular filtration rate has worsened rapidly
- the person is systemically ill.

R98   Discuss the significance of a finding of abnormal albumin excretion rate, and its trend over time, with the individual concerned.

R99   Start ACE inhibitors with the usual precautions and titrate to full dose in all individuals with confirmed raised albumin excretion rate (>2.5 mg/mmol for men, >3.5 mg/mmol for women).

R100   Have an informed discussion before starting an ACE inhibitor in a woman for whom there is a possibility of pregnancy, assessing the relative risks and benefits of the use of the ACE inhibitor.

R101   Substitute an angiotensin II-receptor antagonist for an ACE inhibitor for a person with an abnormal albumin:creatinine ratio if an ACE inhibitor is poorly tolerated.

R102   For a person with an abnormal albumin:creatinine ratio, maintain blood pressure below 130/80 mmHg.

R103   Agree referral criteria for specialist renal care between local diabetes specialists and nephrologists.

17 | Eye damage

Diabetes eye damage is the single largest cause of blindness before old age with a progressive incidence in people with Type 2 diabetes.[346] The success of laser therapy in the treatment of sight-threatening retinopathy is an accepted part of ophthalmological care and has not been assessed for this guideline.

Appropriate clinical questions to be addressed are, however, how people with developing retinopathy can be selected for ophthalmological referral in time for optimal treatment, and whether preventative therapy other than good blood glucose, good blood pressure, and good blood lipid control can be useful in people with Type 2 diabetes.

17.1.1 Methodological introduction

It was noted that management in this area was largely determined by practice for all people with diabetes and not just those with Type 2 diabetes. Indeed retinopathy screening programmes to be provided on a local community basis were a key early target of the National Service Framework (NSF) for diabetes, and since that time the UK National Screening Programme has published and updated a workbook on 'Essential elements in developing a diabetic retinopathy screening programme' for the guidance of health authorities and primary care trusts in England (fourth edition, January 2007).[347]

These observations, and a lack of awareness amongst experts of new publications that might affect recommendations on retinopathy screening, led to the conclusion that recommendations for people with Type 2 diabetes should closely follow those for Type 1 diabetes (NICE guideline 2004),[26] which themselves were largely based on generic evidence independent of type of diabetes.

Accordingly the recommendations of the Type 1 diabetes guidelines, and the evidence statements underlying them were reviewed, together with the national screening document. There are no significant changes from the Type 1 diabetes recommendations.

RECOMMENDATIONS

R104   Arrange or perform eye screening at, or around, the time of diagnosis. Arrange repeat of structured eye surveillance annually.

R105   Explain the reasons for and success of eye surveillance systems to the individual and ensure attendance is not reduced by ignorance of need, or fear of outcome.

R106   Use mydriasis with tropicamide when photographing the retina, after prior informed agreement following discussion of the advantages and disadvantages. Discussions should include precautions for driving.

R107   Use a quality assured digital retinal photography programme using appropriately trained staff.

R108   Perform visual acuity testing as a routine part of eye surveillance programmes.

R109 Repeat structured eye surveillance according to the findings by:
- routine review in 1 year, or
- earlier review, or
- referral to an ophthalmologist.

R110 Arrange emergency review by an ophthalmologist for:
- sudden loss of vision
- rubeosis iridis
- pre-retinal or vitreous haemorrhage
- retinal detachment.

R111 Arrange rapid review by an ophthalmologist for new vessel formation.

R112 Refer to an ophthalmologist in accordance with the National Screening Committee criteria and timelines if any of these features is present:
- referable maculopathy:
  - exudate or retinal thickening within one disc diameter of the centre of the fovea
  - circinate or group of exudates within the macula (the macula is defined here as a circle centred on the fovea, with a diameter the distance between the temporal border of the optic disc and the fovea)
  - any microaneurysm or haemorrhage within one disc diameter of the centre of the fovea, only if associated with deterioration of best visual activity to 6/12 or worse.
- referable pre-proliferative retinopathy (if cotton wool spots are present, look carefully for the following features, but cotton wool spots themselves do not define pre-proliferative retinopathy):
  - any venous beading
  - any venous loop or reduplication
  - any intraretinal microvascular abnormalities
  - multiple deep, round or blot haemorrhages
- any unexplained drop in visual acuity.

18 | Nerve damage

18.1 Diabetic neuropathic pain management

18.1.1 Clinical introduction

Neuropathic pain is a troublesome symptom of chronic exposure to poor blood glucose control that cannot be managed acutely by restoration of blood glucose control. It can take many forms, and is often distressing and sometimes depressing, particularly if symptoms are predominantly nocturnal and disturb sleep. People with diabetes may be reluctant to report the symptoms to those with expertise in diabetes care, because of lack of awareness that the problem is diabetes related. A number of drug and non-drug approaches to management are available, this diversity reflecting that none of them are fully effective.

Clinically the issues are when to start specific drug therapy for neuropathic pain, which medications to use, and in what order to try them.

18.1.2 Methodological introduction

▷ Tricyclics

There were nine studies identified in this area. All five studies included were double-blind, crossover studies. One study compared desipramine, amitriptyline and active placebo* (benzotropine to mimic dry mouth).[348] One study compared clomipramine with desipramine.[349] One study compared imipramine with mianserin (60 mg/day).[350] One study considered amitriptyline with gabapentin,[351] and the last study compared amitriptyline with lamotrigine.[352] Four studies were excluded for methodological reasons.[353,354,355,356]

One study specified the proportion of patients with Type 2 diabetes, 88%,[351] and a second study was conducted only in patients with Type 2 diabetes.[352]

The different drug and dose comparisons prevented a direct comparison between the studies.

▷ Duloxetine

There were six RCTs and one meta-analysis identified in this area.[357–363] The meta-analysis was excluded for methodological reasons.[360]

Two double-blind studies compared patients on duloxetine 60 mg/day and duloxetine 60 mg twice daily with placebo,[358,362] and a further study compared patients on duloxetine 20 mg/day, 60 mg/day or 60 mg twice daily with placebo[359] all over a 12-week study duration. There were two open-label long-term efficacy studies of 52-weeks duration comparing duloxetine 60 mg twice daily with routine care,[357,363] although in one of these studies the dose of duloxetine could be reduced to 60 mg/day in cases of poor tolerability. Additional medications were allowed in both studies; including gabapentin, amitriptyline, venlafaxine extended release and

---

* Based on the results of two studies amitriptyline compared with desipramine and fluoxetine compared with placebo (N=52).

acetaminophene,[357] and paracetamol, non-steroidal anti-inflammatory drugs (NSAIDS) or opioids.[363] The final study compared duloxetine 60 mg twice daily with duloxetine 120 mg once daily in an open-label study over 28 weeks.[361]

The majority of study participants had Type 2 diabetes; between approximately 88–94% in all studies.[357–359,361–363]

▷ Gabapentin

There were five studies identified in this area, four of these were RCTs and one was an open-label study.[364]

One study[365] was excluded for methodological reasons.

Two studies compare gabapentin with placebo,[366,367] (the study by Simpson DA[367] reported on a three-phase study. Phases two and three included gabapentin compared with venlafaxine and therefore only phase one, gabapentin compared with placebo, has been included here). One study considered gabapentin and amitriptyline in a crossover study.[351]

The open-label study considered a fixed dose of gabapentin compared with a titrating dose which was titrated until it was perceived to have reached clinical effect – that was a ≥50% reduction in pain.[364]

The majority of study participants had Type 2 diabetes; approximately 75%,[366] 89%,[364] 88%,[351] and 82%.[367]

▷ Pregabalin

There were three studies identified in this area, all were RCTs comparing varying doses of pregabalin (75 mg/day to 600 mg/day) with placebo for those with both Type 1 and Type 2 diabetes, N=729.[368–370]

The majority of the participants in each study were those with Type 2 diabetes; 90.1%,[368] 91%,[369] and 87%.[370]

There were no studies which considered pregabalin in comparison with other treatments for painful diabetic neuropathy. The included studies were all of short duration (6–9 weeks) and there were no studies which considered longer-term effectiveness.

▷ Carbamazepine

There were a limited number of studies identified in this area. It should be noted that studies looking at oxcarbazepine, a new form of carbamazepine which has the same indications but seems to be better tolerated, were also included. All the studies were conducted in diabetic patients.

In relation to carbamazepine, we found three small RCTs with a crossover design. Two of them compared carbamazepine against placebo.*[371,372] The third RCT[373] compared carbamazepine monotherapy with the combination of nortriptyline-fluphenazine.

---

* These two studies were published more than 30 years ago (1969, 1974) reflecting the fact that carbamazepine was one of the first interventions studied for treatment of painful diabetic neuropathy.

There were some methodological quality issues with the two placebo-controlled studies[371,372] which often involved a short follow-up and the absence of a washout period.

Three RCTs were identified comparing oxcarbazepine with placebo using a parallel design.[374–376] One of these studies was excluded due to a high dropout rate.[376]

18.1.3 Health economic methodological introduction

Three papers were identified from the literature search. One paper was excluded because it was a review and did not include economic evidence. The other two papers were excluded for methodological reasons.[377–379]

18.1.4 Evidence statements

▷ Tricyclics

Outcomes

Pain related outcomes were measured using either a six-item neuropathy scale,[349,350] or a pain diary.[348]

Mean pain score

Overall, the results indicate that all of the drugs, with the exception of mianserin,[350] produced reduction in pain scores compared to placebo. However, there are no statistically significant differences between the individuals.[348,349,351] **Level 1+**

There was a significant reduction on the observer and the self-rating neuropathy scale in favour of clomipramine ($p<0.05$) and desipramine ($p<0.05$ and $p<0.01$) both compared to placebo ($p<0.05$). There were no statistically significant differences between the two treatments. The median reduction as compared with placebo was on cloimpramine 39% (95% CI 27 to 79%) and desipramine 32% (0 to 46%).[349] **Level 1+**

Desipramine and amitriptyline resulted in an equivalent reduction in mean pain scores and pain intensity. Both treatments were superior to placebo on mean pain score (mean change 0.47 and 0.35 vs 0.15, $p<0.05$ for both) and pain intensity* (–0.48 and –0.48 vs –0.15, $p<0.05$, one-tailed Dunnett's test).[348] **Level 1+**

There was a significant difference in favour of imipramine compared to placebo ($p=0.03$) and compared to mianserin ($p=0.033$) on the observer-rated score but not the self-rated score. There was no significant difference between mianserin and placebo.[350] **Level 1+**

Although both gabapentin and amitriptyline showed significant reductions in pain intensity scores there was no significant difference between the drugs, this was also found for global pain score.[351] **Level 1+**

Both amitriptyline and lamotrigine resulted in improvements in pain relief on several pain measures, although there was no significant difference between the treatments.[352] **Level 1+**

---

* The data has been extracted from a graphical representation of the results.

Adverse events and dropout rates

The total side-effect score was significantly higher for clomimpramine (median 4.0) and desipramine (median 4.5) than during placebo (median 0.02, p< 0.05 for both). There were no statistically significant differences between cloimpramine and desipramine. The most common side effects were dry mouth, sweating, orthostatic dizziness and fatigue. Six patients withdrew from the study all due to side effects (three each during clomimpramine and desipramine).[349] **Level 1+**

The proportion of patients who experienced any side effects associated with amitriptyline, desipramine or placebo treatments was 81%, 76% and 68% respectively. Seven patients withdrew whilst on amitriptyline and seven whilst on desipramine, all due to drug-associated side effects.[348] **Level 1+**

The total adverse effect scores were significantly higher during mianserin (median 2.03, p=0.0093) and imipramine (median 4.00, p=0.0001) than during placebo (median, 0.98) but there were no significant differences between the two active treatments. The most common side effects were dry mouth, orthostatic dizziness and fatigue. One patient withdrew due to side effects whilst taking imipramine.[350] **Level 1+**

With the exception of weight gain with amitriptyline (p<0.03) there was no significant difference in occurrence of adverse events (AEs) between amitriptyline and gabapentin. Adverse effects included sedation, dry mouth, dizziness, postural hypotension, weight gain, ataxia and lethargy. Two patients (one from each group) crossed over early due to AEs and completed the study.[351] **Level 1+**

Amiptriptyline resulted in significantly more AEs overall than lamotrigine (p<0.001), the major side effect being an increase in sleep. More patients discontinued treatment while on amitriptyline (19/46) than while on lamotrigine (8/46).[352] **Level 1+**

▷ Duloxetine

Pain

Pain-related outcomes were measured throughout the papers using recognised and validated tools.

Overall, duloxetine 60 and 120 mg/day (delivered as 60 mg twice daily) were associated with significant reductions in measures of pain (24-hour average pain, brief pain inventory (BPI) and Short-form McGill Pain Questionnaire (SF-MPQ)) when compared with placebo.[358,359,362] Two studies found greater improvements in all pain measures in the duloxetine 120 mg/day arm,[359,362] while the other study found greater improvements in the duloxetine 120 mg daily arm in selected pain measures (BPI interference scores and SF-MPQ).[358] **Level 1++** and **level 1+**

One study found a significantly lower dose of concomitant analgesics (acetaminophen) used in the duloxetine 120 mg daily arm than either the duloxetine 60 mg daily arm (p<0.05) or the placebo arm (p<0.001).[362] **Level 1+**

Table 18.1 Pain related and quality of life measures (mean change (standard error)) for duloxetine 60 mg daily vs duloxetine 120 mg daily (given as 60 mg twice daily)

Measure	Goldstein (2005)[359]	Raskin (2005)[358]	Wernicke (2006)[362]
24-hour average pain	Duloxetine 60 mg vs placebo −1.17 (95% CI −1.84 to −0.50) p≤0.001 Duloxetine 120 mg vs placebo −1.45 (95% CI −2.13 to −0.78) p≤0.001	Duloxetine 60 mg vs placebo −2.50 (0.18) vs −1.60 (0.18) p<0.001 Duloxetine 120 mg vs placebo −2.45 (0.18) vs −1.60 (0.18) p<0.001	Duloxetine 60 mg vs placebo −2.72 (0.22) vs −1.39 (0.23) p<0.001 Duloxetine 120 mg vs placebo −2.84 (0.23) vs −1.39 (0.23) p<0.001
BPI	Duloxetine 60 mg vs placebo −2.81 (0.21) vs −2.40 (0.21) p≤0.01 Duloxetine 120 mg vs placebo −3.07 (0.22) vs −2.40 (0.21) p≤0.001	Duloxetine 60 mg vs placebo −2.65 (0.19) vs −1.82 (0.19) p<0.01 Duloxetine 120 mg vs placebo −2.62 (0.19) vs −1.82 (0.19) p<0.01	Duloxetine 60 mg vs placebo −2.66 (0.23) vs −1.48 (0.23) p<0.001 Duloxetine 120 mg vs placebo −3.05 (0.24) vs −1.48 (0.23) p<0.001
BPI interference	–	Duloxetine 60 mg vs placebo −2.43 (0.18) vs −1.56 (0.18) p<0.001 Duloxetine 120 mg vs placebo −2.54 (0.18) vs −1.56 (0.18) p<0.001	Duloxetine 60 mg vs placebo −2.36 (0.19) vs −1.72 (0.19) p<0.05 Duloxetine 120 mg vs placebo −2.79 (0.19) vs −1.72 (0.19) p<0.001
SF-MPQ	Duloxetine 20 mg vs placebo −8.25 (0.65) vs −5.369 (0.66) p≤0.05 Duloxetine 60 mg vs placebo −8.25 (0.65) vs −5.39 (0.66) p≤0.001 Duloextine 120 mg vs placebo −9.18 (0.64) vs −5.39 (0.66) p≤0.001	Duloxetine 60 mg vs placebo −7.47 (0.61) vs −4.96 (0.60) p<0.01 Duloxetine 120 mg vs placebo −7.82 (0.61) vs −4.96 (0.60) p<0.001	Duloxetine 60 mg vs placebo −7.23 (0.70) vs −4.18 (0.73) p<0.01 Duloxetine 120 mg vs placebo −7.98 (0.71) vs −4.18 (0.73) p<0.001
CGI – severity score	Duloxetine 20 mg vs placebo −1.28 (0.11) vs −0.83 (0.12) p≤0.05 Duloxetine 60 mg vs placebo −1.42(0.12) vs −0.83 (0.12) p≤0.001 Duloxetine 120 mg vs placebo −1.70 (0.012) vs −0.83 (0.12) p≤0.001	Duloxetine 60 mg vs placebo −1.42 (0.09) vs −0.3 (0.09) p<0.001 Duloxetine 120 mg vs placebo −1.40 (0.10) vs −0.3 (0.09) p<0.001	Duloxetine 60 mg vs placebo −1.37 (0.11) vs −0.98 (0.12) p<0.05 Duloxetine 120 mg vs placebo −1.47 (0.12) vs −0.98 (0.12) p<0.01
PGI – improvement score	Duloxetine 60 mg/d vs placebo 2.21 (0.12) vs 2.91(0.12) p≤0.001) Duloxetine 120 mg/d vs placebo 2.24 (0.12) vs 2.91(0.12) p≤0.01	Duloxetine 60 mg vs placebo 2.50 (0.10) vs 3.04 (0.10) p<0.001 Duloxetine 120 mg vs placebo 2.54 (0.10) vs 3.04 (0.10) p<0.001	Duloxetine 60 mg vs placebo 2.61 (1.44) vs 3.17 (1.44) p<0.01 Duloxetine 120 mg vs placebo 2.40 (1.29) vs 3.17 (1.44) p<0.001
SF-36	Duloxetine 60 mg vs placebo Bodily pain 18.00 (1.89) vs 10.32 (1.89) p≤0.01 Mental health 2.99 (1.65) vs −2.63 (1.69); p≤0.05 Duloxetine 120 mg/d vs placebo Mental 1.84 (0.75) vs −1.09 (0.75) p≤0.01 Bodily pain 18.32 (0.88) vs 10.32 (1.89) p≤0.01 General health perceptions 9.56 (1.62) vs 2.03 (1.61) p≤0.001 Mental health 5.14 (1.62) vs −2.63 (1.69) p≤0.001	–	Duloxetine 60 mg vs placebo Physical functioning 11.96 (1.81) vs 3.64 (1.90) p<0.01 Vitality 8.47 (1.73) vs 2.79 (1.78) p<0.05 Physical component score 6.85 (0.76) vs 3.67 (0.78) p<0.01 Duloxetine 120 mg vs placebo Physical functioning 11.20 (1.86) vs 3.64 (1.90) p<0.01 Physical component score 7.46 (0.77) vs 3.67 (0.78) p<0.001 Bodily pain 20.59(2.04) vs 12.17(2.10) p<0.01 General health perceptions 7.73 (1.39) vs 2.39(1.42) p<0.01 Mental health 3.82 (1.49) vs −0.31 (1.52) p<0.05
EQ-5D	Duloxetine 60 mg and 120 mg vs placebo 0.13 (0.02) vs 0.08 (0.02) p≤0.05		Duloxetine 60 mg and 120 mg vs placebo 0.15 (0.02) vs 0.08 (0.02) p<0.05

CGI, clinical global impression; EQ-SD, EuroQol 5-Dimensional outcomes questionnaire; PGI, patient global impression; SF-36, short-form 36

CGI, PGI and quality of life

Overall, duloxetine 60 and 120 mg/day were associated with significant improvements on the CGI and PGI compared with placebo-treated patients.[358,359,362] **Level 1++** and **level 1+**

Two studies reported a significant improvement in favour of duloxetine 60 and 120 mg/day compared to placebo on the SF-36 and EQ-5D.[359,362] **Level 1++** and **level 1+**

One long-term efficacy study reported no significant differences between duloxetine and routine care on the SF-36 or EQ-5D.[357] The other study found significant differences between duloxetine and routine care arms in SF-36 bodily pain (p=0.021) and in the EQ-5D (p=0.001).[363] **Level 1+**

A 28-week open-label study comparing duloxetine 60 mg twice daily with 120 mg once daily found that both treatment groups showed improvement from baseline to endpoint on all subscales of the BPI and clinical global impression of change score (CGIC-S) (p<0.001 for both). (Results taken from graph.)[361] **Level 1+**

Adverse events

Three studies reported higher treatment-related AEs and discontinuation rate due to AEs, in duloxetine dose treatment arms compared with placebo or routine care.[358,359,362] Two studies reported higher AEs in the routine care or placebo arms, which was significant in one of the studies,[357] although both these studies also reported higher discontinuation due to AEs in the duloxetine arm.[357,363] **Level 1++** and **level 1+**

Three studies reported significant differences in treatment-emergent AEs in duloxetine groups compared with placebo.[358,359,362] In these studies the following treatment-emergent AEs were reported to occur significantly more in one or both duloxetine groups (60 mg daily or 60 mg twice daily); nausea, somnolence, increased sweating, dizziness, constipation, fatigue, insomnia, vomiting, dry mouth, anorexia and decreased appetite. Most AEs were mild or moderate. **Level 1++** and **level 1+**

In three studies, including the two studies with 52 weeks of follow-up,[357,363] there were no treatment related AEs that were reported to occur significantly more in the duloxetine group than in routine care groups. Most AEs were moderate or mild. **Level 1++** and **level 1+**

▷ Gabapentin

Outcomes

Pain-related outcomes were measured throughout the papers using recognised and validated tools.

Mean pain score

Both placebo-based studies found significant decreases in pain score with gabapentin compared with placebo; −1.2 (−1.9 to −0.6), p<0.001[366] and −2 vs −0.5, p<0.01.[367]

For the titration to clinical effect doses (range from 900–3600 mg/day) gabapentin showed significantly greater reductions in final mean pain scores than the fixed dose of 900 mg/day, 53.6% vs 43.3%, p=0.009.[364]

Although both gabapentin and amitriptyline showed significant reductions in pain intensity scores there was no significant difference between the drugs, this was also found for global pain score.[351] **Level 1+**

Short-form McGill pain questionnaire

There was a significant decrease in total SF-MPQ scores for gabapentin compared with placebo, −5.9 (−8.8 to −3.1), p<0.001 which was also noted in the VAS, −16.9 (−25.3 to −8.4), p<0.001 and the present pain intensity score (PPI), −0.6 (−0.9 to −0.3), p<0.001.[366] This significant difference between gabapentin and placebo for the total SF-MPQ was also noted in the other placebo-based study, though further detail was not reported.[367]

The titration to clinical effect group showed a significant decrease in the short-form McGill Pain Questionnaire visual analogue scale (SF-MPQ VAS) compared with fixed dose (p<0.001) but was not significant in the total or PPI scores.[364] **Level 1+**

Sleep interference

There was a significant decrease in sleep interference, at endpoint, compared with placebo for gabapentin, −1.47 (−2.2 to −0.8), p<0.001.[366] Changes in sleep interference also showed significant improvement in the gabapentin-treated group against placebo, further details were not reported.[367]

The titration to clinical effect study showed significant improvements in sleep interference compared with the fixed dose group (57% vs 37.2%, p=0.013).[364] **Level 1+**

Short-form 36

The gabapentin compared with placebo studies showed significant increases (denotes improvement) in SF-36 results for; bodily pain 7.8 (1.8–13.8), p=0.01; mental health 5.4 (0.5–10.3), p=0.03 and vitality 9.7 (3.9–5.5), p=0.001.[366] Again, Simpson DA[367] stated there had been significant differences without further details.

There was no significant differences found in the SF-36 results for the titration to clinical effect compared with fixed-dose study.[364] **Level 1+**

PGIC and CGIC

Gabapentin compared with placebo showed significant improvements in pain for both the patient perception score and the clinician perception score (p=0.001).[366] Differences were also identified for PGIC and CGIC in the other placebo-based study with 55.5% in the much/moderately improved category for gabapentin compared with 25.9% for placebo. Significance not reported.[367]

The titration to clinical effect group identified a significant improvement in the clinician assessed score CGIC compared with the fixed dose, p=0.02. However, there was no significant difference found between the two groups in the PGIC.[364] **Level 1+**

Adverse events and dropout rates

There were a significantly higher number of AEs of dizziness and somnolence experienced by those in the gabapentin group than with placebo.[366]

The titration to clinical effect group showed higher occurrences of somnolence (20.1% vs 15.3%) and dizziness (16.6% vs 13.5%) than those in the fixed-dose group.[364]

For gabapentin compared with amitriptyline there was no significant difference in the occurrence of the main AEs, such as sedation, dry mouth and dizziness.

▷ Pregabalin

Outcomes

Pain-related outcomes were measured throughout the papers using recognised and validated tools.

Mean pain score (recorded via pain diaries)

Pregabalin was significantly effective in reducing the mean pain score at the 300 mg/day and 600 mg/day doses compared with placebo, this effect was seen from the end of the first week of treatment and throughout the studies, this was identified in all three studies.[368–370] **Level 1++**

For those studies which included lower doses, 75 mg/day[368] and 150 mg/day,[369] there was no significant decrease in mean pain score found. **Level 1++**

Short-form McGill pain questionnaire

Significant decreases were identified with pregabalin 300 and 600 mg/day, compared with placebo but not with the lower doses (see table 18.2). **Level 1++**

Table 18.2 Pregablin 300 and 600 mg/day compared to placebo				
	Study	**Total**	**VAS**	**PPI**
Pregabalin 75 mg/day	Lesser (2004)[368]	NS	NS	NS
Pregabalin 150 mg/day	Richter (2005)[369]	NS	NS	NS
Pregabalin 300 mg/day	Lesser (2004)[368]	−4.89 (−7.29 to −2.48) p=0.0001	−16.09 (−23.11 to −9.08) p=0.0001	−1.59 (−0.88 to −0.30) p=0.0001
	Rosenstock (2004)[370]	−4.41 (−732 to −1.49) p=0.033	−16.19 (−24.52 to −7.86) p=0.0002	−0.37 (−0.72 to −0.02) p=0.0364
Pregabalin 600 mg/day	Lesser (2004)[368]	−5.18 (−7.58 to −2.79) p=0.0001	−19.01 (−26.00 to −12.01) p=0.0001	−0.61 (−0.90 to −0.32) p=0.0001
	Richter (2005)[369]	−5.83 (−8.43 to −3.23) p=0.002	−14.67 (−21.92 to −7.41) p=0.0002	−0.66 (−0.97 to −0.35) p=0.0002

Sleep interference

There was a significant reduction in sleep interference at the 300 mg/day and 600 mg/day doses compared with placebo; p=0.001 for both,[368] 600 mg/day –1.152 (–1.752 to –0.551), p=0.0004[369] and p<0.0001, 300 mg/day.[370] Again there was no significant reduction in sleep interference for the 75 and 150 mg/day groups.[368,369] **Level 1++**

Short-form 36

This efficacy parameter was used in two of the papers and identified that there were significant improvements in the vitality domain for the 75 mg/day (p<0.02) and 300 mg/day (p<0.01) compared with placebo, while in the social functioning and bodily pain domains there were significant improvements in the 300 mg/day (p<0.05 and p=0.005) and 600 mg/day (p<0.01 and p<0.0005) groups.[368] For 300 mg/day compared with placebo,[370] improvements were identified in the bodily pain domain, 6.87 (0.70 to 13.04, p=0.0294). No significant changes were found in the other domains. **Level 1++**

Patient global impression of change

There were significant improvements in the patient perception for 300 mg/day and 600 mg/day, compared with placebo:
- 300 mg/day (p=0.001, both studies)[368,370]
- 600 mg/day (p=0.001,[368] p=0.002).[370]

Level 1++

Clinical global impression of change

Results showed that clinician perceptions echoed those of the patients:
- 300 mg/day (p=0.001 both studies)[368,370]
- 600 mg/day (p=0.001,[368] p=0.004).[370]

Level 1++

Adverse events and dropout rates

There were no major differences in the AE and dropout rates between the drug dosages than placebo. AEs did occur more frequently in the treatment groups, with the most common being dizziness and somnolence.

▷ Carbamazepine

One RCT[372] reported a significant relief of pain in patients treated with carbamazepine compared to those receiving placebo (p<0.05). No significant differences were found in terms of ability to sleep and reduction of numbness when the two groups were compared. Another RCT[371] showed that carbamazepine users experienced greater relief of pain compared to placebo-treated patients. However, no statistical analysis was performed. **Level 1+**

The study comparing carbamazepine monotherapy with the combination of nortriptyline–fluphenazine[373] showed that both interventions produced significant reductions of pain and paraesthesia. However, the study did not find a significant difference between the two interventions. **Level 1+**

▷ Oxcarbazepine

One RCT[375] with a sample size of 146 reported that patients treated with oxcarbazepine experienced a significantly larger decrease from baseline in average VAS-pain scores compared with placebo (p=0.0108). The study also found a significantly greater number of oxcarbazepine-treated patients reporting some improvement from baseline on the patient's global assessment of therapeutic effect, compared to those receiving placebo (p=0.0003). No significant differences were found in terms of quality of life. **Level 1+**

In contrast, the other RCT[374] with a sample size of 347, did not find any significant difference between oxcarbazepine (600 mg, 1,200 mg and 1,800 mg) and placebo in terms of pain (VAS scale), assessment of therapeutic efficacy and quality of life. **Level 1+**

All five studies[371–375] demonstrated a higher incidence of AEs reported by patients receiving the active intervention (carbamazepine or oxcarbazepine) compared to placebo. The most common AEs reported were dizziness, headache and somnolence. No statistical analyses were performed. **Level 1+**

18.1.5 From evidence to recommendations

The evidence reported suggested that tricyclic drugs, duloxetine, gabapentin, and pregabalin, were all effective in at least some people with neuropathic pain of diabetes origin. The evidence included very few comparative studies, and what there was suggested no advantage for the newer drugs over the tricyclics. Clinical experience confirmed both the limited efficacy of all of the drugs in some people, but also that failure with tricyclics did not often predict failure with other drugs. In these circumstances, and given that side effects were a common problem with all drugs, the GDG felt that first-line specific therapy should be with a tricyclic drug on cost grounds, but that lack of necessary efficacy or problematic side effects should then lead onto a trial of a new drug, with a trial of a third drug if side effects again intervened. The GDG felt that carbamazepine should not be offered to patients due to the drug interactions and intolerance. It was noted that these drug interactions make it difficult for prescribers to monitor patients safely.

It was noted that for milder problems simple analgesia was sometimes all that is needed, and that local measures including contact materials or relief from beddings were sometimes helpful. Specific topical creams were not formally appraised, but it was noted these had not entered widespread use.

A more holistic approach was often needed at discovery of the problem in helping people to understand it, where secondary psychological problems occurred, and when onward referral was needed to specialist pain teams for lack of response to conventional measures.

RECOMMENDATIONS

For the management of foot problems relating to Type 2 diabetes, follow recommendations in 'Type 2 diabetes: prevention and management of foot problems'.[380]

R113   Make a formal enquiry annually about the development of neuropathic symptoms causing distress.

- Discuss the cause and prognosis (including possible medium-term remission) of troublesome neuropathic symptoms, if present (bearing in mind alternative diagnoses).
- Agree appropriate therapeutic options and review understanding at each clinical contact.

R114   Be alert to the psychological consequences of chronic painful diabetic neuropathy and offer psychological support according to the needs of the individual.

R115   Use a tricyclic drug to treat neuropathic discomfort (start with low doses, titrated as tolerated) if standard analgesic measures have not worked, timing the medication to be taken before the time of day when the symptoms are troublesome; advise that this is a trial of therapy.

R116   Offer a trial of duloxetine, gabapentin or pregabalin if a trial of tricyclic drug does not provide effective pain relief. The choice of drug should be determined by current drug prices. Trials of these therapies should be stopped if the maximally tolerated drug dose is ineffective. If side effects limit effective dose titration, try another one of the drugs.

R117   Consider a trial of opiate analgesia if severe chronic pain persists despite trials of other measures. If there is inadequate relief of the pain associated with diabetic neuropathic symptoms, seek the assistance of the local chronic pain management service following a discussion with the person concerned.

R118   If drug management of diabetic neuropathic pain has been successful, consider reducing the dose and stopping therapy following discussion and agreement with the individual.

R119   If neuropathic symptoms cannot be controlled adequately, it may be helpful to further discuss:

- the reasons for the problem
- the likelihood of remission in the medium term
- the role of improved blood glucose control.

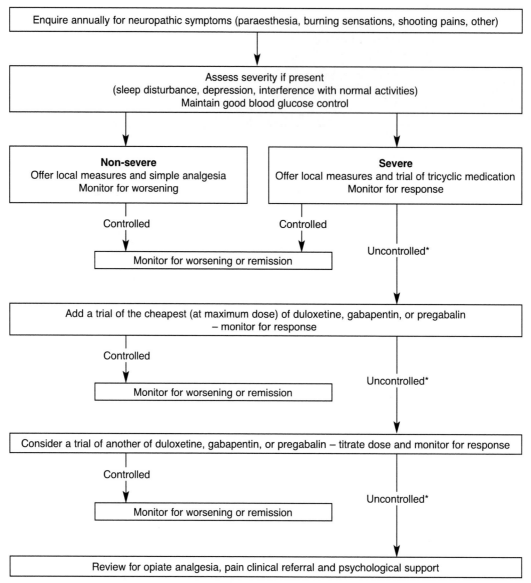

Figure 18.1 Diabetic symptomatic neuropathy management – a therapeutic summary
*Where neuropathic symptoms cannot be adequately controlled it is useful, to help individuals cope, to explain the reasons for the problem, the likelihood of remission in the medium term, the role of improved blood glucose control

18.2 Autonomic neuropathy

18.2.1 Clinical introduction

There are many manifestations of autonomic neuropathy as a complication of long-term hyperglycaemia. These include gastroparesis, diarrhoea, faecal incontinence, erectile dysfunction, bladder disturbance, orthostatic hypotension, gustatory and other sweating disorders, dry feet, and unexplained ankle oedema.

It was identified that two aspects of autonomic neuropathy, erectile dysfunction and gastroparesis, raised significant therapeutic issues; these were subject to formal evidence review. For other aspects only opinion-based recommendations were presented in the NICE Type 1 diabetes guideline,[26] and these were reviewed by the GDG.

18.3 Gastroparesis

18.3.1 Clinical introduction

Gastroparesis can be one of the more devastating complications of autonomic neuropathy. While it can present as bloating, nausea and fullness on eating, severe intermittent hypoglycaemia can be a major problem for people on glucose-lowering therapy, while vomiting may be intermittent and sudden or occasionally severe and protracted.

The clinical questions addressed include in whom to suspect gastroparesis might be present, what medications might help, and what other measures might be taken.

18.3.2 Methodological introduction

Eight studies were identified in this area all of which involved domperidone, metoclopramide or erythromycin. Two studies were excluded for methodological reasons.[381,382]

The remaining six studies comprised four RCTs of the drug against placebo; erythromycin vs placebo,[383] metoclopramide vs placebo,[384,385] domperidone vs placebo,[386] and two direct drug RCT comparisons; metoclopramide vs erythromycin,[387] and domperidone vs metoclopramide.[388]

There were methodological quality issues with these studies, which often involved small numbers of participants with a range of demographic and clinical details. Furthermore, although symptom scores were used as measures in three studies,[384,385,388] these were not based on a recognised or validated scale and were not consistent in the measures they recorded or in the scoring system allotted to the measures. The remaining three studies used the SF-36 health-related quality of life tool,[386] gastric emptying using a γ-camera[387] and scintigraphic studies.[383]

18.3.3 Health economic methodological introduction

No health economic papers were identified.

18.3.4 Evidence statements

▷ Drug vs placebo

Erythromycin

One crossover study with 10 participants with diabetes and known prolonged gastric emptying were given 200 mg of IV erythromycin or IV placebo.[383] Ten age and sex matched health participants were also used as a comparator group. This study used scintigraphic studies and found that for 60 and 120 minutes IV erythromycin significantly increased gastric emptying, (measured as the mean percentage simultaneously ingested food retained in the stomach, for solids), compared with placebo (21 ± 5 vs 85 ± 7, $p<0.0005$ and 4 ± 1 vs 63 ± 9, $p<0.0005$ respectively).

For liquids the mean percentage retained was significantly lower for the IV erythromycin compared with placebo again at both 60 and 120 minutes (22 ± 5 vs 54 ± 5, $p<0.0005$ and 9 ± 3 vs 32 ± 4, $p<0.005$ respectively).

IV erythromycin was also found to have increased gastric emptying for solids at 60 minutes when compared with healthy subjects in the comparator group ($p < 0.05$).

There were no AEs found with this study, this study had a further open-label phase with oral erythromycin, not reported here. **Level 1+**

Metoclopramide

Two studies,[384,385] one of which was a crossover study,[384] were identified comparing oral metoclopramide 10 mg QID and placebo, both studies used the diary recording of symptoms and though the scales used were broadly similar they were not identical, there were no major AEs identified in either study.*

One study identified that the mean symptom scores for the 3-week treatment phase was significantly less for metoclopramide than for placebo; 26.5 ± 3.7 vs 45.3 ± 7.8, $p < 0.01$. This study also found that the mean individual scores for 4/5 symptoms (fullness, pressure and bloating, nausea, vomiting, anorexia) showed that metoclopramide significantly reduced the symptoms compared with placebo ($p < 0.05$).[385]

The crossover study found that symptom improvement was significantly greater for metoclopramide than placebo for nausea at weeks 1 and 3 ($p < 0.05$). This was also found for fullness at weeks 2 and 3 ($p < 0.05$). Changes found for other symptoms were not significantly improved for metoclopramide compared with placebo.[384] **Level 1+**

Domperidone

One study[386] considered domperidone vs placebo, this study combined a 4-week period where participants took 20 mg domperidone QID (single-blind phase) orally, followed by a 4-week period of 20 mg domperidone QID or placebo (double-blind phase). Entry into the second phase was dependent on a decrease on the baseline symptom score, those classed as responders, following completion of the single-blind phase.

Single-blind phase: significant symptomatic improvement was found at the end of the single-blind phase ($p < 0.0001$). Improvements were also noted in the health-related quality of life measured on the SF-36 scale (all domains $p < 0.001$, except physical functioning, $p < 0.01$).

Double-blind phase: symptom severity increased with both domperidone and placebo, though they did not return to baseline levels, this increase in severity was greater for placebo compared with domperidone ($p < 0.05$). AEs were not reported. **Level 1+**

▷ Head-to-head comparisons

Metoclopramide vs erythromycin

One crossover study with 13 participants considered erythromycin 250 mg TID with metoclopramide 10 mg TID.

---

* The crossover study[384] also included an IM metoclopramide injection prior to the double-blind phase and the option to enter an open-label phase at the end of the double-blind; neither of these is reported here.

Gastric empting was considered at 60 and 90 minutes and while significant improvements were found for both drugs there was no significant difference found between the effects between erythromycin and metoclopramide.

The symptom score was significantly less for erythromycin; 2(0–5), than for metoclopramide; 3(0–11), p<0.05.

No serious AEs were noted, though N=2 of the patients did have weakness, sedation and leg cramps with metoclopramide. **Level 1+**

Domperidone vs metoclopramide

One study with 95 participants considered domperidone 20 mg QID with metoclopramide 10 mg QID. Gastroparetic symptoms and tolerability were assessed, it should be noted for tolerability assessment participants were specifically asked about central nervous system (CNS) associated side effects; these have previously been identified in association with metoclopramide.

Although significant reductions in symptoms were found with both domperidone and metoclopramide, there was no significant difference found between the two treatments.

For tolerability, at week 2 the severity of somnolence (p<0.001), akathisia (p=0.03), anxiety (p=0.02) and depression (p=0.05) were significantly greater for metoclopramide than for domperidone (p<0.001-0.05). While at week 4 this was found for severity of somnolence (p=0.03) and reduced mental acuity (p=0.04). **Level 1+**

18.3.5 From evidence to recommendations

The evidence reported had methodological limitations, notably studies of small sample sizes. The GDG agreed that there is a poor evidence base for the treatment of gastroparesis. Nevertheless they noted that the evidence reported suggested that the prokinetic drugs, metoclopramide, domperidone, along with erythromycin, were all effective in at least some people with gastroparesis resulting from autonomic neuropathy. On consideration of the evidence it was not possible to distinguish usefully between the prokinetic drugs. The group agreed that choice of initial therapy should be based on tolerability issues, including drug interactions. It was noted that differential diagnosis can be difficult, and the diagnostic tests not secure, while serious prolonged vomiting could become a medical emergency. Accordingly referral beyond diabetes services is sometimes indicated.

While the group gave priority to medication for the management of this condition, clinical experience suggested that non-pharmacological approaches including postural advice and timing of ingestion of fluids and solids could prove useful to some people.

RECOMMENDATIONS

R120   Consider the diagnosis of gastroparesis in an adult with erratic blood glucose control or unexplained gastric bloating or vomiting, taking into consideration possible alternative diagnoses.

R121   Consider a trial of metoclopramide, domperidone, or erythromycin for an adult with gastroparesis.

R122   If gastroparesis is suspected, consider referral to specialist services if:
- the differential diagnosis is in doubt, or
- persistent or severe vomiting occurs.

18.4 Erectile dysfunction

18.4.1 Clinical introduction

Erectile dysfunction in men with diabetes is common, and to a greater extent than in the matched general population.[389] There have been dramatic changes in the approach to male erectile dysfunction in recent years, stimulated by the advent of the phosphodiesterase type 5 (PDE-5) inhibitors.

This review deals only with care that would routinely be provided within diabetes services, and not with that normally provided by other specialist services. The clinical questions thus related to the effectiveness and relative effectiveness of the PDE-5 inhibitor drugs in people with Type 2 diabetes.

18.4.2 Methodological introduction

Eleven studies were identified in this area all of which involved the PDE-5 inhibitors licensed for the treatment of erectile dysfunction (sildenafil, tadalafil or vardenafil). One study was excluded for methodological reasons.[390]

One meta-analysis (Vardi) reviewed the effect of the PDE-5 inhibitors as a group for the management of erectile dysfunction in diabetic men. This paper included several of the studies that have also been evaluated individually (Bolton 2001, Escobar-Jimenez 2002, Goldstein 2003, Price 1998, Rendell 1999, Saenz de Tejada 2002, Saferinejad 2004, Stuckey 2003). Eight of the remaining nine RCTs were studies conducted in diabetic populations (Type 1 and Type 2) comparing a PDE-5 inhibitor versus placebo and with a follow-up of at least 12 weeks.[391–398] An additional post hoc sub-analysis was also identified.[399] This study evaluated the efficacy and safety of tadalafil 20 mg taken on demand or three times per week and its effect on the sexual activity in a subpopulation of patients with diabetes mellitus and erectile dysfunction.

It should be noted that this topic (i.e. erectile dysfunction) was not covered in detail by the previous guideline thus the studies were searched for from 1965. Nevertheless, all the studies identified were published after 1999.*

The efficacy of the placebo and PDE-5 inhibitors was assessed using responses to the questions from the self-administered International Index of Erectile Function (IIEF), a 15-question, validated measure of erectile dysfunction. The index has five separate response domains; erectile function, orgasmic function, sexual desire, intercourse satisfaction, and overall satisfaction.

Each patient also responded to a global efficacy question ('did the treatment improve your erections?') and maintained an event log, in which was recorded the date of the medication taken, the presence of sexual stimulation, the hardness of erection on a 4-point scale, the

---

* The first PDE-5 inhibitor (sildenafil) was licensed in 1998 by the Food and Drug Administration.

number of attempts at sexual intercourse, and the number of attempts that were successful. Some studies also used the Sexual Encounter Profile (SEP) questions 2 and 3. This is a diary maintained by men after each sexual attempt consisting of a series of yes/no questions regarding overall responses concerning 'success in penetration' (SEP-Q2), 'success in maintaining erection during intercourse' (SEP-Q3).

▷ Meta-analysis

Efficacy

Based on data from five studies (Boulton 2001, Escobar-Jimenez 2002, Rendell 1999, Safarinejad 2004, Stuckey 2003), there was a significant difference in mean scores for question 3 and question 4 of the IIEF in favour of the PDE-5 inhibitors as a group. **Level 1++**

Based on data from seven studies (Boulton 2001, Escobar-Jimenez 2002, Goldstein 2003, Rendell 1999, Saenz de Tejada 2002, Safarinejad 2004, Stuckey 2003) there was a significant improvement in the IIEF erectile function domain in the PDE-5 inhibitor treated group. **Level 1++**

There was a significantly higher risk of a positive response to the global efficacy question (GEQ) ('has treatment improved your erections') in patients treated with PDE-5 inhibitors compared to those receiving placebo. However, there was significant heterogeneity found between studies. **Level 1++**

Based on data from four studies (Boulton 2001, Goldstein 2003, Saenz de Tejada 2002, Stuckey 2003) patients treated with PDE-5 inhibitors reported a higher mean percentage increase in successful intercourse attempts per participant. **Level 1++**

Two studies assessing the effects of sildenafil reported quality of life measures and in the meta-analysis showed significantly improved scores for sexual life. There were no statistically significant results in any other quality of life domains. **Level 1++**

Adverse events

No studies reported on mortality. One study reported on cardiovascular morbidity (Safarinejad 2004) which is detailed further under the sildenafil AEs section. In the meta-analysis the overall risk ratio for developing any AE was 4.8 (95% CI 3.74 to 6.16) in the PDE-5 inhibitors arm compared to control.

Sildenafil

There were four studies looking at sildenafil, three of them had a follow-up of 12 weeks and compared 50 mg of sildenafil with placebo.[391,392,395,396] The remaining study[396] had a follow-up of 16 weeks and compared sildenafil 100 mg with placebo.

Across the four sildenafil-studies, the primary efficacy assessment consisted of responses to question three (Q3; achieving an erection) and question four (Q4; maintaining an erection) from the IIEF. The secondary efficacy assessments included: an event log of erectile function, a global efficacy question asked at the end of the study and other IIEF domains.

18.4.3 Health economic methodological introduction

No health economic papers were identified.

18.4.4 Evidence statements

▷ Efficacy

All four RCTs[391,392,395,396] reported that improvements in mean scores from baseline to end of treatment for IIEF Q3 and Q4 were significantly greater in patients receiving sildenafil compared with those receiving placebo. **Level 1+**

Similarly, the four RCTs showed a significantly higher proportion of men reporting successful attempts at sexual intercourse in the sildenafil group compared to placebo-treated patients. **Level 1+**

Three RCTs[391,392,396] reported a significantly higher number of positive responses to the GEQ ('has treatment improved your erections') in patients treated with sildenafil compared to those receiving placebo. **Level 1+**

Finally, two RCTs[391,396] concluded that sildenafil significantly improved erectile function across all the efficacy variables regardless of patient age, the duration of ED, and the duration of diabetes. **Level 1++**

The other two RCTs concluded that when efficacy was analysed for patients with different HbA$_{1c}$ baseline levels ($<8\%$ or $\geq 8\%$)[395] ($\leq 8.3\%$ of $>8.3\%$)[392] no significant differences were found in end-of-treatment score for any of the efficacy parameters. **Level 1+**

▷ Adverse events

The most common treatment-related AEs across the four RCTs included headache, flushing, dyspepsia and respiratory tract disorders. The incidence of these AEs was higher in patients receiving sildenafil.

Only one RCT[396] performed a statistical analysis for AEs and reported a significantly higher incidence in sildenafil-treated patients in comparison with the placebo group ($p<0.001$). The same RCT showed that the incidence of cardiovascular events were significantly much higher ($p<0.001$) in the patients taking sildenafil compared with patients taking placebo.* **Level 1++**

Vardenafil

There were three RCTs comparing vardenafil with placebo in patients with diabetes. Two RCTs were three-arm studies in which patients were randomised to receive vardenafil 10 mg, 20 mg or placebo.[394,397] The other RCT[398] compared placebo with a flexible-dose (5–20 mg) of vardenafil. All the three studies had a follow-up of 12 weeks.

---

* The overall incidence of cardiovascular adverse effects other than flushing occurred in 7% of patients taking sildenafil vs 0% of patients taking placebo. In the sildenafil group, four patients had new chest pain of whom two manifested an ST elevation >3 mm with documented MI. Other cardiovascular events in the sildenafil group were two congestive heart failures and four hypertensions.

Across the three vardenafil-studies the measures of efficacy were the erectile function domain of the validated IIEF questionnaire (the sum of question 1–5 plus question 15), overall responses on the patient's diary concerning 'success in penetration' (SEP-Q2), 'success in maintaining erection during intercourse' (SEP-Q3) and other IIEF domain scores.

▷ Efficacy

All RCTs[394,397,398] reported that patients receiving vardenafil significantly improved the erectile function domain (IIEF questionnaire) score compared with those treated with placebo (p<0.0001). **Level 1+**

One RCT[394] also showed a significant greater improvement in the erectile function domain score (IIEF questionnaire) in patients receiving 20 mg of vardenafil compared with those receiving 10 mg (p=0.03). The same RCT reported a significantly higher number of positive responses to the GEQ ('has treatment improved your erections') in patients treated with vardenafil compared to those receiving placebo (p<0.0001). Again, the response rate at 20 mg was also significantly higher than at 10 mg (p≤0.02). **Level 1++**

All RCTs found that the rate of successful insertion (SEP-Q2) with vardenafil was significantly increased at all time points compared with placebo (p<0.0001). In addition, the mean rate of maintained erections allowing successful intercourse (SEP-Q3) was also significantly increased compared with placebo-treated patients (p<0.0001). **Level 1+**

One RCT[397] found a significantly higher percentage of positive answers to the questions SEP2 and SEP3 in the group of patients receiving 20 mg of vardenafil compared with the 10 mg group (p<0.005). **Level 1+**

Finally, two RCTs reported that the improvement in erectile function with vardenafil was not affected by the level of glycaemic control.[394,398] **Level 1+**

▷ Adverse events

The most common treatment-related AEs across the three RCTs were headache and flushing. The incidence of these AEs was higher in patients receiving vardenafil compared to those receiving placebo. No statistical analysis was performed

Tadalafil

There were two RCTs identified for tadalafil.[393,399] One study[393] with a follow-up of 12 weeks, compared tadalafil (10–20 mg) with placebo. The other study,[399] was a post hoc sub-analysis which identified 762 patients with Type 1 and Type 2 diabetes from the SURE* cohort. The sub-analysis reported data on the efficacy and safety of tadalafil 20 mg taken on demand or three times per week in this diabetic subpopulation.

---

* The scheduled use vs on demand regimen evaluation (SURE) was a randomised, crossover, open-label study with 4,262 patients in 14 European countries at 392 sites. Briefly the study population included male patients ≥18 years of age who had at least a 3-month history of erectile dysfunction of any severity (mild, moderate, or severe) or aetiology (psychogenic, organic, or mixed).

▷ Efficacy

Tadalafil 10–20 mg vs placebo

The RCT,[393] reported that treatment with tadalafil (particularly at 20 mg) significantly enhanced erectile function across all efficacy outcomes variables: IIEF erectile function domain, erection vaginal penetration rates (SEP-Q2), successful intercourse rates (SEP-Q3) and global assessment question (all $p<0.001$). **Level 1+**

Finally, the RCT also reported that treatment with tadalafil at 10 and 20 mg improved efficacy outcomes regardless of baseline HbA_{1c}, type of diabetes or type of diabetes treatment. **Level 1+**

Tadalafil 20 mg. On-demand regimen vs three times per week regimen

The subpopulation analysis[399] reported a slightly higher IIEF score in patients on the three times per week regimen compared to those taking tadalafil on demand. However, no statistical analysis was reported. Furthermore, the sub-analysis showed significantly higher results for the SEP (SEP Q1 to Q5) in favour of the three times per week over the on-demand regimen ($p<0.05$ for SEP 1–5). **Level 1+**

This study also reported a significant difference in terms of treatment preference. 57.2% of diabetic patients preferred the on-demand regimen and 42.8% of patients preferred the three times per week treatment ($p<0.001$). The result was similar to the overall treatment preference in the SURE study. **Level 1+**

▷ Adverse events

Both studies[393,399] reported that the most common treatment-emergent events in the tadalafil groups were dyspepsia, back pain and flushing. **Level 1+**

Only the incidence of dyspepsia was significantly different across treatment groups in the placebo-controlled study.[393] Approximately 1% in either the 10 or 20 mg group, compared with 0% in the placebo arm ($p=0.005$). **Level 1+**

18.4.5 From evidence to recommendations

The group noted that erectile dysfunction is a traumatic complication for some men with Type 2 diabetes. They noted that it is sometimes not adequately discussed and that the issue of erectile dysfunction should be explored regularly where appropriate, with explanation that it can be a complication of the diabetes, and might be amenable to treatment. Professionals needed to be alert to secondary issues such as relationship breakdown.

There were no studies of head-to-head comparisons of PDE-5 inhibitors. All studies included were against placebo. The evidence appeared to suggest that the PDE-5 inhibitors, sildenafil, vardenafil, and tadalafil, were all effective in the treatment of erectile dysfunction in people with Type 2 diabetes. The evidence was not found sufficient to distinguish between the PDE-5 inhibitors. There was no evidence on the use of second-line PDE-5 inhibitor therapies if the initial drug had proved ineffective.

Other medical and surgical treatment options should be discussed if PDE-5 inhibitors prove ineffective, and onward referral made if appropriate.

Concern was expressed at cardiovascular safety issues associated with the use of these drugs, even after careful exclusion of nitrate therapy.

RECOMMENDATIONS

R123   Review the issue of erectile dysfunction with men annually.

R124   Provide assessment and education for men with erectile dysfunction to address contributory factors and treatment options.

R125   Offer a phosphodiesterase-5 inhibitor (choosing the drug with the lowest acquisition cost), in the absence of contraindications, if erectile dysfunction is a problem.

R126   Following discussion, refer to a service offering other medical, surgical, or psychological management of erectile dysfunction if phosphodiesterase-5 inhibitors have been unsuccessful.

18.5 Other aspects of autonomic neuropathy

18.5.1 Clinical introduction

Other aspects of autonomic neuropathy, including diarrhoea, faecal incontinence, bladder disturbance, orthostatic hypotension, gustatory and other sweating disorders, dry feet, and unexplained ankle oedema, can offer diagnostic and management problems, and on occasion be very disabling.

Alternatively symptoms may be vague and may present insidiously without realisation that they are diabetes-related, while nerve damage can be also be found in asymptomatic people. A mixed presentation is common, may be exacerbated by other drug therapy (e.g. tricyclic drugs), and may give troublesome hypoglycaemia. People with advanced autonomic neuropathy may also have advanced retinopathy, nephropathy, and somatic neuropathy.

18.5.2 From evidence to recommendations

The GDG reviewed the opinion-based recommendations made in the NICE Type 1 diabetes guideline.[26] They were found for the most part appropriate, and are reproduced with some editorial change only. It was recognised that these recommendations are for the most part identification and diagnostic issues, and that specialist management where required would often lie outside diabetes services.

RECOMMENDATIONS

R127   Consider the possibility of contributory sympathetic nervous system damage for a person who loses the warning signs of hypoglycaemia.

R128   Consider the possibility of autonomic neuropathy affecting the gut in an adult with unexplained diarrhoea, particularly at night.

R129   When using tricyclic drugs and antihypertensive medications in people with autonomic neuropathy, be aware of the increased likelihood of side effects such as orthostatic hypotension.

R130   Investigate a person with unexplained bladder-emptying problems for the possibility of autonomic neuropathy affecting the bladder.

R131   Include in the management of autonomic neuropathy symptoms the specific interventions indicated by the manifestations (for example, for abnormal sweating or nocturnal diarrhoea).

19 | Areas for future research

Metformin: confirmatory studies of the advantage in terms of cardiovascular outcome studies.

Studies of the role of sulfonylureas when starting a pre-mix.

Longer term studies of the role of self-monitoring as part of an integrated package with patient education and therapies used to target.

The use of ACEI and A2RBS in combination in early diabetic nephropathy.

Comparison studies on tricyclics, duloxetine, gabapentin, and pregabalin.

References

1 National Institute for Health and Clinical Excellence. *Guidelines manual.* London: NICE, 2006.

2 International Diabetes Federation. *Definition and diagnosis of diabetes mellitus and immediate hyperglycemia: report of a WHO/IDF consultation.* Geneva: World Health Organisation, 2006.

3 Department of Health. *Health survey for England 2004.* London: DH, 2005.

4 International Diabetes Federation. *Diabetes atlas.* Brussels: IDF, 2006.

5 Morgan CL, Currie CJ, Peters JR. Relationship between diabetes and mortality: a population study using record linkage. *Diabetes Care* 2000;23(8):1103–1107.

6 Anon. *British National Formulary for Children* (3). UK: BMJ Publishing Group Ltd and RPS Publishing, 2007. http://bnfc.org/bnfc

7 National Collaborating Centre for Chronic Conditions. *Type 2 diabetes: methodology pack.* London: NCC-CC, 2006.

8 Healthcare Commission. *Managing diabetes: improving services for people with diabetes.* London: Commission for Healthcare Audit and Inspection, 2007.

9 Christensen NK, Williams P, Pfister R. Cost savings and clinical effectiveness of an extension service diabetes program. *Diabetes Spectrum* 2004;17(3):171–175.

10 Mortimer D, Kelly J. Economic evaluation of the good life club intervention for diabetes self-management. *Australian Journal of Primary Health* 2006;12(1):91–100.

11 Connor H, Annan F, Bunn E et al. The implementation of nutritional advice for people with diabetes. *Diabetic Medicine* 2003;20(10):786–807.

12 National Institute for Health and Clinical Excellence. *Obesity: the prevention, identification, assessment and management of overweight and obesity in adults and children* (CG43). London: NICE, 2006.

13 Li Z, Hong K, Saltsman P et al. Long-term efficacy of soy-based meal replacements vs an individualized diet plan in obese type II DM patients: Relative effects on weight loss, metabolic parameters, and C-reactive protein. *European Journal of Clinical Nutrition* 2005;59(3):411–418.

14 Barnard ND, Cohen J, Jenkins DJA et al. A low-fat vegan diet improves glycemic control and cardio-vascular risk factors in a randomized clinical trial in individuals with type 2 diabetes. *Diabetes Care* 2006; 29(8):1777–1783.

15 Brinkworth GD, Noakes M. Long-term effects of advice to consume a high-protein, low-fat diet, rather than a conventional weight-loss diet, in obese adults with type 2 diabetes: one-year follow-up of a randomised trial. *Diabetologia* 2004;47(10):1677–1686.

16 Daly ME, Paisey R. Short-term effects of severe dietary carbohydrate-restriction advice in Type 2 diabetes – a randomized controlled trial. *Diabetic Medicine* 2006;23(1):15–20.

17 Redmon JB, Susan KR, Kristell PR et al. One-year outcome of a combination of weight loss therapies for subjects with type 2 diabetes: A randomized trial. *Diabetes Care* 2003;26(9):2505.

18 Stern L, Iqbal N, Seshadri P et al. The effects of low-carbohydrate versus conventional weight loss diets in severely obese adults: one-year follow-up of a randomized trial. *Annals of Internal Medicine* 2004; 140(10):778–785.

19 The Diabetes and Nutrition Study Group of the Spanish Diabetes Association (GSEDNu). Diabetes nutrition and complications trial: adherence to the ADA nutritional recommendations, targets of metabolic control, and onset of diabetes complications. A 7-year, prospective, population-based, observational multicenter study. *Journal of Diabetes & its Complications* 2006;20(6):361–366.

20 Van ST, Van de Laar FA, Van Leeuwe JF et al. The dieting dilemma in patients with newly diagnosed type 2 diabetes: does dietary restraint predict weight gain 4 years after diagnosis? *Health Psychology* 2007; 26(1):105–112.

21 Anderson RJ, Freedland KE, Clouse RE et al. The prevalence of comorbid depression in adults with diabetes: a meta-analysis. *Diabetes Care* 2001;24(6):1069–1078.

22 Rubin RR, Ciechanowski P, Egede LE et al. Recognizing and treating depression in patients with diabetes. *Current Diabetes Reports* 2004;4(2):119–125.

23 de Groot M, Anderson R, Freedland KE et al. Association of depression and diabetes complications: a meta-analysis. *Psychosomatic Medicine* 2001;63(4):619–630.

24 Lin EH, Katon W, Von KM et al. Relationship of depression and diabetes self-care, medication adherence, and preventive care. *Diabetes Care* 2004;27(9):2154–2160.

25 Egede LE, Zheng D, Simpson K. Comorbid depression is associated with increased health care use and expenditures in individuals with diabetes. *Diabetes Care* 2002;25(3):464–470.

26 National Institute for Health and Clinical Excellence. *Diagnosis and management of type 1 diabetes in children, young people and adults* (CG15). London: NICE, 2004.

27 National Institute for Clinical Excellence. *Depression: management of depression in primary and secondary care* (CG23). London: NICE, 2004.

28 Stratton IM, Adler AI, Neil HA et al. Association of glycaemia with macrovascular and microvascular complications of type 2 diabetes (UKPDS 35): prospective observational study. *British Medical Journal* 2000;321(7258):405–412.

29 Selvin E, Marinopoulos S, Berkenblit G et al. Meta-analysis: glycosylated hemoglobin and cardiovascular disease in diabetes mellitus. *Annals of Internal Medicine* 2004;141(6):421–431.

30 Gerstein HC, Pogue J. The relationship between dysglycaemia and cardiovascular and renal risk in diabetic and non-diabetic participants in the HOPE study: a prospective epidemiological analysis. *Diabetologia* 2005;48(9):1749–1755.

31 Iribarren C, Karter AJ, Go AS et al. Glycemic control and heart failure among adult patients with diabetes. *Circulation* 2001;103(22):2668–2673.

32 Oglesby AK, Secnik K, Barron J, Al-Zakwani I, Lage MJ. The association between diabetes related medical costs and glycemic control: A retrospective analysis. *Cost Effectiveness & Resource Allocation* 2006;4:1.

33 Clarke PM, Gray AM, Briggs A et al. Cost-utility analyses of intensive blood glucose and tight blood pressure control in type 2 diabetes (UKPDS 72). *Diabetologia* 2005;48(5):868–877.

34 Clarke P, Gray A, Adler A et al. Cost-effectiveness analysis of intensive blood-glucose control with metformin in overweight patients with type II diabetes (UKPDS no. 51). *Diabetologia* 2001;44(3):298–304.

35 ACCORD. *ACCORD Study Announcement* www.accordtrial.org. Date of message: 6 February 2008.

36 Sarol JN, Nicodemus NA, Tan KM et al. Self-monitoring of blood glucose as part of a multi-component therapy among non-insulin requiring type 2 diabetes patients: a meta-analysis (1966–2004). *Current Medical Research & Opinion* 2005;21(2):173–184.

37 Welschen LM, Bloemendal E, Nijpels G et al. Self-monitoring of blood glucose in patients with type 2 diabetes who are not using insulin: a systematic review. *Diabetes Care* 2005;28(6):1510–1517.

38 Welschen LM, Bloemendal E, Nijpels G et al. Self-monitoring of blood glucose in patients with type 2 diabetes who are not using insulin. *Cochrane Database of Systematic Reviews* 2005;(2):CD005060.

39 Jansen JP. Self-monitoring of glucose in type 2 diabetes mellitus: a Bayesian meta-analysis of direct and indirect comparisons. *Current Medical Research & Opinion* 2006;22(4):671–681.

40 Farmer A, Wade A, French DP et al. The DiGEM trial protocol: a randomised controlled trial to determine the effect on glycaemic control of different strategies of blood glucose self-monitoring in people with type 2 diabetes. *BMC Family Practice* 2005;6(25)

41 Moreland EC, Volkening LK, Lawlor MT et al. Use of a blood glucose monitoring manual to enhance monitoring adherence in adults with diabetes: a randomized controlled trial. *Archives of Internal Medicine* 2006;166(6):689–695.

42 Siebolds M, Gaedeke O, Schwedes U et al. Self-monitoring of blood glucose – psychological aspects relevant to changes in HbA1c in type 2 diabetic patients treated with diet or diet plus oral antidiabetic medication. *Patient Education & Counseling* 2006;62(1):104–110.

43 Karter AJ, Chan J, Parker MM et al. Longitudinal study of new and prevalent use of self-monitoring of blood glucose. *Diabetes Care* 2006;29(8).

44 Martin S, Schneider B, Heinemann L et al. Self-monitoring of blood glucose in type 2 diabetes and long-term outcome: an epidemiological cohort study. *Diabetologia* 2006;49(2):271–278.

45 Wen L, Parchman ML, Linn WD et al. Association between self-monitoring of blood glucose and glycemic control in patients with type 2 diabetes mellitus. *American Journal of Health-System Pharmacy* 2004; 61(22):2401–2405.

46 Davis WA, Bruce DG, Davis TM. Is self-monitoring of blood glucose appropriate for all type 2 diabetic patients? The Fremantle Diabetes Study. *Diabetes Care* 2006;29(8):1764–1770.

47 Schutt M, Kern W, Krause U et al. Is the frequency of self-monitoring of blood glucose related to long-term metabolic control? Multicenter analysis including 24,500 patients from 191 centers in Germany and Austria. *Experimental & Clinical Endocrinology & Diabetes* 2006;114(7):384–388.

48 Kalergis M, Nadeau J, Pacaud D et al. Accuracy and reliability of reporting self-monitoring of blood glucose results in adults with type 1 and type 2 diabetes. *Canadian Journal of Diabetes* 2006;30(3):241–247.

49 Lawton J, Peel E, Douglas M et al. 'Urine testing is a waste of time': newly diagnosed type 2 diabetes patients' perceptions of self-monitoring. *Diabetic Medicine* 2004;21(9):1045–1048.

50 Peel E, Parry O, Douglas M et al. Blood glucose self-monitoring in non-insulin-treated type 2 diabetes: a qualitative study of patients' perspectives. *British Journal of General Practice* 2004;54(500):183–188.

51 Palmer AJ, Dinneen S, Gavin JR, III et al. Cost-utility analysis in a UK setting of self-monitoring of blood glucose in patients with type 2 diabetes. *Current Medical Research & Opinion* 2006;22(5):861–872.

52 Gray A, Clarke P, Farmer A et al. Implementing intensive control of blood glucose concentration and blood pressure in type 2 diabetes in England: Cost analysis (UKPDS 63). *British Medical Journal* 2002; 325(7369):860–863.

53 UK Prospective Diabetes Study Group. Intensive blood-glucose control with sulphonylureas or insulin compared with conventional treatment and risk of complications in patients with type 2 diabetes (UKPDS 33). UKPDS Group. *Lancet* 1998;352(9131):837–853.

54 Kahn SE, Haffner SM, Heise MA et al. Glycemic durability of rosiglitazone, metformin, or glyburide monotherapy. *New England Journal of Medicine* 2006;355(23):2427–2443.

55 UK Prospective Diabetes Study Group. UK prospective diabetes study 16. Overview of 6 years' therapy of type II diabetes: a progressive disease. *Diabetes* 1995;44(11):1249–1258.

56 Saenz A, Fernandez-Esteban I, Mataix A et al. Metformin monotherapy for type 2 diabetes mellitus. *Cochrane Database of Systematic Reviews* 2005;(3):CD002966.

57 Salpeter S, Greyber E, Pasternak G et al. Risk of fatal and nonfatal lactic acidosis with metformin use in type 2 diabetes mellitus. *Cochrane Database of Systematic Reviews* 2003;(2):CD002967.

58 Cryer DR, Nicholas SP, Henry DH et al. Comparative outcomes study of metformin intervention versus conventional approach the COSMIC Approach Study. *Diabetes Care* 2005;28(3):539–543.

59 Schernthaner G, Matthews DR, Charbonnel B et al. Efficacy and safety of pioglitazone versus metformin in patients with type 2 diabetes mellitus: a double-blind, randomized trial. *Journal of Clinical Endocrinology & Metabolism* 2004;89(12):6068–6076.

60 Derosa G, Franzetti I, Gadaleta G et al. Metabolic variations with oral antidiabetic drugs in patients with type 2 diabetes: comparison between glimepiride and metformin. *Diabetes, Nutrition & Metabolism – Clinical & Experimental* 2004;17(3):143–150.

61 Weissman P, Goldstein BJ, Rosenstock J et al. Effects of rosiglitazone added to submaximal doses of metformin compared with dose escalation of metformin in type 2 diabetes: the EMPIRE Study. *Current Medical Research & Opinion* 2005;21(12):2029–2035.

62 Bailey CJ, Bagdonas A, Rubes J et al. Rosiglitazone/metformin fixed-dose combination compared with uptitrated metformin alone in type 2 diabetes mellitus: a 24-week, multicenter, randomized, double-blind, parallel-group study. *Clinical Therapeutics* 2005;27(10):1548–1561.

63 Marre M, Van GL, Usadel KH et al. Nateglinide improves glycaemic control when added to metformin monotherapy: results of a randomized trial with type 2 diabetes patients. *Diabetes, Obesity & Metabolism* 2002;4(3):177–186.

64   Kvapil M, Swatko A, Hilberg C et al. Biphasic insulin aspart 30 plus metformin: an effective combination in type 2 diabetes. *Diabetes, Obesity & Metabolism* 2006;8(1):39–48.

65   Fujioka K, Pans M, Joyal S. Glycemic control in patients with type 2 diabetes mellitus switched from twice-daily immediate-release metformin to a once-daily extended-release formulation. *Clinical Therapeutics* 2003;25(2):515–529.

66   Fujioka K, Brazg RL, Raz I et al. Efficacy, dose-response relationship and safety of once-daily extended-release metformin (Glucophage XR) in type 2 diabetic patients with inadequate glycaemic control despite prior treatment with diet and exercise: results from two double-blind, placebo-controlled studies. *Diabetes, Obesity & Metabolism* 2005;7(1):28–39.

67   Blonde L, Dailey G, Jabbour SA et al. Gastrointerstinal tolerability of extended-release metformin tablets compared to immediate-release metformin tablets: results of a retrospective cohort study. *Current Medical Research & Opinion* 2006;20(4):565–572.

68   Mohammad F, Fenna I, Leong K et al. Audit of metformin sustained release (SR) in patients intolerant of immediate release metformin. *Diabetic Medicine* 2006;23(Suppl 2):111.

69   Nagle A, Brake J, Hopkins M et al. Glucophage SR. Can it really make a difference? *Diabetic Medicine* 2006;23(Suppl 2):110.

70   Thomas Z, Phillips SM, Hogan D et al. The tolerability of prolonged-release metformin (Glucophage SR) in previously metformin intolerant patients – review of local experience. *Diabetic Medicine* 2006; 23(Suppl 2):111.

71   Yousseif A, Roberts S, Malik S et al. Patient reported side effects and compliance with Glucophage SR. *Diabetic Medicine* 2006;23(Suppl 2):111.

72   Palmer AJ, Roze S, Lammert M et al. Comparing the long-term cost-effectiveness of repaglinide plus metformin versus nateglinide plus metformin in type 2 diabetes patients with inadequate glycaemic control: an application of the CORE Diabetes Model in type 2 diabetes. *Current Medical Research & Opinion* 2004;20(Suppl 1):S41–S51.

73   Salas M, Ward A, Caro J. Health and economic effects of adding nateglinide to metformin to achieve dual control of glycosylated hemoglobin and postprandial glucose levels in a model of type 2 diabetes mellitus. *Clinical Therapeutics* 2002;24(10):1690–1705.

74   Ward AJ, Salas M, Caro JJ, Owens D. Health and economic impact of combining metformin with nateglinide to achieve glycemic control: comparison of the lifetime costs of complications in the UK. *Cost Effectiveness & Resource Allocation* 2004;2:2.

75   Caro JJ, Salas M, Ward AJ et al. Combination therapy for type 2 diabetes: what are the potential health and cost implications in Canada? *Canadian Journal of Diabetes* 2003;27(1):33–41.

76   Alvarsson M, Sundkvist G, Lager I et al. Beneficial effects of insulin versus sulphonylurea on insulin secretion and metabolic control in recently diagnosed type 2 diabetic patients. *Diabetes Care* 2003; 26(8):2231–2237.

77   Tong PC, Chow CC, Jorgensen LN et al. The contribution of metformin to glycaemic control in patients with type 2 diabetes mellitus receiving combination therapy with insulin. *Diabetes Research & Clinical Practice* 2002;57(2):93–98.

78   Inukai K, Watanabe M, Nakashima Y et al. Efficacy of glimepiride in Japanese type 2 diabetic subjects. *Diabetes Research & Clinical Practice* 2005;68(3):250–257.

79   Jibran R, Suliman MI, Qureshi F et al. Safety and efficay of repaglinide compared with glibenclamide in the management of type 2 diabetic Pakistani patients. *Pakistan Journal of Medical Sciences* 2006;22(4): 385–390.

80   Saloranta C, Hershon K, Ball M et al. Efficacy and safety of nateglinide in type 2 diabetic patients with modest fasting hyperglycemia. *Journal of Clinical Endocrinology & Metabolism* 2002;87(9):4171–4176.

81   Bengel FM, Abletshauser C, Neverve J et al. Effects of nateglinide on myocardial microvascular reactivity in type 2 diabetes mellitus: a randomized study using positron emission tomography. *Diabetic Medicine* 2005;22(2):158–163.

82 Moses RG, Gomis R, Frandsen KB et al. Flexible meal-related dosing with repaglinide facilitates glycemic control in therapy-naive type 2 diabetes. *Diabetes Care* 2001;24(1):11–15.

83 Rosenstock J, Hassman DR, Madder RD et al. Repaglinide versus nateglinide monotherapy: a randomized, multicenter study. *Diabetes Care* 2004;27(6):1265–1270.

84 Derosa G, Mugellini A, Ciccarelli L et al. Comparison between repaglinide and glimepiride in patients with type 2 diabetes mellitus: a one-year, randomized, double-blind assessment of metabolic parameters and cardiovascular risk factors. *Clinical Therapeutics* 2003;25(2):472–484.

85 Madsbad S, Kilhovd B, Lager I et al. Comparison between repaglinide and glipizide in type 2 diabetes mellitus: a 1-year multicentre study. *Diabetic Medicine* 2001;18(5):395–401.

86 Esposito K, Giugliano D, Nappo F et al. Regression of carotid atherosclerosis by control of postprandial hyperglycemia in type 2 diabetes mellitus. *Circulation* 2004;110(2):214–219.

87 Furlong NJ, Hulme SA, O'Brien SV et al. Comparison of repaglinide vs. gliclazide in combination with bedtime NPH insulin in patients with type 2 diabetes inadequately controlled with oral hypoglycaemic agents. *Diabetic Medicine* 2003;20(11):935–941.

88 Raskin P, Klaff L, McGill J et al. Efficacy and safety of combination therapy: repaglinide plus metformin versus nateglinide plus metformin. *Diabetes Care* 2003;26(7):2063–2068.

89 Gerich J, Raskin P, Jean LL et al. PRESERVE-beta: two-year efficacy and safety of initial combination therapy with nateglinide or glyburide plus metformin. *Diabetes Care* 2005;28(9):2093–2099.

90 Ristic S, ColloberMaugeais C, Pecher E et al. Comparison of nateglinide and gliclazide in combination with metformin, for treatment of patients with type 2 diabetes mellitus inadequately controlled on maximum doses of metformin alone. *Diabetic Medicine* 2006;23(7):757–762.

91 Horton ES, Foley JE, Shen SG et al. Efficacy and tolerability of initial combination therapy with nateglinide and metformin in treatment-naive patients with type 2 diabetes. *Current Medical Research & Opinion* 2004;20(6):883–889.

92 Dashora UK, Sibal L, Ashwell SG et al. Insulin glargine in combination with nateglinide in people with type 2 diabetes: a randomized placebo-controlled trial. *Diabetic Medicine* 2007;24(4):344–349.

93 Schernthaner G, Grimaldi A, Di MU et al. GUIDE study: double-blind comparison of once-daily gliclazide MR and glimepiride in type 2 diabetic patients. *European Journal of Clinical Investigation* 2004;34(8): 535–542.

94 Lu CH, Chang CC, Chuang LM et al. Double-blind, randomized, multicentre study of the efficacy and safety of gliclazide-modified release in the treatment of Chinese type 2 diabetic patients. *Diabetes, Obesity & Metabolism* 2006;8(2):184–191.

95 Charpentier G, Fleury F, Kabir M et al. Improved glycaemic control by addition of glimepiride to metformin monotherapy in type 2 diabetic patients. *Diabetic Medicine* 2001;18(10):828–834.

96 Forst T, Eriksson JW, Strotmann HJ et al. Metabolic effects of mealtime insulin lispro in comparison to glibenclamide in early type 2 diabetes. *Experimental & Clinical Endocrinology & Diabetes* 2003;111(2): 97–103.

97 Wright AD, Cull CA, Macleod KM et al. Hypoglycemia in type 2 diabetic patients randomized to and maintained on monotherapy with diet, sulfonylurea, metformin, or insulin for 6 years from diagnosis (UKPDS 73). *Journal of Diabetes & its Complications* 2006;20(6):395–401.

98 Gray A, Raikou M, McGuire A et al. Cost effectiveness of an intensive blood glucose control policy in patients with type 2 diabetes: Economic analysis alongside randomised controlled trial (UKPDS 41). *British Medical Journal* 2000;320(7246):1373–1378.

99 Van de Laar FA, Lucassen PL, Akkermans RP et al. Alpha-glucosidase inhibitors for type 2 diabetes mellitus. *Cochrane Database of Systematic Reviews* 2005;(2):CD003639.

100 Ko GTC, Tsang CC, Ng CW et al. Effects on blood pressure of the a-glucosidase inhibitor acarbose compared with the insulin enhancer glibenclamide in patients with hypertension and type 2 diabetes mellitus. *Clinical Drug Investigation* 2001;21(6):401–408.

101 Goke B, German Pioglitazone Study Group. Effects on blood pressure of the a-glucosidase inhibitor acarbose compared with the insulin enhancer glibenclamide in patients with hypertension and type 2 diabetes mellitus. *Treatments in Endocrinology* 2002;1(5):329–336.

102 Feinbock C, Luger A, Klingler A et al. Effects on blood pressure of the a-glucosidase inhibitor acarbose compared with the insulin enhancer glibenclamide in patients with hypertension and type 2 diabetes mellitus. *Diabetes, Nutrition & Metabolism - Clinical & Experimental* 2003;16(4):214–221.

103 Hwu CM, Ho LT, Fuh MM et al. Effects on blood pressure of the a-glucosidase inhibitor acarbose compared with the insulin enhancer glibenclamide in patients with hypertension and type 2 diabetes mellitus. *Diabetes Research & Clinical Practice* 2003;60(2):111–118.

104 Phillips P, Karrasch J, Scott R et al. Effects on blood pressure of the a-glucosidase inhibitor acarbose compared with the insulin enhancer glibenclamide in patients with hypertension and type 2 diabetes mellitus. *Diabetes Care* 2003;26(2):269–273.

105 Bachmann W, Petzinna D, Raptis SA et al. Effects on blood pressure of the a-glucosidase inhibitor acarbose compared with the insulin enhancer glibenclamide in patients with hypertension and type 2 diabetes mellitus. *Clinical Drug Investigation* 2003;23(10):679–686.

106 Lin BJ, Wu HP, Huang HS et al. Effects on blood pressure of the a-glucosidase inhibitor acarbose compared with the insulin enhancer glibenclamide in patients with hypertension and type 2 diabetes mellitus. *Journal of Diabetes & its Complications* 2003;17(4):179–185.

107 Segal P, Eliahou HE, Petzinna D et al. Effects on blood pressure of the a-glucosidase inhibitor acarbose compared with the insulin enhancer glibenclamide in patients with hypertension and type 2 diabetes mellitus. *Clinical Drug Investigation* 2005;25(9):589–595.

108 White TJ, Vanderplas A, Chang E et al. The costs of non-adherence to oral antihyperglycemic medication in individuals with diabetes mellitus and concomitant diabetes mellitus and cardiovascular disease in a managed care environment. *Disease Management and Health Outcomes* 2004;12(3):181–188.

109 Quilici S, Chancellor J, Maclaine G et al. Cost-effectiveness of acarbose for the management of impaired glucose tolerance in Sweden. *International Journal of Clinical Practice* 2005;59(10):1143–1152.

110 Huang ES, Shook M, Jin L et al. The impact of patient preferences on the cost-effectiveness of intensive glucose control in older patients with new-onset diabetes. *Diabetes Care* 2006;29(2):259–264.

111 Johnson JA, Simpson SH, Toth EL et al. Reduced cardiovascular morbidity and mortality associated with metformin use in subjects with type 2 diabetes. *Diabetic Medicine* 2005;22(4):497–502.

112 Evans JMM, Ogston SA, EmslieSmith A et al. Risk of mortality and adverse cardiovascular outcomes in type 2 diabetes: A comparison of patients treated with sulfonylureas and metformin. *Diabetologia* 2006;49(5):930–936.

113 National Institute for Health and Clinical Excellence. *Glitazones in the treatment of type 2 diabetes (Review of TA9 and TA21)*. (TA63). London: NICE, 2003.

114 European Medicines Agency. 2007. www.emea.europa.eu

115 Nissen SE, Wolski K. Effect of rosiglitazone on the risk of myocardial infarction and death from cardiovascular causes. *New England Journal of Medicine* 2007;356(24):2457–2471.

116 Home PD, Pocock SJ, Beck-Nielsen H et al. Rosiglitazone evaluated for cardiovascular outcomes – an interim analysis. *New England Journal of Medicine* 2007;357(1):28–38.

117 Lincoff AM, Wolski K, Nicholls SJ et al. Pioglitazone and risk of cardiovascular events in patients with type 2 diabetes mellitus: a meta-analysis of randomized trials. *The Journal of the American Medical Association* 2007;298(10):1180–1188.

118 Diamond GA, Bax L, Kaul S. Uncertain effects of rosiglitazone on the risk for myocardial infarction and cardiovascular death. *Annals of Internal Medicine* 2007;147(8):578–581.

119 Singh S, Loke YK, Furberg CD. Long-term risk of cardiovascular events with rosiglitazone: a meta-analysis [see comment]. *The Journal of the American Medical Association* 2007;298(10):1189–1195.

120 Lago RM, Singh PP, Nesto RW. Congestive heart failure and cardiovascular death in patients with prediabetes and type 2 diabetes given thiazolidinediones: a meta-analysis of randomised clinical trials. *Lancet* 2007;370(9593):1129–1136.

121 GlaxoSmithKline. Coronary heart disease outcomes in patients receiving antidiabetic agents. Uxbridge, Middlesex: GlaxoSmithKline, 2008.

122 Richter B, Bandeira-Echtler E, Bergerhoff K et al. Rosiglitazone for type 2 diabetes mellitus. *Cochrane Database of Systematic Reviews* 2007;(3):CD006063.

123 Derosa G, Gaddi AV, Piccinni MN et al. Differential effect of glimepiride and rosiglitazone on metabolic control of type 2 diabetic patients treated with metformin: a randomized, double-blind, clinical trial. *Diabetes, Obesity & Metabolism* 2006;8(2):197–205.

124 Rosenstock J, Goldstein BJ, Vinik AI et al. Effect of early addition of rosiglitazone to sulphonylurea therapy in older type 2 diabetes patients (>60 years): the Rosiglitazone Early vs. SULphonylurea Titration (RESULT) study. *Diabetes, Obesity & Metabolism* 2006;8(1):49–57.

125 Raskin P, McGill J, Saad MF et al. Combination therapy for type 2 diabetes: repaglinide plus rosiglitazone. *Diabetic Medicine* 2004;21(4):329–335.

126 Bakris GL, Ruilope LM, McMorn SO et al. Rosiglitazone reduces microalbuminuria and blood pressure independently of glycemia in type 2 diabetes patients with microalbuminuria. *Journal of Hypertension* 2006;24(10):2047–2055.

127 Vongthavaravat V, Wajchenberg BL, Waitman JN et al. An international study of the effects of rosiglitazone plus sulphonylurea in patients with type 2 diabetes. *Current Medical Research & Opinion* 2002;18(8):456–461.

128 St John SM, Rendell M, Dandona P et al. A comparison of the effects of rosiglitazone and glyburide on cardiovascular function and glycemic control in patients with type 2 diabetes. *Diabetes Care* 2002;25(11):2058–2064.

129 Hanefeld M, Patwardhan R, Jones NP et al. A one-year study comparing the efficacy and safety of rosiglitazone and glibenclamide in the treatment of type 2 diabetes. *Nutrition Metabolism & Cardiovascular Diseases* 2007;17(1):13–23.

130 Kerenyi Z, Samer H, James R et al. Combination therapy with rosiglitazone and glibenclamide compared with upward titration of glibenclamide alone in patients with type 2 diabetes mellitus. *Diabetes Research & Clinical Practice* 2004;63(3):213–223.

131 Derosa G, Gaddi AV, Piccinni MN et al. Antithrombotic effects of rosiglitazone-metformin versus glimepiride-metformin combination therapy in patients with type 2 diabetes mellitus and metabolic syndrome. *Pharmacotherapy* 2005;25(5):637–645.

132 Baksi A, James RE, Zhou B et al. Comparison of uptitration of gliclazide with the addition of rosiglitazone to gliclazide in patients with type 2 diabetes inadequately controlled on half-maximal doses of a sulphonylurea. *Acta Diabetologica* 2004;41(2):63–69.

133 Derosa G, D'Angelo A, Ragonesi PD et al. Metabolic effects of pioglitazone and rosiglitazone in patients with diabetes and metabolic syndrome treated with metformin. *Internal Medicine Journal* 2007;37(2):79–86.

134 Rosenstock J, Rood J, Cobitz A et al. Initial treatment with rosiglitazone/metformin fixed-dose combination therapy compared with monotherapy with either rosiglitazone or metformin in patients with uncontrolled type 2 diabetes. *Diabetes, Obesity & Metabolism* 2006;8(6):650–660.

135 Stewart MW, Cirkel DT, Furuseth K et al. Effect of metformin plus roziglitazone compared with metformin alone on glycaemic control in well-controlled type 2 diabetes. *Diabetic Medicine* 2006;23(10):1069–1078.

136 Home PD, Jones NP, Pocock SJ et al. Rosiglitazone RECORD study: glucose control outcomes at 18 months. *Diabetic Medicine* 2007;24(6):626–634.

137 Raskin P, Rendell M, Riddle MC et al. A randomized trial of rosiglitazone therapy in patients with inadequately controlled insulin-treated type 2 diabetes. *Diabetes Care* 2001;24(7):1226–1232.

138 Home PD, Bailey CJ, Donaldson J et al. A double-blind randomized study comparing the effects of continuing or not continuing rosiglitazone + metformin therapy when starting insulin therapy in people with type 2 diabetes. *Diabetic Medicine* 2007;24(6):618–625.

139 Rosenstock J, Sugimoto D, Strange P et al. Triple therapy in type 2 diabetes: insulin glargine or rosiglitazone added to combination therapy of sulfonylurea plus metformin in insulin-naive patients. *Diabetes Care* 2006;29(3):554–559.

140 Vinik AI, Zhang Q. Adding insulin glargine versus rosiglitazone: health-related quality-of-life impact in type 2 diabetes. *Diabetes Care* 2007;30(4):795–800.

141 Richter B, Bandeira-Echtler E, Bergerhoff K et al. Pioglitazone for type 2 diabetes mellitus. *Cochrane Database of Systematic Reviews* 2006;(4):CD006060.

142 Dormandy JA. PROactive study. *Lancet* 2006;367(9405):26–27.

143 Yudkin J.S., Freemantle N. PROactive study. *Lancet* 2006;367(3504):24–25.

144 PROactive Study Executive Committee and Data and Safety Monitoring Committee. PROactive study. *Lancet* 2006;367(9515):982.

145 Mattoo V, Eckland D, Widel M et al. Metabolic effects of pioglitazone in combination with insulin in patients with type 2 diabetes mellitus whose disease is not adequately controlled with insulin therapy: results of a six-month, randomized, double-blind, prospective, multicenter, parallel-group study. *Clinical Therapeutics* 2005;27(5):554–567.

146 Davidson JA, Perez A, Zhang J. Addition of pioglitazone to stable insulin therapy in patients with poorly controlled type 2 diabetes: results of a double-blind, multicentre, randomized study. *Diabetes, Obesity & Metabolism* 2006;8(2):164–174.

147 Raz I, Stranks S, Filipczak R et al. Efficacy and safety of biphasic insulin aspart 30 combined with pioglitazone in type 2 diabetes poorly controlled on glibenclamide (glyburide) monotherapy or combination therapy: an 18-week, randomized, open-label study. *Clinical Therapeutics* 2005;27(9):1432–1443.

148 Charbonnel B, Schernthaner G, Brunetti P et al. Long-term efficacy and tolerability of add-on pioglitazone therapy to failing monotherapy compared with addition of gliclazide or metformin in patients with type 2 diabetes. *Diabetologia* 2005;48(6):1093–1104.

149 Jain R, Osei K, Kupfer S et al. Long-term safety of pioglitazone versus glyburide in patients with recently diagnosed type 2 diabetes mellitus. *Pharmacotherapy* 2006;26(10):1388–1395.

150 Erdmann E, Dormandy JA, Charbonnel B et al. The effect of pioglitazone on recurrent myocardial infarction in 2,445 patients with type 2 diabetes and previous myocardial infarction: results from the PROactive (PROactive 05) Study. *Journal of the American College of Cardiology* 2007;49(17):1772–1780.

151 Mazzone T, Meyer PM, Feinstein SB et al. Effect of pioglitazone compared with glimepiride on carotid intima-media thickness in type 2 diabetes: a randomized trial. *The Journal of the American Medical Association* 2006;296(21):2572–2581.

152 Wilcox R, Bousser MG, Betteridge DJ et al. effects of pioglitazone in patients with type 2 diabetes with or without previous stroke: results from PROactive (PROspective pioglitAzone Clinical Trial In macroVascular Events 04). *Stroke* 2007;38(3):865–873.

153 Berlie HD, Kalus JS, Jaber LA. Thiazolidinediones and the risk of edema: a meta-analysis. *Diabetes Research & Clinical Practice* 2007;76(2):279–289.

154 Czoski-Murray C, Warren E, Chilcott J et al. Clinical effectiveness and cost-effectiveness of pioglitazone and rosiglitazone in the treatment of type 2 diabetes: a systematic review and economic evaluation (structured abstract). *Health Technology Assessment* 2004;8(13)

155 National Institute for Health and Clinical Excellence. *Diabetes (type 2) – pioglitazone (replaced by TA63)* (TA21). London: NICE, 2001.

156 Beale S, Bagust A, Shearer AT et al. Cost-effectiveness of rosiglitazone combination therapy for the treatment of type 2 diabetes mellitus in the UK. *Pharmacoeconomics* 2006;24(Suppl 1):21–34.

157 Tilden DP, Mariz S, O'BryanTear G et al. A lifetime modelled economic evaluation comparing pioglitazone and rosiglitazone for the treatment of type 2 diabetes mellitus in the UK. *Pharmacoeconomics* 2007;25(1):39–54.

158 Dormandy JA, Charbonnel B, Eckland DJ et al. Secondary prevention of macrovascular events in patients with type 2 diabetes in the PROactive Study (PROspective pioglitAzone Clinical Trial In macroVascular Events): a randomised controlled trial. *Lancet* 2005;366(9493):1279–1289.

159 Buse JB, Henry RR, Han J et al. Effects of exenatide (exendin-4) on glycemic control over 30 weeks in sulfonylurea-treated patients with type 2 diabetes. *Diabetes Care* 2004;27(11):2628–2635.

160 DeFronzo RA, Ratner RE, Han J et al. Effects of exenatide (exendin-4) on glycemic control and weight over 30 weeks in metformin-treated patients with type 2 diabetes. *Diabetes Care* 2005;28(5):1092–1100.

161 Kendall DM, Riddle MC, Rosenstock J et al. Effects of exenatide (exendin-4) on glycemic control over 30 weeks in patients with type 2 diabetes treated with metformin and a sulfonylurea. *Diabetes Care* 2005;28(5):1083–1091.

162 Blonde L, Klein EJ, Han J et al. Interim analysis of the effects of exenatide treatment on A1C, weight and cardiovascular risk factors over 82 weeks in 314 overweight patients with type 2 diabetes. *Diabetes, Obesity & Metabolism* 2006;8(4):436–447.

163 Poon T, Nelson P, Shen L et al. Exenatide improves glycemic control and reduces body weight in subjects with type 2 diabetes: a dose-ranging study. *Diabetes Technology & Therapeutics* 2005;7(3):467–477.

164 Heine RJ, Van Gaal LF, Johns D et al. Exenatide versus insulin glargine in patients with suboptimally controlled type 2 diabetes: a randomized trial. *Annals of Internal Medicine* 2005;143(8):559–569.

165 Secnik BK, Matza LS, Oglesby A et al. Patient-reported outcomes in a trial of exenatide and insulin glargine for the treatment of type 2 diabetes. *Health & Quality of Life Outcomes* 2006;4(80).

166 Nauck MA, Duran S, Kim D et al. A comparison of twice-daily exenatide and biphasic insulin aspart in patients with type 2 diabetes who were suboptimally controlled with sulfonylurea and metformin: a non-inferiority study. *Diabetologia* 2007;50(2):259–267.

167 Zinman B, Hoogwerf BJ, Duran GS et al. The effect of adding exenatide to a thiazolidinedione in suboptimally controlled type 2 diabetes: a randomized trial. *Annals of Internal Medicine* 2007;146(7): 477–485.

168 European Medicines Agency. *EPARs for authorised medicinal products for human use.* Available from: www.emea.europa.eu. Last accessed on: 19 January 2008.

169 Ray JA, Boye KS, Yurgin N et al. Exenatide versus insulin glargine in patients with type 2 diabetes in the UK: a model of long-term clinical and cost outcomes. *Current Medical Research & Opinion* 2007;23(3): 609–622.

170 Goudswaard AN, Furlong NJ, Rutten GE et al. Insulin monotherapy versus combinations of insulin with oral hypoglycaemic agents in patients with type 2 diabetes mellitus. *Cochrane Database of Systematic Reviews* 2004;(4):CD003418.

171 Kokic SB. Lispro insulin and metformin versus other combination in the diabetes mellitus type 2 management after secondary oral antidiabetic drug failure. *Collegium Antropologicum* 2003;27(1):181–187.

172 Olsson PO, Lindstrom T. Combination-therapy with bedtime nph insulin and sulphonylureas gives similar glycaemic control but lower weight gain than insulin twice daily in patients with type 2 diabetes. *Diabetes & Metabolism* 2002;28(4:Pt 1):272–277.

173 Altuntas Y, Ozen B, Ozturk B et al. Comparison of additional metformin or NPH insulin to mealtime insulin lispro therapy with mealtime human insulin therapy in secondary OAD failure. *Diabetes, Obesity & Metabolism* 2003;5(6):371–378.

174 Kabadi MU, Kabadi UM. Efficacy of sulfonylureas with insulin in type 2 diabetes mellitus. *Annals of Pharmacotherapy* 2003;37(11):1572–1576.

175 Zargar AH, Masoodi SR, Laway BA et al. Response of regimens of insulin therapy in type 2 diabetes mellitus subjects with secondary failure. *Journal of the Association of Physicians of India* 2002;50(5):641–646.

176 Douek IF, Allen SE, Ewings P et al. Continuing metformin when starting insulin in patients with type 2 diabetes: a double-blind randomized placebo-controlled trial. *Diabetic Medicine* 2005;22(5):634–640.

177 Goudswaard AN, Stolk RP, Zuithoff P et al. Starting insulin in type 2 diabetes: continue oral hypoglycemic agents? A randomized trial in primary care. *Journal of Family Practice* 2004;53(5):393–399.

178 Janka HU, Plewe G, Riddle MC et al. Comparison of basal insulin added to oral agents versus twice-daily premixed insulin as initial insulin therapy for type 2 diabetes. *Diabetes Care* 2005; 28(2):254–259.

179 Stehouwer MH, DeVries JH, Lumeij JA et al. Combined bedtime insulin – daytime sulphonylurea regimen compared with two different daily insulin regimens in type 2 diabetes: effects on HbA1c and hypo-glycaemia rate – a randomised trial. *Diabetes/Metabolism Research and Reviews* 2003;19(2):148–152.

180 Lechleitner M, Roden M, Haehling E et al. Insulin glargine in combination with oral antidiabetic drugs as a cost-equivalent alternative to conventional insulin therapy in type 2 diabetes mellitus. *Wiener Klinische Wochenschrift* 2005;117(17):593–598.

181 Drummond M, O'Brien B, Stoddart G, Torrance G. *Methods for economic evaluation of health care programmes,* 2nd edn. Oxford: Oxford University Press, 2003.

182 Christiansen JS, Vaz JA, Metelko Z. Twice daily biphasic insulin aspart improves postprandial glycaemic control more effectively than twice daily NPH insulin, with low risk of hypoglycaemia, in patients with type 2 diabetes. *Diabetes, Obesity & Metabolism* 2003;5(6):446–454.

183 Kilo C, Mezitis N, Jain R et al. Starting patients with type 2 diabetes on insulin therapy using once-daily injections of biphasic insulin aspart 70/30, biphasic human insulin 70/30, or NPH insulin in combination with metformin. *Journal of Diabetes & its Complications* 2003;17(6):307–313.

184 Ceriello A, Del PS, Bue VJ et al. Premeal insulin lispro plus bedtime NPH or twice-daily NPH in patients with type 2 diabetes: acute postprandial and chronic effects on glycemic control and cardiovascular risk factors. *Journal of Diabetes & its Complications* 2007;21(1):20–27.

185 Siebenhofer A, Plank J, Berghold A et al. Short acting insulin analogues versus regular human insulin in patients with diabetes mellitus. *Cochrane Database of Systematic Reviews* 2006;(2):CD003287.

186 Boehm BO, Home PD, Behrend C et al. Premixed insulin aspart 30 vs. premixed human insulin 30/70 twice daily: a randomized trial in type 1 and type 2 diabetic patients [erratum appears in *Diabetic Medicine.* 2002 Sep;19(9):797]. *Diabetic Medicine* 2002;19(5):393–399.

187 Boehm BO, Vaz JA, Brondsted L et al. Long-term efficacy and safety of biphasic insulin aspart in patients with type 2 diabetes. *European Journal of Internal Medicine* 2004;15(8):496–502.

188 Abrahamian H, Ludvik B, Schernthaner G et al. Improvement of glucose tolerance in type 2 diabetic patients: traditional vs. modern insulin regimens (results from the Austrian Biaspart Study). *Hormone & Metabolic Research* 2005;37(11):684–689.

189 Schernthaner G, Kopp HP, Ristic S et al. Metabolic control in patients with type 2 diabetes using Humalog Mix50 injected three times daily: crossover comparison with human insulin 30/70. *Hormone & Metabolic Research* 2004;36(3):188–193.

190 Ligthelm RJ, Mouritzen U, Lynggaard H et al. Biphasic insulin aspart given thrice daily is as efficacious as a basal-bolus insulin regimen with four daily injections: a randomised open-label parallel group four months comparison in patients with type 2 diabetes. *Experimental & Clinical Endocrinology & Diabetes* 2006;114(9):511–519.

191 Joshi SR, Kalra S, Badgandi M et al. Designer insulins regimens in clinical practice – pilot multicenter Indian study. *Journal of the Association of Physicians of India* 2005;53(Sept):775–779.

192 Davies M, Storms F, Shutler S. Initiation of Insulin Glargine in type 2 patients with suboptimal glycaemic control on twice-daily premix insulin: results from the AT.LANTUS trial. *Diabetologia* 2004;47(Suppl 1): 319.

193 National Institute for Clinical Excellence. *The clinical effectiveness and cost effectiveness of long acting insulin analogues for diabetes* (TA53). London: NICE, 2002.

194 Rosenstock J, Dailey G, Massi-Benedetti M et al. Reduced hypoglycemia risk with insulin glargine: a meta-analysis comparing insulin glargine with human NPH insulin in type 2 diabetes. *Diabetes Care* 2005; 28(4):950–955.

195 Horvath K, Jeitler K, Berghold A et al. Long-acting insulin analogues versus NPH insulin (human isophane insulin) for type 2 diabetes mellitus. *Cochrane Database of Systematic Reviews* 2007;(2):CD005613.

196 Yki JH, Kauppinen MR, Tiikkainen M et al. Insulin glargine or NPH combined with metformin in type 2 diabetes: the LANMET study. *Diabetologia* 2006;49(3):442–451.

197 Herman WH, Ilag LL, Johnson SL et al. A clinical trial of continuous subcutaneous insulin infusion versus multiple daily injections in older adults with type 2 diabetes. *Diabetes Care* 2005;28(7):1568–1573.

198 Raskin P, Allen E, Hollander P et al. Initiating insulin therapy in type 2 diabetes: a comparison of biphasic and basal insulin analogs. *Diabetes Care* 2005;28(2):260–265.

199 Eliaschewitz FG, Calvo C, Valbuena H et al. Therapy in type 2 diabetes: insulin glargine vs. NPH insulin both in combination with glimepiride. *Archives of Medical Research* 2006;37(4):495–501.

200 Rosskamp R. Safety and efficacy of insulin glargine (HOE 901) versus NPH insulin in combination with oral treatment in type 2 diabetic patients. *Diabetic Medicine* 2003;20(7):545–551.

201 Malone JK, Kerr LF, Campaigne BN et al. Combined therapy with insulin lispro mix 75/25 plus metformin or insulin glargine plus metformin: a 16-week, randomized, open-label, crossover study in patients with type 2 diabetes beginning insulin therapy. *Clinical Therapeutics* 2004;26(12):2034–2044.

202 Malone JK, Bai S, Campaigne BN et al. Twice-daily pre-mixed insulin rather than basal insulin therapy alone results in better overall glycaemic control in patients with type 2 diabetes. *Diabetic Medicine* 2005;22(4): 374–381.

203 Jacober SJ, Scism BJ, Zagar AJ. A comparison of intensive mixture therapy with basal insulin therapy in insulin-naive patients with type 2 diabetes receiving oral antidiabetes agents. *Diabetes, Obesity & Metabolism* 2006;8(4):448–455.

204 Kann PH, Wascher T, Zackova V et al. Starting insulin therapy in type 2 diabetes: twice-daily biphasic insulin aspart 30 plus metformin versus once-daily insulin glargine plus glimepiride. *Experimental & Clinical Endocrinology & Diabetes* 2006;114(9):527–532.

205 Kazda C, Hulstrunk H, Helsberg K et al. Prandial insulin substitution with insulin lispro or insulin lispro mid mixture vs. basal therapy with insulin glargine: a randomized controlled trial in patients with type 2 diabetes beginning insulin therapy. *Journal of Diabetes & its Complications* 2006;20(3):145–152.

206 Pan CY, Sinnassamy P, Chung KD et al. Insulin glargine versus NPH insulin therapy in Asian type 2 diabetes patients. *Diabetes Research & Clinical Practice* 2007;76(1):111–118.

207 Raskin PR, Hollander PA, Lewin A et al. Basal insulin or premix analogue therapy in type 2 diabetes patients. *European Journal of Internal Medicine* 2007;18(1):56–62.

208 Yokoyama H, Tada J, Kamikawa F et al. Efficacy of conversion from bedtime NPH insulin to morning insulin glargine in type 2 diabetic patients on basal-prandial insulin therapy. *Diabetes Research & Clinical Practice* 2006;73(1):35–40.

209 Standl E, Maxeiner S, Raptis S et al. Once-daily insulin glargine administration in the morning compared to bedtime in combination with morning glimepiride in patients with type 2 diabetes: an assessment of treatment flexibility. *Hormone & Metabolic Research* 2006;38(3):172–177.

210 Gerstein HC, Yale JF, Harris SB et al. A randomized trial of adding insulin glargine vs. avoidance of insulin in people with type 2 diabetes on either no oral glucose-lowering agents or submaximal doses of metformin and/or sulphonylureas. The Canadian INSIGHT (Implementing New Strategies with Insulin Glargine for Hyperglycaemia Treatment) Study. *Diabetic Medicine* 2006;23(7):736–742.

211 Fritsche A, Schweitzer MA, Haring HU et al. Glimepiride combined with morning insulin glargine, bedtime neutral protamine hagedorn insulin, or bedtime insulin glargine in patients with type 2 diabetes. A randomized, controlled trial. *Annals of Internal Medicine* 2003;138(12):952–959.

212 Massi BM, Humburg E, Dressler A et al. A one-year, randomised, multicentre trial comparing insulin glargine with NPH insulin in combination with oral agents in patients with type 2 diabetes. *Hormone & Metabolic Research* 2003;35(3):189–196.

213 Riddle MC, Rosenstock J, Gerich J et al. The treat-to-target trial: randomized addition of glargine or human NPH insulin to oral therapy of type 2 diabetic patients. *Diabetes Care* 2003;26(11):3080–3086.

214 Rosenstock J, Schwartz SL, Clark CM Jr et al. Basal insulin therapy in type 2 diabetes: 28-week comparison of insulin glargine (HOE 901) and NPH insulin. *Diabetes Care* 2001;24(4):631–636.

215 Warren E, Weatherley-Jones E, Chilcott J et al. Systematic review and economic evaluation of a long-acting insulin analogue, insulin glargine. *Health Technology Assessment* 2004;8(45):iii, 1–57.

216 McEwan P, Poole CD, Telow T et al. Evaluation of the cost-effectiveness of insulin glargine versus NPH insulin for the treatment of type 1 diabetes in the UK. *Current Medical Research & Opinion* 2007;23(1): S7–S19.

217 National Institute for Health and Clinical Excellence. *The clinical effectiveness and cost effectiveness of insulin pump therapy* (TA57). London: NICE, 2003.

218 Little RR, Rohilfing CL, Wiedmeyer HM et al. The National Glycohaemoglobin Standardization Program (NGSP): a five-year progress report. *Clinical Chemistry* 2001;47:1985–1992.

219 Coscelli C. Safety, efficacy, acceptability of a pre-filled insulin pen in diabetic patients over 60 years old. *Diabetes Research & Clinical Practice* 1995;28(3):173–177.

220 Fox C, McKinnon C, Wall A et al. Ability to handle, and patient preference for, insulin delivery devices in visually impaired patients with type 2 diabetes. *Practical Diabetes International* 2002;19(4):104–107.

221 Kadiri A, Chraibi A, Marouan F et al. Comparison of NovoPen 3 and syringes/vials in the acceptance of insulin therapy in NIDDM patients with secondary failure to oral hypoglycaemic agents. *Diabetes Research & Clinical Practice* 1998;41(1):15–23.

222 Korytkowski M, Bell D, Jacobsen C et al. A multicenter, randomized, open-label, comparative, two-period crossover trial of preference, efficacy, and safety profiles of a prefilled, disposable pen and conventional vial/syringe for insulin injection in patients with type 1 or 2 diabetes mellitus. *Clinical Therapeutics* 2003;25(11):2836–2848.

223 Shelmet J. Preference and resource utilization in elderly patients: InnoLet versus vial/syringe. *Diabetes Research & Clinical Practice* 2004;63(1):27–35.

224 Stockl K, Ory C, Vanderplas A et al. An evaluation of patient preference for an alternative insulin delivery system compared to standard vial and syringe. *Current Medical Research & Opinion* 2007;23(1):133–146.

225 Asakura T, Seino H. Assessment of dose selection attributes with audible notification in insulin pen devices. *Diabetes Technology & Therapeutics* 2005;7(4):620–626.

226 Turner R, Holman R, Stratton I et al. Tight blood pressure control and risk of macrovascular and microvascular complications in type 2 diabetes (UKPDS 38). *British Medical Journal* 1998;317:703–713.

227 Sibal L, Law HN, Gebbie J et al. Cardiovascular risk factors predicting the development of distal symmetrical polyneuropathy in people with type 1 diabetes: A 9-year follow-up study. *Annals of the New York Academy of Sciences* 2006;1084:304–318.

228 Pohl MA, Blumenthal S, Cordonnier DJ et al. Independent and additive impact of blood pressure control and angiotensin II receptor blockade on renal outcomes in the irbesartan diabetic nephropathy trial: clinical implications and limitations. *Journal of the American Society of Nephrology* 2005;16(10):3027–3037.

229 Berl T, Hunsicker LG, Lewis JB et al. Impact of achieved blood pressure on cardiovascular outcomes in the Irbesartan Diabetic Nephropathy Trial. *Journal of the American Society of Nephrology* 2005;16(7):2170–2179.

230 Matthews DR, Stratton IM, Aldington SJ et al. Risks of progression of retinopathy and vision loss related to tight blood pressure control in type 2 diabetes mellitus (UKPDS 69). *Archives of Opthalmology* 2004;122(11):1631–1640.

231 Bakris GL, Weir MR, Shanifar S et al. Effects of blood pressure level on progression of diabetic nephropathy: results from the RENAAL study. *Archives of Internal Medicine* 2003;163(13):1555–1565.

232 Estacio RO, Coll JR, Tran ZV et al. Effect of intensive blood pressure control with valsartan on urinary albumin excretion in normotensive patients with type 2 diabetes. *American Journal of Hypertension* 2006;19(12):1241–1248.

233 Schrier RW, Estacio RO, Esler A et al. Effects of aggressive blood pressure control in normotensive type 2 diabetic patients on albuminuria, retinopathy and strokes. *Kidney International* 2002;61(3):1086–1097.

234 Turnbull F, Neal B, Algert C et al. Effects of different blood pressure-lowering regimens on major cardiovascular events in individuals with and without diabetes mellitus: results of prospectively designed overviews of randomized trials. *Archives of Internal Medicine* 2005;165(12):1410–1419.

235 Torffvit O, Agardh CD. A blood pressure cut-off level identified for renal failure, but not for macro-vascular complications in type 2 diabetes: a 10-year observation study. *Hormone & Metabolic Research* 2002;34(1):32–35.

236 Strippoli GF, Craig M, Craig JC. Antihypertensive agents for preventing diabetic kidney disease. *Cochrane Database of Systematic Reviews* 2005;(4):CD004136.

237 Strippoli GF, Bonifati C, Craig M et al. Angiotensin converting enzyme inhibitors and angiotensin II receptor antagonists for preventing the progression of diabetic kidney disease. *Cochrane Database of Systematic Reviews* 2006;(4):CD006257.

238 Casas JP, Chua W, Loukogeorgakis S et al. Effect of inhibitors of the renin-angiotensin system and other antihypertensive drugs on renal outcomes: systematic review and meta-analysis. *Lancet* 2005;366(9502): 2026–2033.

239 Mann JF, Gerstein HC, Yi QL et al. Progression of renal insufficiency in type 2 diabetes with and without microalbuminuria: results of the Heart Outcomes and Prevention Evaluation (HOPE) randomized study. *American Journal of Kidney Diseases* 2003;42(5):936–942.

240 Mann JF, Gerstein HC, Yi QL et al. Development of renal disease in people at high cardiovascular risk: results of the HOPE randomized study. *Journal of the American Society of Nephrology* 2003;14(3):641–647.

241 Bosch J. Long-term effects of ramipril on cardiovascular events and on diabetes: results of the HOPE study extension. *Circulation* 2005;112(9):1339–1346.

242 Barnett AH, Bain SC, Bouter P et al. Angiotensin-receptor blockade versus converting-enzyme inhibition in type 2 diabetes and nephropathy. *New England Journal of Medicine* 2004;351(19):1952–1961.

243 Sengul AM, Altuntas Y, Kurklu A et al. Beneficial effect of lisinopril plus telmisartan in patients with type 2 diabetes, microalbuminuria and hypertension. *Diabetes Research & Clinical Practice* 2006;71(2):210–219.

244 Dalla VM, Pozza G, Mosca A et al. Effect of lercanidipine compared with ramipril on albumin excretion rate in hypertensive type 2 diabetic patients with microalbuminuria: DIAL study (diabete, ipertensione, albuminuria, lercanidipina). *Diabetes, Nutrition & Metabolism – Clinical & Experimental* 2004;17(5):259–266.

245 Fogari R, Preti P, Zoppi A et al. Effects of amlodipine fosinopril combination on microalbuminuria in hypertensive type 2 diabetic patients. *American Journal of Hypertension* 2002;15(12):1042–1049.

246 Ruggenenti P, Perna A, Ganeva M et al. Impact of blood pressure control and angiotensin-converting enzyme inhibitor therapy on new-onset microalbuminuria in type 2 diabetes: a post hoc analysis of the BENEDICT trial. *Journal of the American Society of Nephrology* 2006;17(12):3472–3481.

247 Whelton PK, Barzilay J, Cushman WC et al. Clinical outcomes in antihypertensive treatment of type 2 diabetes, impaired fasting glucose concentration, and normoglycemia: Antihypertensive and Lipid-Lowering Treatment to Prevent Heart Attack Trial (ALLHAT). *Archives of Internal Medicine* 2005;165(12): 1401–1409.

248 Fernandez R, Puig JG, Rodriguez PJ et al. Effect of two antihypertensive combinations on metabolic control in type-2 diabetic hypertensive patients with albuminuria: a randomised, double-blind study. *Journal of Human Hypertension* 2001;15(12):849–856.

249 Holzgreve H, Nakov R, Beck K et al. Antihypertensive therapy with verapamil SR plus trandolapril versus atenolol plus chlorthalidone on glycemic control. *American Journal of Hypertension* 2003;16(5:Pt 1):381–386.

250 Derosa G, Cicero AF, Gaddi A et al. Effects of doxazosin and irbesartan on blood pressure and metabolic control in patients with type 2 diabetes and hypertension. *Journal of Cardiovascular Pharmacology* 2005;45(6):599–604.

251 Derosa G, Cicero AF, Bertone G et al. Comparison of the effects of telmisartan and nifedipine gastrointestinal therapeutic system on blood pressure control, glucose metabolism, and the lipid profile in patients with type 2 diabetes mellitus and mild hypertension: a 12-month, randomized, double-blind study. *Clinical Therapeutics* 2004;26(8):1228–1236.

252 Viberti G, Wheeldon NM, MicroAlbuminuria Reduction With VALsartan (MARVAL) Study Investigators. Microalbuminuria reduction with valsartan in patients with type 2 diabetes mellitus: a blood pressure-independent effect. *Circulation* 2002;106(6):672–678.

253 Appel GB, Radhakrishnan J, Avram MM et al. Analysis of metabolic parameters as predictors of risk in the RENAAL study. *Diabetes Care* 2003;26(5):1402–1407.

254 Remuzzi G, Ruggenenti P, Perna A et al. Continuum of renoprotection with losartan at all stages of type 2 diabetic nephropathy: a post hoc analysis of the RENAAL trial results. *Journal of the American Society of Nephrology* 2004;15(12):3117–3125.

255 Andersen S, Bröchner-Mortensen J, Parving HH et al. Kidney function during and after withdrawal of long-term irbesartan treatment in patients with type 2 diabetes and microalbuminuria. *Diabetes Care* 2003;26(12):3296–3302.

256 Lindholm LH, Ibsen H. Cardiovascular morbidity and mortality in patients with diabetes in the Losartan Intervention For Endpoint reduction in hypertension study (LIFE): a randomised trial against atenolol. *Lancet* 2002;359(9311):1004–1010.

257 Lewis EJ, Hunsicker LG, Clarke WR et al. Renoprotective effect of the angiotensin-receptor antagonist irbesartan in patients with nephropathy due to type 2 diabetes. *New England Journal of Medicine* 2001; 345(12):851–860.

258 Zanchetti A, Julius S, Kjeldsen S et al. Outcomes in subgroups of hypertensive patients treated with regimens based on valsartan and amlodipine: an analysis of findings from the VALUE trial. *Journal of Hypertension* 2006;24(11):2163–2168.

259 Pepine CJ, Handberg EM, Cooper-DeHoff RM et al. A calcium antagonist vs a non-calcium antagonist hypertension treatment strategy for patients with coronary artery disease. The International Verapamil-Trandolapril Study (INVEST): a randomized controlled trial. *The Journal of the American Medical Association* 2003;290(21):2805–2816.

260 Bakris GL, Fonseca V. Metabolic effects of carvedilol vs metoprolol in patients with type 2 diabetes mellitus and hypertension: a randomized controlled trial. *The Journal of the American Medical Association* 2004;292(18):2227–2236.

261 Black HR, Elliott WJ, Grandits G et al. Principal results of the Controlled Onset Verapamil Investigation of Cardiovascular End Points (CONVINCE) trial. *The Journal of the American Medical Association* 2003; 289(16):2073–2082.

262 Dahlöf B. Prevention of cardiovascular events with an antihypertensive regimen of amlodipine adding perindopril as required versus atenolol adding bendroflumethiazide as required, in the Anglo-Scandinavian Cardiac Outcomes Trial-Blood Pressure Lowering Arm (ASCOT-BPLA): a multicentre randomised controlled trial. *Lancet* 2005;366(9489):895–906.

263 Beard SM, Gaffney L, Backhouse ME. An economic evaluation of ramipril in the treatment of patients at high risk for cardiovascular events due to diabetes mellitus (structured abstract). *Journal of Medical Economics* 2001;4:199–205.

264 Schadlich PK, Brecht JG, Rangoonwala B et al. Cost effectiveness of ramipril in patients at high risk for cardiovascular events: economic evaluation of the HOPE (Heart Outcomes Prevention Evaluation) study for Germany from the Statutory Health Insurance perspective. *Pharmacoeconomics* 2004;22(15):955–973.

265 Gray A, Clarke P, Raikou M et al. An economic evaluation of atenolol vs. captopril in patients with type 2 diabetes (UKPDS 54). *Diabetic Medicine* 2001;18(6):438–444.

266 Palmer AJ, Annemans L, Roze S et al. An economic evaluation of the Irbesartan in Diabetic Nephropathy Trial (IDNT) in a UK setting. *Journal of Human Hypertension* 2004;18:733–738.

267 Rodby RA, Chiou CF, Borenstein J et al. The cost-effectiveness of irbesartan in the treatment of hypertensive patients with type 2 diabetic nephropathy. *Clinical Therapeutics* 2003;25(7):2102–2119.

268 Coyle D, Rodby RA. Economic evaluation of the use of irbesartan and amlodipine in the treatment of diabetic nephropathy in patients with hypertension in Canada. *Canadian Journal of Cardiology* 2004;20(1):71–79.

269 Vora J, Carides G, Robinson P. Effects of losartan-based therapy on the incidence of end-stage renal disease and associated costs in type 2 diabetes mellitus: A retrospective cost-effectiveness analysis in the United Kingdom. *Current Therapeutic Research, Clinical & Experimental* 2005;66(6):475–485.

270 Smith DG, Nguyen AB, Peak CN et al. Markov modeling analysis of health and economic outcomes of therapy with valsartan versus amlodipine in patients with type 2 diabetes and microalbuminuria. *Journal of Managed Care Pharmacy* 2004;10(1):26–32.

271 *International currency rates.* Available from: *Financial Times.* Last accessed on: 13 March 2007.

272 National Institute for Health and Clinical Excellence. *Hypertension: management of hypertension in adults in primary care* (CG34). London: NICE, 2006.

273 Haffner SM, Lehto S, Ronnemaa T et al. Mortality from coronary heart disease in subjects with type 2 diabetes and in nondiabetic subjects with and without prior myocardial infarction. *New England Journal of Medicine* 1998;339(4):229–234.

274 Eddy DM, Schlessinger L. Validation of the archimedes diabetes model. *Diabetes Care* 2003;26(11): 3102–3110.

275 Song SH, Brown PM. Coronary heart disease risk assessment in diabetes mellitus: comparison of UKPDS risk engine with Framingham risk assessment function and its clinical implications. *Diabetic Medicine* 2004;21(3):238–245.

276 Stephens JW, Ambler G, Vallance P et al. Cardiovascular risk and diabetes. Are the methods of risk prediction satisfactory? *European Journal of Cardiovascular Prevention and Rehabilitation* 2004;11(6): 521–528.

277 Guzder RN, Gatling W, Mullee MA et al. Prognostic value of the Framingham cardiovascular risk equation and the UKPDS risk engine for coronary heart disease in newly diagnosed type 2 diabetes: results from a United Kingdom study. *Diabetic Medicine* 2005;22(5):554–562.

278 Coleman RL, Stevens RJ, Renakaran R et al. Framington, SCORE and DECODE do not provide reliable cardiovascular risk estimates in type 2 diabetes. *Diabetes Care* 2007;30(5):1292–1293.

279 Stevens RJ, Kothari V, Adler AI et al. The UKPDS risk engine: a model for the risk of coronary heart disease in type II diabetes (UKPDS 56). *Clinical Science* 2001;101(6):671–679.

280 Tuomilehto J, Rastenyte D. Epidemiology of macrovascular disease and hypertension in diabetes mellitus. *International textbook of diabetes mellitus*, 2nd edn. Chichester: John Wiley, 1997: 1559–1583.

281 Baigent C, Keech A, Kearney PM et al. Efficacy and safety of cholesterol-lowering treatment: prospective meta-analysis of data from 90,056 participants in 14 randomised trials of statins. *Lancet* 2005;366(9493): 1267–1278.

282 Vijan S, Hayward RA, American College of Physicians. Pharmacologic lipid-lowering therapy in type 2 diabetes mellitus: background paper for the American College of Physicians. *Annals of Internal Medicine* 2004;140(8):650–658.

283 National Institute for Health and Clinical Excellence. *Statins for the prevention of cardiovascular events in patients at increased risk of developing cardiovascular disease or those with established cardiovascular disease* (TA94). London: NICE, 2006.

284 National Institute for Health and Clinical Excellence. *Ezetimibe for the treatment of primary (heterozygous familial and non-familial) hypercholesterolaemia* (TA132). London: NICE, 2007.

285 Insull W, Kafonek S, Goldner D et al. Comparison of efficacy and safety of atorvastatin (10mg) with simvastatin (10mg) at six weeks. ASSET Investigators. *American Journal of Cardiology* 2001;87(5):554–559.

286 van Venrooij FV, van de Ree MA, Bots ML et al. Aggressive lipid lowering does not improve endothelial function in type 2 diabetes: the Diabetes Atorvastatin Lipid Intervention (DALI) Study: a randomized, double-blind, placebo-controlled trial. *Diabetes Care* 2002;25(7):1211–1216.

287 Miller M, Dobs A, Yuan Z et al. Effectiveness of simvastatin therapy in raising HDL-C in patients with type 2 diabetes and low HDL-C. *Current Medical Research & Opinion* 2004;20(7):1087–1094.

288 Berne C, Siewert DA, URANUS study investigators. Comparison of rosuvastatin and atorvastatin for lipid lowering in patients with type 2 diabetes mellitus: results from the URANUS study. *Cardiovascular Diabetology* 2005;4:7.

289 Colhoun HM, Betteridge DJ, Durrington PN et al. Rapid emergence of effect of atorvastatin on cardiovascular outcomes in the Collaborative Atorvastatin Diabetes Study (CARDS). *Diabetologia* 2005;48(12):2482–2485.

290 Sever PS, Poulter NR, Dahlof B et al. Reduction in cardiovascular events with atorvastatin in 2,532 patients with type 2 diabetes: Anglo-Scandinavian Cardiac Outcomes Trial – lipid-lowering arm (ASCOT-LLA). *Diabetes Care* 2005;28(5):1151–1157.

291 Shepherd J, Barter P, Carmena R et al. Effect of lowering LDL cholesterol substantially below currently recommended levels in patients with coronary heart disease and diabetes: the Treating to New Targets (TNT) study. *Diabetes Care* 2006;29(6):1220–1226.

292 Steiner G, Hamsten A, Hosking J et al. Effect of fenofibrate on progression of coronary-artery disease in type 2 diabetes: the Diabetes Atherosclerosis Intervention Study, a randomised study. *Lancet* 2001; 357(9260):905–910.

293 Vakkilainen J, Steiner G, Ansquer JC et al. Relationships between low-density lipoprotein particle size, plasma lipoproteins, and progression of coronary artery disease: the Diabetes Atherosclerosis Intervention Study (DAIS). *Circulation* 2003;107(13):1733–1737.

273

294 Keech A, Simes R, Barter P et al. Effects of long–term fenofibrate therapy on cardiovascular events in 9795 people with type 2 diabetes mellitus (the FIELD study): Randomised controlled trial. *Lancet* 2005; 366(9500):1849–1861.

295 Derosa G, Cicero AE, Bertone G et al. Comparison of fluvastatin + fenofibrate combination therapy and fluvastatin monotherapy in the treatment of combined hyperlipidemia, type 2 diabetes mellitus, and coronary heart disease: a 12-month, randomized, double-blind, controlled trial. *Clinical Therapeutics* 2004;26(10):1599–1607.

296 Athyros VG, Papageorgiou VV, Athyrou DS et al. Atorvastatin and micronized fenofibrate alone and in combination, in type-2 diabetes mellitus with combined hyperlipidemia. *Atherosclerosis* 2002;3(2):70.

297 Durrington PN, Tuomilehto J, Hamann A et al. Rosuvastatin and fenofibrate alone and in combination in type 2 diabetes patients with combined hyperlipidaemia. *Diabetes Research & Clinical Practice* 2004;64(2):137–151.

298 Muhlestein JB, May HT, Jensen JR et al. The reduction of inflammatory biomarkers by statin, fibrate, and combination therapy among diabetic patients with mixed dyslipidemia: the DIACOR (Diabetes and Combined Lipid Therapy Regimen) study. *Journal of the American College of Cardiology* 2006;48(2):396–401.

299 Rubins HB, Robins SJ, Collins D et al. Diabetes, plasma insulin, and cardiovascular disease: subgroup analysis from the Department of Veterans Affairs High-Density Lipoprotein Intervention Trial (VA-HIT). *Archives of Internal Medicine* 2002;162(22):2597–2604.

300 Ashraf R, Amir K, Shaikh AR. Comparison between duration dependent effects of simvastatin and gemfibrozil on dyslipidemia in patients with type 2 diabetes. *Journal of the Pakistan Medical Association* 2005;55(8):324–327.

301 Schweitzer M, Tessier D, Vlahos WD et al. A comparison of pravastatin and gemfibrozil in the treatment of dyslipoproteinemia in patients with non-insulin-dependent diabetes mellitus. *Atherosclerosis* 2002;162(1):201–210.

302 Wagner AM, Jorba O, Bonet R et al. Efficacy of atorvastatin and gemfibrozil, alone and in low dose combination, in the treatment of diabetic dyslipidemia. *Journal of Clinical Endocrinology & Metabolism* 2003;88(7):3212–3217.

303 Feher MD, Langley-Hawthorne CE, Byrne CD. Cost-outcome benefits of fibrate therapy in type 2 diabetes. *British Journal of Diabetes & Vascular Disease* 2003;3(2):124–130.

304 Elam MB, Hunninghake DB, Davis KB et al. Effect of niacin on lipid and lipoprotein levels and glycemic control in patients with diabetes and peripheral arterial disease: the ADMIT study: a randomized trial. Arterial Disease Multiple Intervention Trial. *The Journal of the American Medical Association* 2000;284(10):1263–1270.

305 Grundy SM, Vega GL, McGovern ME et al. Efficacy, safety, and tolerability of once-daily niacin for the treatment of dyslipidemia associated with type 2 diabetes: results of the assessment of diabetes control and evaluation of the efficacy of niaspan trial. *Archives of Internal Medicine* 2002;162(14):1568–1576.

306 Garg A, Grundy SM. Nicotinic acid as therapy for dyslipidemia in non-insulin-dependent diabetes mellitus. *The Journal of the American Medical Association* 1990;264(6):723–726.

307 Tsalamandris C, Panagiotopoulos S, Sinha A et al. Complementary effects of pravastatin and nicotinic acid in the treatment of combined hyperlipidaemia in diabetic and non-diabetic patients. *Journal of Cardiovascular Risk* 1994;1(3):231–239.

308 Armstrong EP, Zachry WM III, Malone DC. Cost-effectiveness analysis of simvastatin and lovastatin/extended-release niacin to achieve LDL and HDL goal using NHANES data. *Journal of Managed Care Pharmacy* 2004;10(3):251–258.

309 Olson BM, Malone DC, Armstrong EP. Modeling the cost-effectiveness of doubling atorvastatin's dose versus adding niacin ER. *Formulary* 2001;36(10):730–746.

310 Roze S, Wierzbicki AS, Liens D et al. Cost-effectiveness of adding prolonged-release nicotinic acid in statin-treated patients who achieve LDL cholesterol goals but remain at risk due to low HDL cholesterol: a UK-based economic evaluation. *British Journal of Cardiology* 2006;13(6):411–418.

311 Farmer A, Montori V, Dinneen S et al. Fish oil in people with type 2 diabetes mellitus. *Cochrane Database of Systematic Reviews* 2001;(3):CD003205.

312 Hartweg J, Farmer AJ, Holman RR et al. Meta-analysis of the effects of n-3 polyunsaturated fatty acids on haematological and thrombogenic factors in type 2 diabetes. *Diabetologia* 2007;50(2):250–258.

313 Jain S, Gaiha M, Bhattacharjee J et al. Effects of low-dose omega-3 fatty acid substitution in type-2 diabetes mellitus with special reference to oxidative stress – a prospective preliminary study. *Journal of the Association of Physicians of India* 2002;50(Aug):1028–1033.

314 Woodman RJ, Mori TA, Burke V et al. Effects of purified eicosapentaenoic and docosahexaenoic acids on glycemic control, blood pressure, and serum lipids in type 2 diabetic patients with treated hypertension. *American Journal of Clinical Nutrition* 2002;76(5):1007–1015.

315 Pedersen H, Petersen M, Major-Pedersen A et al. Influence of fish oil supplementation on in vivo and in vitro oxidation resistance of low-density lipoprotein in type 2 diabetes. *European Journal of Clinical Nutrition* 2003;57(5):713–720.

316 Petersen M, Pedersen H, Major-Pedersen A et al. Effect of fish oil versus corn oil supplementation on LDL and HDL subclasses in type 2 diabetic patients. *Diabetes Care* 2002;25(10):1704–1708.

317 Dunstan DW, Mori TA, Puddey IB et al. Exercise and fish intake: effects on serum lipids and glycemic control for type 2 diabetics. *Cardiology Review* 1998;15(8):34–37.

318 Hooper L, Thompson RL, Harrison RA et al. Risks and benefits of omega 3 fats for mortality, cardiovascular disease, and cancer: systematic review. *British Medical Journal* 2006;332(7544):752–760.

319 Wood D, Durrington P, McInnes G et al. Joint British recommendations on prevention of coronary heart disease in clinical practice. *Heart* 1998;80(Suppl 2):1S–29S.

320 McIntosh A, Hutchinson A, Home PD, Brown F, Bruce A. *Clinical guidelines and evidence review for type 2 diabetes: management of blood glucose.* Sheffield: School of Health and Related Research, 2001.

321 National Institute for Health and Clinical Excellence. *Clopidogrel and modified release dipyridamole in the prevention of occlusive vascular events.* (TA90). London: NICE, 2005.

322 Khajehdehi P, Roozbeh J, Mostafavi H. A comparative randomized and placebo-controlled short-term trial of aspirin and dipyridamole for overt type-2 diabetic nephropathy. *Scandinavian Journal of Urology & Nephrology* 2002;36(2):145–148.

323 Sacco M, Pellegrini F, Roncaglioni MC et al. Primary prevention of cardiovascular events with low-dose aspirin and vitamin E in type 2 diabetic patients: results of the Primary Prevention Project (PPP) trial. *Diabetes Care* 2003;26(12):3264–3272.

324 Neri Serneri GG, Coccheri S, Marubini E et al. Picotamide, a combined inhibitor of thromboxane A2 synthase and receptor, reduces 2-year mortality in diabetics with peripheral arterial disease: The DAVID study. *European Heart Journal* 2004;25(20):1845–1852.

325 Diener HC, Bogousslavsky J, Brass LM et al. Aspirin and clopidogrel compared with clopidogrel alone after recent ischaemic stroke or transient ischaemic attack in high-risk patients (MATCH): randomised, double-blind, placebo-controlled trial. *Lancet* 2004;364(9431):331–337.

326 Bhatt DL, Marso SP, Hirsch AT et al. Amplified benefit of clopidogrel versus aspirin in patients with diabetes mellitus. *American Journal of Cardiology* 2002;90(6):625–628.

327 Yusuf S, Zhao F, Mehta SR et al. Effects of clopidogrel in addition to aspirin in patients with acute coronary syndromes without ST-segment elevation. *New England Journal of Medicine* 2001;345(7): 494–502.

328 Bhatt DL, Fox KA, Hacke W et al. Clopidogrel and aspirin versus aspirin alone for the prevention of atherothrombotic events. *New England Journal of Medicine* 2006;354(16):1706–1717.

329 Steinhubl SR, Berger PB, Mann JT III et al. Early and sustained dual oral antiplatelet therapy following percutaneous coronary intervention: a randomized controlled trial. *The Journal of the American Medical Association* 2002;288(19):2411–2420.

330 Mehta SR, Yusuf S, Peters RJ et al. Effects of pretreatment with clopidogrel and aspirin followed by long-term therapy in patients undergoing percutaneous coronary intervention: the PCI-CURE study. *Lancet* 2001;358(9281):527–533.

331 Jonsson B, Hansson L, Stalhammar NO. Health economics in the Hypertension Optimal Treatment (HOT) study: costs and cost-effectiveness of intensive blood pressure lowering and low-dose aspirin in patients with hypertension. *Journal of Internal Medicine* 2003;253(4):472–480.

332 National Institute for Health and Clinical Excellence. *Clopidogrel in the treatment of non-ST-segment-elevation acute coronary syndrome.* (TA80). London: NICE, 2004.

333 Weintraub WS, Mahoney EM, Lamy A et al. Long-term cost-effectiveness of clopidogrel given for up to one year in patients with acute coronary syndromes without ST-segment elevation. *Journal of the American College of Cardiology* 2005;45(6):838–845.

334 Ringborg A, Lindgren P, Jonsson B. The cost-effectiveness of dual oral antiplatelet therapy following percutaneous coronary intervention: a Swedish analysis of the CREDO trial. *European Journal of Health Economics* 2005;6(4):354–362.

335 Cowper PA, Udayakumar K, Sketch MH Jr et al. Economic effects of prolonged clopidogrel therapy after percutaneous coronary intervention. *Journal of the American College of Cardiology* 2005;45(3):369–376.

336 Harvey JN. Trends in the prevalence of diabetic nephropathy in type 1 and type 2 diabetes. *Current Opinion in Nephrology & Hypertension* 2003;12(3):317–322.

337 Banerjee S, Ghosh US, Saha SJ. Role of GFR estimation in assessment of the status of nephropathy in type 2 diabetes mellitus. *Journal of the Association of Physicians of India* 2005;53:181–4.

338 Baskar V, Venugopal H, Holland MR et al. Clinical utility of estimated glomerular filtration rates in predicting renal risk in a district diabetes population. *Diabetic Medicine* 2006;23(10):1057–1060.

339 Cortes SL, Martinez RH, Hernandez JL et al. Utility of the Dipstick Micraltest II in the screening of microalbuminuria of diabetes mellitus type 2 and essential hypertension. *Revista de Investigacion Clinica* 2006;58(3):190–197.

340 Incerti J, Zelmanovitz T, Camargo JL et al. Evaluation of tests for microalbuminuria screening in patients with diabetes. *Nephrology Dialysis Transplantation* 2005;20(11):2402–2407.

341 MacIsaac RJ, Tsalamandris C, Panagiotopoulos S et al. Nonalbuminuric renal insufficiency in type 2 diabetes. *Diabetes Care* 2004;27(1):195–200.

342 Middleton RJ, Foley RN, Hegarty J et al. The unrecognized prevalence of chronic kidney disease in diabetes. *Nephrology Dialysis Transplantation* 2006;21(1):88–92.

343 Parikh CR, Fischer MJ, Estacio R et al. Rapid microalbuminuria screening in type 2 diabetes mellitus: simplified approach with Micral test strips and specific gravity [erratum appears in *Nephrol Dial Transplant* 2004;19(9):2425]. *Nephrology Dialysis Transplantation* 2004;19(7):1881–1885.

344 Poggio ED, Wang X, Greene T et al. Performance of the modification of diet in renal disease and Cockcroft-Gault equations in the estimation of GFR in health and in chronic kidney disease. *Journal of the American Society of Nephrology* 2005;16(2):459–466.

345 Rigalleau V, Lasseur C, Perlemoine C et al. A simplified Cockcroft-Gault formula to improve the prediction of the glomerular filtration rate in diabetic patients. *Diabetes & Metabolism* 2006;32(1):56–62.

346 Younis N, Broadbent DM, Vora JP et al. Incidence of sight-threatening retinopathy in patients with type 2 diabetes in the Liverpool Diabetic Eye Study: a cohort study. *Lancet* 2003;361(9353):195–200.

347 UK National Screening Committee. *Essential elements in developing a diabetic retinopathy screening programme.* Workbook 4:(1–79). Available from: UK National Screening Committee.

348 Max MB, Lynch SA, Muir J et al. Effects of desipramine, amitriptyline, and fluoxetine on pain in diabetic neuropathy. *New England Journal of Medicine* 1992;326(19):1250–1256.

349 Sindrup SH, Gram LF, Skjold T et al. Clomipramine vs desipramine vs placebo in the treatment of diabetic neuropathy symptoms. A double-blind cross-over study. *British Journal of Clinical Pharmacology* 1990;30(5):683–691.

350 Sindrup SH, Tuxen C. Lack of effect of mianserin on the symptoms of diabetic neuropathy. *European Journal of Clinical Pharmacology* 1992;43(3):251–255.

351 Morello CM, Leckband SG, Stoner CP et al. Randomized double-blind study comparing the efficacy of gabapentin with amitriptyline on diabetic peripheral neuropathy pain. *Archives of Internal Medicine* 1999;159(16):1931–1937.

352 Jose VM, Bhansali A, Hota D et al. Randomized double-blind study comparing the efficacy and safety of lamotrigine and amitriptyline in painful diabetic neuropathy. *Diabetic Medicine* 2007;24(4):377–383.

353 Kvinesdal B, Molin J, Froland A et al. Imipramine treatment of painful diabetic neuropathy. *The Journal of the American Medical Association* 1984;251(13):1727–1730.

354 Max MB, Kishore KR, Schafer SC et al. Efficacy of desipramine in painful diabetic neuropathy: a placebo-controlled trial. *Pain* 1991;45(1):3–9.

355 Max MB, Culnane M, Schafer SC et al. Amitriptyline relieves diabetic neuropathy pain in patients with normal or depressed mood. *Neurology* 1987;37(4):589–596.

356 Sindrup SH, Ejlertsen B. Imipramine treatment in diabetic neuropathy: relief of subjective symptoms without changes in peripheral and autonomic nerve function. *European Journal of Clinical Pharmacology* 1989;37(2):151–153.

357 Raskin J, Smith TR, Wong K et al. Duloxetine versus routine care in the long-term management of diabetic peripheral neuropathic pain. *Journal of Palliative Medicine* 2006;9(1):29–40.

358 Raskin J, Pritchett YL, Wang F et al. A double-blind, randomized multicenter trial comparing duloxetine with placebo in the management of diabetic peripheral neuropathic pain. *Pain Medicine* 2005;6(5):346–356.

359 Goldstein DJ, Lu Y, Detke MJ et al. Duloxetine vs. placebo in patients with painful diabetic neuropathy. *Pain* 2005;116(1–2):109–118.

360 Hardy T, Sachson R, Shen S et al. Does treatment with duloxetine for neuropathic pain impact glycemic control? *Diabetes Care* 2007;30(1):21–26.

361 Raskin J, Wang F, Pritchett YL et al. Duloxetine for patients with diabetic peripheral neuropathic pain: a 6-month open-label safety study. *Pain Medicine* 2006;7(5):373–385.

362 Wernicke JF, Pritchett YL, D'Souza DN et al. A randomized controlled trial of duloxetine in diabetic peripheral neuropathic pain. *Neurology* 2006;67(8):1411–1420.

363 Wernicke JF, Raskin J, Rosen A et al. Duloxetine in the long-term management of diabetic peripheral neuropathic pain: An open-label, 52-week extension of a randomized controlled clinical trial. *Current Therapeutic Research, Clinical & Experimental* 2006;67(5):283–304.

364 Gomez-Perez FJ, PerezMonteverde A, Nascimento O et al. Gabapentin for the treatment of painful diabetic neuropathy: dosing to achieve optimal clinical response. *British Journal of Diabetes & Vascular Disease* 2004;4(3):173–178.

365 Gorson KC, Schott C, Herman R et al. Gabapentin in the treatment of painful diabetic neuropathy: a placebo controlled, double blind, crossover trial. *Journal of Neurology, Neurosurgery, and Psychiatry* 1999;66(2):251–252.

366 Backonja M, Beydoun A, Edwards KR et al. Gabapentin for the symptomatic treatment of painful neuropathy in patients with diabetes mellitus: a randomized controlled trial. *The Journal of the American Medical Association* 1998;280(21):1831–1836.

367 Simpson DA. Gabapentin and venlafaxine for the treatment of painful diabetic neuropathy. *Journal of Clinical Neuromuscular Disease* 2001;3(2):53–62.

368 Lesser H, Sharma U, Lamoreaux L et al. Pregabalin relieves symptoms of painful diabetic neuropathy: a randomized controlled trial. *Neurology* 2004;63(11):2104–2110.

369 Richter RW, Portenoy R, Sharma U et al. Relief of painful diabetic peripheral neuropathy with pregabalin: a randomized, placebo-controlled trial. *Journal of Pain* 2005;6(4):253–260.

370 Rosenstock J, Tuchman M, Lamoreaux L et al. Pregabalin for the treatment of painful diabetic peripheral neuropathy: a double-blind, placebo-controlled trial. *Pain* 2004;110(3):628–638.

371 Rull JA, Quibrera R, Gonzalez MH et al. Symptomatic treatment of peripheral diabetic neuropathy with carbamazepine (Tegretol): double blind crossover trial. *Diabetologia* 1969;5(4):215–218.

372 Wilton TD. Tegretol in the treatment of diabetic neuropathy. *South African Medical Journal* 1974;48(20):869–872.

373 Gomez-Perez FJ, Choza R, Rios JM et al. Nortriptyline-fluphenazine vs. carbamazepine in the symptomatic treatment of diabetic neuropathy. *Archives of Medical Research* 1996;27(4):525–529.

374 Beydoun A, Kobetz SA, Carrazana EJ. Efficacy of oxcarbazepine in the treatment of painful diabetic neuropathy. *Clinical Journal of Pain* 2004;20(3):174–178.

375 Dogra S, Beydoun S, Mazzola J et al. Oxcarbazepine in painful diabetic neuropathy: a randomized, placebo-controlled study. *European Journal of Pain* 2005;9(5):543–554.

376 Grosskopf J, Mazzola J, Wan Y et al. A randomized, placebo-controlled study of oxcarbazepine in painful diabetic neuropathy. *Acta Neurologica Scandinavica* 2006;114(3):177–180.

377 Cepeda MS, Farrar JT. Economic evaluation of oral treatments for neuropathic pain. *Journal of Pain* 2006;7(2):119–128.

378 Maizels M, McCarberg B. Antidepressants and antiepileptic drugs for chronic non-cancer pain. *American Family Physician* 2005;71(3):483–490.

379 Wu EQ, Birnbaum HG, Mareva MN et al. Cost-effectiveness of duloxetine versus routine treatment for U.S. patients with diabetic peripheral neuropathic pain. *Journal of Pain* 2006;7(6):399–407.

380 National Institute for Health and Clinical Excellence. *Type 2 diabetes: prevention and management of foot problems* (CG10). London: NICE, 2004.

381 Braun AP. Domperidone in the treatment of symptoms of delayed gastric emptying in diabetic patients. *Advances in Therapy* 1989;6(2):51–62.

382 Samsom M. Effects of oral erythromycin on fasting and postprandial antroduodenal motility in patients with type I diabetes, measured with an ambulatory manometric technique. *Diabetes Care* 1997; 20(2):129–134.

383 Janssens J, Peeters TL, Vantrappen G et al. Improvement of gastric emptying in diabetic gastroparesis by erythromycin. Preliminary studies. *New England Journal of Medicine* 1990;322(15):1028–1031.

384 McCallum RW, Ricci DA, Rakatansky H et al. A multicenter placebo-controlled clinical trial of oral metoclopramide in diabetic gastroparesis. *Diabetes Care* 1983;6(5):463–467.

385 Ricci DA, Saltzman MB, Meyer C et al. Effect of metoclopramide in diabetic gastroparesis. *Journal of Clinical Gastroenterology* 1985;7(1):25–32.

386 Farup CE, Leidy NK, Murray M et al. Effect of domperidone on the health-related quality of life of patients with symptoms of diabetic gastroparesis. *Diabetes Care* 1998;21(10):1699–1706.

387 Erbas T, Varoglu E, Erbas B et al. Comparison of metoclopramide and erythromycin in the treatment of diabetic gastroparesis. *Diabetes Care* 1993;16(11):1511–1514.

388 Patterson D, Abell T, Rothstein R et al. A double-blind multicenter comparison of domperidone and metoclopramide in the treatment of diabetic patients with symptoms of gastroparesis. *American Journal of Gastroenterology* 1999;94(5):1230–1234.

389 McCulloch DK, Campbell IW, Wu FC et al. The prevalence of diabetic impotence. *Diabetologia* 1980;18(4):279–283.

390 Price DE, Gingell JC, Gepi AS et al. Sildenafil: study of a novel oral treatment for erectile dysfunction in diabetic men. *Diabetic Medicine* 1998;15(10):821–825.

391 Rendell MS, Rajfer J. Sildenafil for treatment of erectile dysfunction in men with diabetes: a randomized controlled trial. Sildenafil Diabetes Study Group. *The Journal of the American Medical Association.* 1999;281(5):421–426.

392 Boulton AJM, Selam JL, Sweeney M et al. Sildenafil citrate for the treatment of erectile dysfunction in men with type II diabetes mellitus. *Diabetologia* 2001;44(10):1296–1301.

393 Saenz de Tejada I, Anglin G, Knight JR et al. Effects of tadalafil on erectile dysfunction in men with diabetes. *Diabetes Care* 2002;25(12):2159–2164.

394 Goldstein I, Young JM, Fischer J et al. Vardenafil, a new phosphodiesterase type 5 inhibitor, in the treatment of erectile dysfunction in men with diabetes: a multicenter double-blind placebo-controlled fixed-dose study. *Diabetes Care* 2003;26(3):777–783.

395 Stuckey BGA, Jadzinsky MN, Murphy LJ et al. Sildenafil citrate for treatment of erectile dysfunction in men with type 1 diabetes: results of a randomized controlled trial. *Diabetes Care* 2003;26(2):279–284.

396 Safarinejad MR. Oral sildenafil in the treatment of erectile dysfunction in diabetic men: a randomized double-blind and placebo-controlled study. *Journal of Diabetes & its Complications* 2004;18(4):205–210.

397 Ishii N, Nagao K, Fujikawa K et al. Vardenafil 20-mg demonstrated superior efficacy to 10-mg in Japanese men with diabetes mellitus suffering from erectile dysfunction. *International Journal of Urology* 2006;13(8):1066–1072.

398 Ziegler D, Merfort F, van Ahlen et al. Efficacy and safety of flexible-dose vardenafil in men with type 1 diabetes and erectile dysfunction. *Journal of Sexual Medicine* 2006;3(5):883–891.

399 Buvat J, van Ahlen, Schmitt H et al. Efficacy and safety of two dosing regimens of tadalafil and patterns of sexual activity in men with diabetes mellitus and erectile dysfunction: scheduled use vs. on-demand regimen evaluation (SURE) study in 14 European countries. *Journal of Sexual Medicine* 2006;3(3):512–520.

400 Weinstein MC, O'Brien B, Hornberger J et al. Principles of good practice for decision analytic modeling in health-care evaluation: report of the ISPOR Task Force on Good Research Practices – Modeling Studies. *Value in Health* 2003;6:9–17.

401 Clarke PM, Gray AM, Briggs A et al. A model to estimate the lifetime health outcomes of patients with type 2 diabetes: the United Kingdom Prospective Diabetes Study (UKPDS) Outcomes Model (UKPDS no. 68). *Diabetologia* 2004;47(10):1747–1759.

402 Clarke P, Gray A, Legood R et al. The impact of diabetes-related complications on healthcare costs: results from the United Kingdom Prospective Diabetes Study (UKPDS Study No. 65). *Diabetic Medicine* 2003; 20(6):442–450.

403 Curtis L, Netten A. *Unit costs of health and social care 2006.* Canterbury: Personal Social Services Research Unit, 2006.

404 Calvert MJ, McManus RJ, Freemantle N. Management of type 2 diabetes with multiple oral hypoglycaemic agents or insulin in primary care: retrospective cohort study. *British Journal of General Practice* 2007; 57(539):455–460.

405 Scottish Medicines Consortium. Glasgow. *New product assessment form – exenatide* 2006. Personal communication.

406 Melanie Davies, 31 May 2007. Personal communication.

407 Warren E. *The cost-effectiveness of long-acting insulin analogue, insulin glargine.* Sheffield: ScHARR, 16 August 2002.

408 Currie CJ, Morgan CL, Poole CD et al. Multivariate models of health-related utility and the fear of hypoglycaemia in people with diabetes. *Current Medical Research & Opinion* 2006;22(8):1523–1534.

409 Anon. Contributed poster presentations. *Value in Health* 2006;9(3):A24–A173.

410 Rowlett R. *How many? A dictionary of units of measurement* 2001.

411 Glenny AM, Altman DG, Song F et al. Indirect comparisons of competing interventions. *Health Technology Assessment* 2005;9(26):1–iv.

412 GlaxoSmithKline. *Rosiglitazone maleate ZM2006/00207/00(meta-analysis)1–8.* GlaxoSmithKline. 27 June 2006.

413 Food and Drug Administration. *Avandia (rosiglitazone maleate)* NDA21-071 supplement 022 FDA. 2007.

414 National Institute for Health and Clinical Excellence. *Management of type 2 diabetes – management of blood pressure and blood lipids* (Guideline H). London: NICE, 2002.